T0259368

Bronchiectasis

Guest Editors

MARK L. METERSKY, MD
ANNE E. O'DONNELL, MD

CLINICS IN
CHEST MEDICINE

www.chestmed.theclinics.com

June 2012 • Volume 33 • Number 2

SAUNDERS an imprint of ELSEVIER, Inc.

W.B. SAUNDERS COMPANY
A Division of Elsevier Inc.

1600 John F. Kennedy Boulevard ● Suite 1800 ● Philadelphia, Pennsylvania 19103

http://www.theclinics.com

CLINICS IN CHEST MEDICINE Volume 33, Number 2
June 2012 ISSN 0272-5231, ISBN-13: 978-1-4557-3843-4

Editor: Katie Hartner
Developmental Editor: Donald E. Mumford

© **2012 Elsevier Inc. All rights reserved.**

This journal and the individual contributions contained in it are protected under copyright by Elsevier, and the following terms and conditions apply to their use:

Photocopying

Single photocopies of single articles may be made for personal use as allowed by national copyright laws. Permission of the Publisher and payment of a fee is required for all other photocopying, including multiple or systematic copying, copying for advertising or promotional purposes, resale, and all forms of document delivery. Special rates are available for educational institutions that wish to make photocopies for non-profit educational classroom use. For information on how to seek permission visit www.elsevier.com/permissions or call: (+44) 1865 843830 (UK)/(+1) 215 239 3804 (USA).

Derivative Works

Subscribers may reproduce tables of contents or prepare lists of articles including abstracts for internal circulation within their institutions. Permission of the Publisher is required for resale or distribution outside the institution. Permission of the Publisher is required for all other derivative works, including compilations and translations (please consult www.elsevier.com/permissions).

Electronic Storage or Usage

Permission of the Publisher is required to store or use electronically any material contained in this journal, including any article or part of an article (please consult www.elsevier.com/permissions). Except as outlined above, no part of this publication may be reproduced, stored in a retrieval system or transmitted in any form or by any means, electronic, mechanical, photocopying, recording or otherwise, without prior written permission of the Publisher.

Notice

No responsibility is assumed by the Publisher for any injury and/or damage to persons or property as a matter of products liability, negligence or otherwise, or from any use or operation of any methods, products, instructions or ideas contained in the material herein. Because of rapid advances in the medical sciences, in particular, independent verification of diagnoses and drug dosages should be made.

Although all advertising material is expected to conform to ethical (medical) standards, inclusion in this publication does not constitute a guarantee or endorsement of the quality or value of such product or of the claims made of it by its manufacturer.

Clinics in Chest Medicine (ISSN 0272-5231) is published quarterly by Elsevier Inc., 360 Park Avenue South, New York, NY 10010-1710. Months of issue are March, June, September, and December. Periodicals postage paid at New York, NY and additional mailing offices. Subscription prices are $316.00 per year (domestic individuals), $506.00 per year (domestic institutions), $151.00 per year (domestic students/residents), $347.00 per year (Canadian individuals), $621.00 per year (Canadian institutions), $431.00 per year (international individuals), $621.00 per year (international institutions), and $211.00 per year (international and Canadian students/residents). International air speed delivery is included in all Clinics subscription prices. All prices are subject to change without notice. **POSTMASTER:** Send address changes to Clinics in Chest Medicine, Elsevier Health Sciences Division, Subscription Customer Service, 3251 Riverport Lane, Maryland Heights, MO 63043. **Customer Service: Telephone: 1-800-654-2452** (U.S. and Canada); **1-314-447-8871** (outside U.S. and Canada). **Fax: 1-314-447-8029. E-mail: journalscustomerservice-usa@elsevier.com** (for print support); **journalsonlinesupport-usa@elsevier.com** (for online support).

Reprints. For copies of 100 or more of articles in this publication, please contact the Commercial Reprints Department, Elsevier Inc., 360 Park Avenue South, New York, NY 10010-1710. Tel.: 212-633-3812; Fax: 212-462-1935; E-mail: reprints@elsevier. com.

Clinics in Chest Medicine is covered in *MEDLINE/PubMed (Index Medicus), Current Contents/Clinical Medicine, EMBASE/ Excerpta Medica, Science Citation Index,* and *ISI/BIOMED.*

Printed and bound by CPI Group (UK) Ltd, Croydon, CR0 4YY

Transferred to Digital Print 2012

Contributors

GUEST EDITORS

MARK L. METERSKY, MD
Professor of Medicine, Director, Center for
Bronchiectasis Care, Division of Pulmonary
and Critical Care Medicine, University of
Connecticut School of Medicine, Farmington,
Connecticut

ANNE E. O'DONNELL, MD
Professor of Medicine, Chief, Division of
Pulmonary, Critical Care and Sleep Medicine,
Georgetown University Hospital,
Washington, DC

AUTHORS

PENNY AGENT, BSc (Hons), MCSP, DMS
Deputy Director of Rehabilitation and
Therapies, Physiotherapy Department,
The Royal Brompton and Harefield NHS
Foundation Trust, Royal Brompton Hospital,
London, United Kingdom

TIMOTHY R. AKSAMIT, MD
Associate Professor of Medicine, Department
of Internal Medicine, Mayo Clinic College of
Medicine, Rochester, Minnesota

SONIA N. BAINS, MD
Assistant Professor of Medicine, Division of
Pulmonary, Critical Care, Allergy & Sleep
Medicine, Medical University of South
Carolina, Charleston, South Carolina

ALAN F. BARKER, MD
Pulmonary and Critical Care Medicine,
Oregon Health and Science University,
Portland, Oregon

DIANA BILTON, MD, FRCP
Consultant Physician, Director of Cystic
Fibrosis, Cystic Fibrosis Unit, Department
of Respiratory Medicine, The Royal Brompton
and Harefield NHS Foundation Trust,
Royal Brompton Hospital, London,
United Kingdom

JOHN BONAVITA, MD, FACR
Department of Radiology, New York
University-Langone Medical Center,
New York, New York

CHARLES L. DALEY, MD
Division of Mycobacterial and Respiratory
Infections, National Jewish Health, Denver,
Colorado

**CHARLES FELDMAN, MB BCh, DSc, PhD,
FRCP, FCP (SA)**
Professor of Pulmonology and Chief Physician,
Division of Pulmonology, Department of
Internal Medicine, Faculty of Health Sciences,
Charlotte Maxeke Johannesburg Academic
Hospital, University of the Witwatersrand,
Johannesburg, South Africa

LIZZIE J. FLUDE, BSc, MCSP
Specialist Physiotherapist Adult Respiratory
Medicine, Physiotherapy Department,
The Royal Brompton and Harefield NHS
Foundation Trust, Royal Brompton Hospital,
London, United Kingdom

ALEXANDRA F. FREEMAN, MD
Staff Clinician, Laboratory of Clinical Infectious
Diseases, National Institute of Allergy and
Infectious Diseases, National Institutes of
Health, Bethesda, Maryland

CHRISTINE M. GOULD, MD
Fellow, Division of Pulmonary & Sleep
Medicine, Children's National Medical Center,
Washington, DC; Staff Pediatric
Pulmonologist, Department of Pediatrics,
Walter Reed National Military Medical Center,
Bethesda, Maryland

DAVID E. GRIFFITH, MD, FACP, FCCP
Professor of Medicine, Edward A. and
Elizabeth B. Moncrief Distinguished Professor;
Chief, Pulmonary and Critical Care Division,
Department of Medicine, University of Texas
Health Science Center, Tyler, Tyler, Texas

ADAM T. HILL, MB ChB, MD, FRCPE
Consultant Respiratory Physician, Department
of Respiratory Medicine, Royal Infirmary of
Edinburgh; Honorary Senior Lecturer,
University of Edinburgh, Edinburgh,
United Kingdom.

JONATHAN S. ILOWITE, MD
Associate Clinical Professor of Medicine,
SUNY Stony Brook, Stony Brook, New York

MICHAEL D. ISEMAN, MD
Division of Mycobacterial and Respiratory
Infections, National Jewish Health, Denver,
Colorado

MARC A. JUDSON, MD
Professor of Medicine; Chief, Division of
Pulmonary and Critical Care Medicine,
Department of Medicine, Albany Medical
College, Albany, New York

NAOTO KEICHO, MD, PhD
Director, Department of Respiratory Diseases,
Research Institute, National Center for Global
Health and Medicine, Shinjuku-ku, Tokyo, Japan

SHOJI KUDOH, MD, PhD
President, Fukujuji Hospital, Japan
Anti-Tuberculosis Association, Tokyo, Japan;
Professor Emeritus, Nippon Medical School,
Sendagi, Bunkyo-ku, Tokyo, Japan

JASON LOBO, MD
Research Fellow, Division of Pulmonary
and Critical Care Medicine, Department
of Medicine, University of North Carolina,
Chapel Hill, North Carolina

DAVID C. MAUCHLEY, MD
Section of General Thoracic Surgery, Division of
Cardiothoracic Surgery, University of Colorado
School of Medicine, Aurora, Colorado

MARK L. METERSKY, MD
Professor of Medicine, Director, Center for
Bronchiectasis Care, Division of Pulmonary
and Critical Care Medicine, University of
Connecticut School of Medicine, Farmington,
Connecticut

JOHN D. MITCHELL, MD
Chief, Section of General Thoracic Surgery,
Division of Cardiothoracic Surgery, University
of Colorado School of Medicine, Aurora,
Colorado

BART C. MOULTON, MD
Pulmonary and Critical Care Medicine, Oregon
Health and Science University, Portland, Oregon

DAVID P. NAIDICH, MD, FACCP
Department of Radiology, New York
University-Langone Medical Center,
New York, New York

GIRISH B. NAIR, MD
Pulmonary and Critical Care Medicine Fellow,
Winthrop University Hospital, Mineola, New York

PEADAR G. NOONE, MD, FCCP, FRCPI
Associate Professor of Medicine, Division
of Pulmonary and Critical Care Medicine,
Department of Medicine, University of
North Carolina, Chapel Hill, North Carolina

ANNE E. O'DONNELL, MD
Professor of Medicine, Chief, Division of
Pulmonary, Critical Care and Sleep Medicine,
Georgetown University Hospital,
Washington, DC

KENNETH N. OLIVIER, MD, MPH
Staff Clinician, Laboratory of Clinical Infectious
Diseases, National Institute of Allergy and
Infectious Diseases, National Institutes of
Health, Bethesda, Maryland

JUAN M. ROJAS-BALCAZAR, MD
Research Fellow, Division of Pulmonary
and Critical Care Medicine, Department
of Medicine, University of North Carolina,
Chapel Hill, North Carolina

MAEVE P. SMITH, MB ChB, MRCP
Respiratory Specialist Registrar, Department
of Respiratory Medicine, Royal Infirmary of
Edinburgh, Edinburgh, United kingdom

GRANT W. WATERER, MD, PhD
Professor of Medicine, University of Western
Australia, Royal Perth Hospital, Perth,
Australia; Adjunct Professor of Medicine,
Northwestern University, Chicago, Illinois

Contents

for measuring response to therapy. The full potential of computed tomography for evaluating airways disease has yet to be fully explored.

Our understanding of the pathologic cycle leading to the development of bronchiectasis is enhanced by greater understanding of the genetic influences contributing to its development. Genome-wide linkage analysis, family-based genetic linkage studies, and the testing of candidate genes have all greatly advanced our understanding of the complexity of the genetic basis of bronchiectasis. This article discusses how allelic variations, gene modifiers, HLA associations, and the interplay of developmental, host, and environmental factors all contribute in lesser and greater degrees, depending on the specific disease, toward the development of bronchiectasis in a spectrum of disease processes.

Allergic bronchopulmonary aspergillosis (ABPA) is caused by an exaggerated T_H2 response to the ubiquitous mold *Aspergillus fumigatus*. ABPA develops in a small fraction of patients with cystic fibrosis and asthma, suggesting that intrinsic host defects play a major role in disease susceptibility. This article reviews current understanding of the immunopathology, clinical and laboratory findings, and diagnosis and management of ABPA. It highlights clinical and laboratory clues to differentiate ABPA from cystic fibrosis and asthma, which are challenging given clinical and serologic similarities. A practical diagnostic algorithm and management scheme to aid in the treatment of these patients is outlined.

Over the last 30 years it has become increasingly clear that nontuberculous mycobacterial (NTM) lung infections and bronchiectasis are closely related disorders. Although incontrovertible proof is lacking, there is a growing consensus of opinion that NTM lung disease characterized by nodules and bronchiectasis (nodular/bronchiectatic NTM lung disease) may be a consequence of preexisting bronchiectasis that predisposes to NTM infection and disease. To use published diagnostic guidelines effectively, physicians must become familiar with the disease-causing potential of individual NTM species. Essentially all NTM patients have bronchiectasis, so optimal overall patient management requires successful therapeutic strategies for both NTM infection and bronchiectasis.

Diffuse panbronchiolitis (DPB) is characterized by chronic airway infection with diffuse bilateral micronodular pulmonary lesions. DPB is mainly distributed in east Asian people. Studies on causes of the disease point to a genetic predisposition unique to Asians. The advent of low-dose, long-term macrolide therapy has changed disease prognosis. The mechanism of action is attributed to anti-inflammatory actions of 14-membered and 15-membered ring macrolides. Recently, the success of macrolide therapy in DPB has extended its application to the treatment of other chronic airway inflammatory diseases.

Cystic fibrosis (CF) is an inherited chronic disease that remains a common cause of morbidity and mortality in affected patients, mostly in the young. A wealth of knowledge has been gained into the genetics, pathophysiology, and clinical manifestation of the disease. In parallel with these new insights into the disease, novel treatments have been developed or are under development that have had a major impact on quality of life and survival. Improvement in the delivery of care to patients in CF centers, using a team-based approach, and constant review of process, and by quality improvement projects, have also had an impact on outcomes in CF.

Long-term treatment goals of bronchiectasis frequently include limiting the bacterial burden and inflammatory insult in the airways with the aim of improving symptoms, reducing exacerbation frequency and severity, and improving health-related quality-of-life. However, few clinical or laboratory markers specifically validated for bronchiectasis exist, and how best to assess the disease and its response to treatment is poorly understood. Pertinent, reliable markers are urgently needed to facilitate effective treatment of bronchiectasis and to ensure ongoing development of future therapies. This article explores the utility of potential end points in evaluating therapies used in the long-term management of stable bronchiectasis.

Bronchiectasis is a persistent and progressive condition characterized by inflammation and infection causing damage that potentiates impaired mucociliary clearance. The rationale for promoting airway clearance is so that purulent secretions are removed from the airways, ameliorating the inflammation and improving control of symptoms such as cough and sputum plugging. Physiotherapists aim to teach patients one of a variety of airway clearance techniques to regularly perform as part of their daily management.

There are no approved pharmacologic agents to enhance mucus clearance in non–cystic fibrosis (CF) bronchiectasis. Evidence supports the use of hyperosmolar agents in CF, and studies with inhaled mannitol and hypertonic saline are ongoing in bronchiectasis. N-acetylcysteine may act more as an antioxidant than a mucolytic in other lung diseases. Dornase α is beneficial to patients with CF, but is not useful in patients with non-CF bronchiectasis. Mucokinetic agents such as β-agonists have the potential to improve mucociliary clearance in normals and many disease states, but have not been adequately studied in patients with bronchiectasis.

Airway inflammation is a major component of disease pathogenesis in bronchiectasis, suggesting that antiinflammatory therapies could be of benefit in treatment. This article addresses the use of anti-inflammatory/immunomodulatory therapies in the management of patients with bronchiectasis and individually discusses the use of corticosteroids, macrolides, and other potential anti-inflammatory agents.

Antibiotics have a role in the management of acute exacerbations of bronchiectasis and may also benefit selected subsets of patients with bronchiectasis as a part of a long-term maintenance strategy. At present, there are no Food and Drug Administration–approved antibiotics for acute or chronic management of bronchiectasis. Clinical trials are underway to determine the efficacy and safety of various inhaled antibiotics for chronic therapy for bronchiectasis. Until those results are available, clinicians need to tailor their therapies to individual patients based on their best clinical judgment and information from data and guidelines currently available in the published literature.

The purpose of this article is to update specialists in pulmonary medicine on the role of surgical resection and lung transplantation for bronchiectasis. The focus is on pre-operative workup, the technical details of surgical resection, complications, and outcomes.

CLINICS IN CHEST MEDICINE

DOWNLOAD
Free App!

Review Articles
THE CLINICS

NOW AVAILABLE FOR YOUR iPhone and iPad

Preface

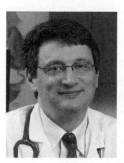 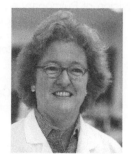

Mark L. Metersky, MD   Anne E. O'Donnell, MD
Guest Editors

Bronchiectasis has long been considered an orphan disease. Neglected by pharmaceutical companies and funding agencies, there are no medications that are FDA approved for its treatment. Interestingly, this is not because bronchiectasis is rare. Although the prevalence may have declined with the introduction of antibiotics in the last century, there are over 110,000 patients with bronchiectasis in the United States alone. The lack of attention to the disease is even more remarkable given pharmaceutical companies' long interest in cystic fibrosis (CF), which has a prevalence about one-third as high as non-CF bronchiectasis. There also has seemed to be a perception among many physicians that there is little that can be done to improve patients' quality of life or alter the course of their disease.

The last 5 to 10 years has brought a significant change in this attitude. Perhaps because of recent studies demonstrating the surprisingly high prevalence of the disease, or perhaps due to advances in the science of aerosolized drug delivery, we are entering a new era of bronchiectasis care. Numerous clinical trials of therapies for bronchiectasis have been recently completed and many more are currently in progress. Agents being investigated include various aerosolized antibiotics, hyperosmolar agents, and anti-inflammatory agents. The expanding therapeutic armamentarium increases the importance of physicians having a firm understanding of the pathophysiology, evaluation, and treatment of bronchiectasis. Therefore, this monograph, devoted entirely to bronchiectasis and related diseases, is being published at a particularly appropriate time.

Dr O'Donnell and I have recruited an international group of experts to write a comprehensive, state-of-the-art review of bronchiectasis and related diseases. We have purposefully chosen authors who have contributed greatly to our knowledge of these diseases and who have extensive experience in caring for affected patients. Because bronchiectasis has received little attention from funding agencies and pharmaceutical companies in the past, we have little high-quality evidence on which to base our clinical decision-making as we care for these patients. Therefore, the clinical expertise of our authors makes them uniquely able to interpret the relevant literature in the context of their experience.

The first two articles review the fundamental scientific underpinnings of airway defense mechanisms and the relationship of host defense to the pathophysiology of bronchiectasis. The next article lays out a suggested approach for the initial evaluation of a patient newly diagnosed with bronchiectasis. A discussion of radiographic techniques for the evaluation of bronchiectasis follows. There are several articles in the monograph devoted to comprehensive reviews of specific causes of bronchiectasis and related diseases, including genetic causes, allergic bronchopulmonary aspergillosis, nontuberculous mycobacterial infection, diffuse panbronchiolitis, and CF. We then turn to articles on treatment-related issues, beginning with an appraisal of a thorny area: the appropriate endpoints for clinical trials of therapies for bronchiectasis. That discussion sets the foundation for the specific treatment articles, which include practical information on chest

Clin Chest Med 33 (2012) xi–xii
doi:10.1016/j.ccm.2012.04.002
0272-5231/12/$ – see front matter © 2012 Elsevier Inc. All rights reserved.

physiotherapy techniques, pharmacologic agents for mucus clearance, the use of anti-inflammatory agents and macrolides, inhaled and systemic antibiotics, and the use of surgical modalities.

We hope that both researchers and clinicians caring for patients with bronchiectasis find this monograph informative. We thank the authors for submitting uniformly excellent articles. Their hard work made our job both easy and enlightening. We would also like to thank Katie Hartner of Elsevier, for her support and patience during the many months of this effort. Finally, Mark would like to thank his wife Karen, and sons Andrew and Joshua, for their understanding as he retired repeatedly to the study to work on this project, and Anne would like to thank her family, friends, and colleagues for their support.

Mark L. Metersky, MD
Center for Bronchiectasis Care
Division of Pulmonary and Critical Care Medicine
University of Connecticut School of Medicine
263 Farmington Avenue
Farmington, CT 06030-1321, USA

Anne E. O'Donnell, MD
Critical Care and Sleep Medicine
Georgetown University Hospital
4 North Main Hospital
3800 Reservoir Road NW
Washington, DC 20007, USA

E-mail addresses:
Metersky@nso.uchc.edu (M.L. Metersky)
odonnela@georgetown.edu (A.E. O'Donnell)

Airway Defense Mechanisms

Grant W. Waterer, MD, PhD[a,b]

KEYWORDS

- Immunity • Airways • Innate

KEY POINTS

- The immune system is complex, with multiple redundancies and overlapping mechanisms; evolution of this complex system is probably a response to the ability of pathogens to develop ways to overcome the immune barriers of their hosts.
- The key role that small proteins and peptides such as defensins, cathelicidins, and collectins play provide major new insights into protection against pathogens.
- These proteins and peptides are an area of new research, particularly intervention with inhaled therapies, including stem cell approaches.

Human airways are regularly in contact with a wide variety of potential pathogens. In response, we have developed strategies to protect ourselves. As many of these organisms have developed mechanisms to help them bypass immune defenses, so has the human immune system developed a complex array of overlapping strategies to counter them.

In bronchiectasis, the balance between host and pathogen has been tipped in favor of the assailants. Not only are there often one or more deficits in the immune response that has led to bronchiectasis, the destruction of normal bronchial architecture leads to a variety of immune deficits in the region of damaged airways. Although the immune response is critical to removing pathogens, inflammation is likely to contribute not only to further lung damage but, at least temporarily, impairs immune response making the host more vulnerable to subsequent infections; the so-called vicious cycle hypothesis in bronchiectasis.[1]

A comprehensive summary of all airway defense mechanisms is a textbook in itself, and far beyond the scope of this article. This article highlights both the key airway defense mechanisms typically compromised in bronchiectasis, as well as key insights into the response to pathogens that have been discovered in the past decade. It focuses particularly on the innate immune system because this is where most of the developments have occurred that are particularly relevant to bronchiectasis.

MECHANICAL DEFENSES
Cilia

Basic mechanical adaptations to protect airways are extremely important. The respiratory tract is for the most part covered with ciliated epithelium. On top of the cilia is a thick mucus blanket ranging from 5 to 10 μm in depth where inhaled particles are deposited.[2] Coordinated movements of the cilia propel microorganisms and other inhaled particles trapped in the mucus blanket. In the upper airways, the cilia propel particles toward the pharynx where they are swallowed; in the lower airway they are propelled toward the trachea where they can be coughed up.

A wide variety of inherited and acquired disorders of cilia numbers and/or function have now been described.[3] The correlation between the degree of impairment of ciliary function and the extent and severity of lung and sinus disease is

[a] University of Western Australia, Royal Perth Hospital, Level 4 MRF Building, GPO Box X2213, Perth 6847, Australia
[b] Northwestern University, Chicago, IL, USA
E-mail address: grant.waterer@uwa.edu.au

Clin Chest Med 33 (2012) 199–209
doi:10.1016/j.ccm.2012.03.003
0272-5231/12/$ – see front matter © 2012 Elsevier Inc. All rights reserved.

evidence of how important this basic defense mechanism is in protecting airways.

Mucus

The mucus layer is composed of a variety of high-molecular-weight glycoproteins (2%–3%), salts (1%), and water (95%), and is produced by goblet cells and by serous and mucus glands in the submucosa.[4] Although the superficial part of the mucus layer is moved by the action of the cilia, the deeper layer of periciliary fluid is not.[2] The salt concentration of the mucus layer is tightly controlled and may be important in limiting bacterial growth. Failure to regulate the salt concentration, as occurs, for example, with defects of the cystic fibrosis transmembrane conductance regulator,[5] causes significant changes in the viscoelastic properties of the mucus, with the potentially devastating effects on mucosal immunity seen in patients with cystic fibrosis.

Apart from glycoproteins, the mucus layer also contains a variety of proteins important in the innate immune response. Although some of these proteins arise by transudation from plasma, others, such as immunoglobulin (Ig) A, lysozyme, and lactoferrin, are actively secreted into the mucus layer.[6]

INNATE IMMUNITY
Toll-like Receptors

Recognition of the specific type of pathogen begins with the toll-like receptors (TLRs), a family of cell surface proteins that help trigger both innate and adaptive immune responses, although they are not obligatory for the latter. Eleven TLRs with differing pathogen specificity are currently recognized (**Table 1**), although the ligand, and therefore specificity, for TLR-10 remains unknown.[7] TLRs are expressed on a variety of cells including neutrophils, macrophages, dendritic cells, regulatory T cells, B-cells, and epithelial cells.[7–9]

The signaling pathways activated by binding of TLR to their ligands have been well characterized, as have disorders of signaling resulting in clinical disease.[7] In general, signaling from TLRs can be divided into MyD88-dependent and MyD88-independent pathways, with the MyD88-dependent route being the main pathway for most TLRs.[7]

There is some evidence that TLR regulation may be different in bronchiectasis, but whether this precedes or is induced by disease is unclear.[10] The primary result of TLR activation is the release of a variety of cytokines that have neutrophils and macrophages as their primary targets.[7] Key cytokines include tumor necrosis factor α, interleukin (IL)-1 β and IL-6.

In addition to initiating an inflammatory cascade, stimulation of TLR2[11] and TLR3[12] induce mucin expression and activate epidermal growth factors.[13] Although these effects should be protective, excess mucus production may have adverse consequences, particularly by impairing neutrophil recruitment.[14]

Non-TLR Recognition of Pathogens and Inflammatory Signaling

TLRs are not the only mechanism by which the immune system recognizes the type of invading pathogen and initiates the most appropriate inflammatory response. The nucleotide oligomerization domain (NOD)–like receptors are a large family of intracellular receptors that sense microbial components in the cytosol. Of the 23

Table 1
Toll-like receptors and their specificity

Toll-like Receptor(s)	Ligand	Pathogen
1, 2, and 6	Lipopeptides	Gram-positive bacteria and fungi
3	Poly I:C, dsDNA	Viruses
4	Lipopolysaccharide	Gram-negative bacteria
5	Flagellin	Bacterial flagellum
7	ssRNA, resiquimod, imiquimod, loxoribine	Viruses
8	ssRNA	Viruses
9	Unmethylated DNA, CPG-DNA	Bacteria, DNA
10	Unknown	unknown
11	Unknown component of uropathic *Escherichia coli*, profilinlike molecule	Uropathic *E coli*,[99] toxoplasma[100]

Abbreviations: CPG, cytosine-phosphate-guanine; dsDNA, double-strand DNA; ssRNA, single-strand RNA.
Data from Moresco EM, LaVine D, Beutler B. Toll-like receptors. Curr Biol 2011;21:R488–93.

NOD-like receptors so far reported, the best-described members of the family are NOD1 and NOD2, both of which recognize bacterial peptidoglycan, although NOD1 is more specific to gram-negative peptidoglycan.[15–17] Stimulation of NOD-like receptors results in increased NF-κB activation via RIP2 kinase.[18]

TNF receptor 1 (TNFR1) is abundant on the surface of many inflammatory cells and the airway epithelium.[19] As well as TNF, TNFR1 also recognizes staphylococcal protein A and seems to be the primary sensing mechanism for *Staphylococcus aureus* in the airways because MyD88, and hence TLR signaling, is not important with this pathogen.[20]

C-type lectins are unusual in that they are focused primarily in the detection of fungi, particularly through binding to carbohydrates such as β-glycans.[21] The C-lectin family, which includes dectin-1, dectin-2 and mincle, have been also been shown to have an important role in detecting carbohydrates from yeast and mycobacteria.[22] Although present in airway epithelial cells,[23] most research has been done in myeloid cells, and their role in resisting airways pathogens is still poorly understood. However, given that C-lectins are expressed on neutrophils[24] and macrophages,[25] it is reasonable to presume that they have an important role in the airways' response to invading fungal and mycobacterial pathogens.

Nonspecific Antimicrobial Agents

A variety of chemical defenses are embedded within the mucus layer of the respiratory epithelium. The first described chemical agent was lysozyme, which has nonspecific antibacterial activity by lysing the cell wall of bacteria and various fungi.[2] Other important molecules include lactoferrin, uric acid, leukoprotease inhibitor, peroxidase, aminopeptidase, secretory phospholipase A2, and defensins. Nitric oxide is also found in both the upper and lower respiratory tract and may have antibacterial activity.

Defensins and Cathelicidins

In the past decade, there has been a significant increase in knowledge of the role of defensins and cathelicidins against a broad range of microbial threats including bacteria, viruses and fungi. Both defensins and cathelicidins are amphipathic peptides, having both hydrophobic and hydrophilic properties that enable them to disrupt microbial membranes. Although many cells seem to have the capacity to produce antimicrobial peptides, the main source seems to be neutrophils and epithelial cells. Although generally thought to

be protective, there is increasing evidence that, in some circumstances, antimicrobial peptides, like many inflammatory molecules, may have adverse effects including impairing neutrophil phagocytosis in patients with bronchiectasis.[26]

Defensins are divided into 2 families: α-defensins and β-defensins. As well as some differences in the pairing of cysteine residues, α-defensins are mainly produced by neutrophils,[27] whereas β-defensins come mainly from epithelial cells.[28] In addition, defensins seem to have a key role in immunity in both the gut[29] and the reproductive tract.[30]

Although at least 4 β-defensins have been well characterized based on their disulfide connectivity (eg, Cys1-Cys5, Cys2-Cys4), many others have been identified by whole-genome screening.[31] The type of β-defensin produced depends on the inflammatory cell of origin.[32]

Cathelicidins are α-helical cationic peptides that are produced as precursors consisting of a cathelin-like domain and the active peptide and hence require proteolytic conversion to the active form.[33] As with defensins, cathelicidins seem to play antimicrobial roles in the respiratory, digestive, and reproductive tracts. The main cathelicidin released by neutrophils, LL-37, displays a wide range of effects beyond antimicrobial activity, including neutralizing microbial products like lipopolysaccharide (LPS), chemoattraction of inflammatory cells, and upregulation of epithelial proliferation and repair activity.[34] Of particular note in the setting of bronchiectasis is that cathelicidins including LL-37 have antibiofilm activity against *Pseudomonas*.[35]

Collectins: Surfactant Protein A and D

Another family of proteins important for opsonizing bacterial pathogens are collectins. Among the collectins are mannose-binding lectin (discussed later) and surfactant A (SP-A) and surfactant D (SP-D), which are lipoproteins synthesized by type II pneumocytes and Clara cells. Although known for a long time to modulate surface tension, more recently the role of surfactant in host defense against infection and inflammation has been discovered.

All collectins share a collagenlike domain that is capable of binding oligosaccharides found on bacterial, nonencapsulated fungal, and some viral envelope surfaces.[36] Both SP-A and SP-D bind to a wide range of pathogens, suppress microbial growth, damage bacterial membranes, and modulate macrophage phagocytosis.[37] Removal and detoxification of LPS by alveolar macrophages is also facilitated by SP-A and SP-D.[38]

Although able to activate several signaling cascades, including TLR2 and TLR4,[37] SP-A and SP-D tend to suppress the production of proinflammatory cytokines by macrophages.[39,40] Consistent with an antiinflammatory regulatory role for SP-A and SP-D, they have also been shown to increase alveolar macrophage production of IL-10 and TGF-β.[41]

Bactericidal/Permeability-Increasing Protein

The role of bactericidal/permeability-increasing protein (BPI), although first described in the 1970s,[42] has been better delineated in the past decade, particularly with respect to its key role in defense against gram-negative bacteria. As well as being found in neutrophil azurophilic granules (discussed later), BPI is also found in eosinophils[43] and epithelial cells,[44] and has emerged as another of the key antimicrobial peptides.

BPI seems to have 2 main functions. First, it binds to and neutralizes LPS with high efficacy, significantly reducing the inflammatory response.[45] This anti-LPS activity makes BPI particularly important against gram-negative pathogens. Second, BPI has innate bactericidal activity, particularly against gram-negative bacteria like *Pseudomonas*.[46,47]

Complement

The complement system is an important component of both the adaptive an innate immune systems. The complement system consists of more than 25 plasma and cell surface proteins with 3 different activation pathways.[48] The main function of the cascade of activity that occurs through activation of one of the pathways is to mark pathogens for destruction by phagocytes. The classic pathway is activated by antigen-antibody complexes. The alternative pathway is activated without antibody by microbial structures. A third pathway is triggered by microbial cell wall components containing mannans and is called the lectin pathway (discussed further later).[49]

Interferons

Interferons (IFN) are an important part of the innate host defense against viruses. Virally infected epithelial cells secrete 2 classes of IFNs. Type I IFNs include IFN-α, IFN-β, INF-κ, IFN-ε, and limitin. The class I IFNs signal via the IFN-α/β receptor and produce their effects via the Janus kinase/signal transducers and activators of transcription (JAK-STAT) pathways.[50] Type III IFNs IFN-λ1 (also known as IL29), IFN-λ2 (also known as IL28A) and IFN-λ3 (also known as IL28B) signal via IL-28R, which is expressed in epithelial cells and

a limited number of other cell types.[51] The products of IFN-induced genes act to limit viral replication and spread by degrading viral RNA, inhibiting cellular translation machinery used for viral replication, and limiting interaction with viral polymerase complexes.[50]

Cytokines

Cytokines are a diverse group of proteins and peptides that can have autocrine, paracrine, and/or endocrine activities that modulate immune function. Although there is an extensive list, the major proinflammatory cytokines that have been extensively studied in humans are TNFα, IL-1β, IL-6, IL-8, IL-12, and IFN-γ. Although some of the functions of these cytokines are addressed elsewhere, TNFα, ILβ, and IL-6 all play an important role in vasodilatation, increasing vascular permeability, and upregulating cellular adhesion molecules. Key antiinflammatory cytokines include IL-10, TGF-β, and IL1-Ra.

Recently, IL-23 has emerged as another key cytokine in innate host defense against bacterial pathogens. IL-23 shares a common p40 subunit with IL-12 but has a unique p19 subunit.[52] IL-23 seems to be predominantly produced by antigen-presenting cells and stimulates the production of IL-17 by TH17 and γδ T cells in a TLR-dependent manner.[53] Several studies have shown that the IL-23/IL-17 response is critical for clearing gram-negative infections such as *Klebsiella pneumoniae*[54] and *Pseudomonas aeruginosa*.[55] IL-17 is a family of 6 related proteins, IL-17 A to F, with IL-17A usually termed IL-17 and IL-17E also known as IL-25.[56] Although most of the IL-17 family have proinflammatory effects, the source and site of action differ.[56] IL-25 is unusual in the IL-17 family in that it inhibits some proinflammatory responses in addition to promoting a Th2-type response.[56]

Chemokines

Chemokines are cytokines that induce leukocyte infiltration into the site of infection. Chemokines are grouped into 4 main types based on the presence of a cysteine toward the N-terminus: C, CC, CXC, and CX3C.[57] A large number of human chemokines have been reported; however, the most important in humans seems to be IL-8.[58]

Neutrophils

Neutrophils are a predominant feature in the airways of patients with bronchiectasis. If containment of pathogens fails by all the mechanism already discussed and the airways' bacterial load is less than 10^6 colony-forming units/mL then a neutrophil inflammatory response is initiated.[59]

The recruitment of these neutrophils to the site of infection is orchestrated by the expression of leukocyte and vascular adhesion molecules combined with the release of chemotaxins like IL-8 and leukotriene B4 (LTB4) into the submucosa.[60,61] In bronchiectasis, there is evidence that IL-8 may be more important for chemotaxis than LTB4, at least in acute exacerbations.[62]

Once in the airways, neutrophils attempt to neutralize the invading pathogen with a combination of phagocytosis and the release of their arsenal of proteolytic enzymes, reactive oxygen species (ROS), and other immunoactive compounds.[63] Neutrophil granules are generally divided into 3 subsets, although it is possible to discern further variations and subsets.[64] Azurophilic granules release myeloperoxidase, elastase, proteinase 3, cathepsin G, defensins, and BPIs, among others. Specific granules contain lactoferrin, cathelicidins, and other antibacterial proteins. Gelatinase granules contain gelatinase acetyltransferase and lysozyme[64] has direct bactericidal activity through its N-terminal domain.[65]

Neutrophil phagocytosis is facilitated by opsonization. Although IgA (discussed later) does promote phagocytosis,[66] IgG is particularly important in this process. Complement activated by IgG (classic pathway) or independently (lectin or alternative pathway) is also important for phagocytosis.[67] Mannose-binding lectin plays a critical role in activating complement through the lectin pathway, which may explain the association between bronchiectasis and low levels of this protein.[68] P aeruginosa has an alkaline protease that blocks complement activation through both the classic and lectin pathways.[69]

The respiratory or oxidative burst is a key mechanism for digesting the contents of phagocytic vacuoles. Production of the ROS in the respiratory burst depends on nicotinamide adenine dinucleotide phosphate (NADPH) oxidase.[70] A genetic disorder of one of the subunits of NADPH leads to an inability to produce ROS, with resulting recurrent bacterial infections and chronic granulomatous disease.[71] Whether respiratory burst is impaired in patients with bronchiectasis is controversial.[72,73]

It was recently recognized that neutrophils have an additional antibacterial function. Neutrophils are able to create extracellular traps capable of trapping and killing extracellular bacteria and fungi.[74] These neutrophil traps are created by expelling decondensed chromatin mixed with antibacterial proteins. Large numbers of neutrophil extracellular traps can be released by the destruction of neutrophils, which seems to be a novel form of cell death compared with the traditional models of apoptosis or necrosis.[75] The formation of extracellular nets is deficient in neonates, which may partially explain their markedly increased susceptibility to infection.[76]

Macrophages

Both macrophages and dendritic cells are derived from common progenitor cells and therefore share several properties including phagocytosis and endocytosis of pathogens, antigen presentation and activation of T cells, secretion of cytokines, and migration to local lymphoid tissue.[77] Although macrophages are an important source of proinflammatory cytokines (particularly TNFα, IL1-β, IFN-α, IFN-β, IL-6, IL-12, and IL-18), it seems that lung alveolar macrophages and dendritic cells are biased toward an immunosuppressive response (eg, with IL-10 and TGFβ) and need a strong inflammatory signal to overcome this predisposition.[78]

Although they have similar functions, macrophages are superior to dendritic cells in their ability to phagocytose and kill bacteria. Alveolar macrophages make up more than 90% of the pulmonary macrophage population,[79] but functionally are similar to other tissue macrophages. Alveolar macrophages predominantly originate from monocytes recruited from blood, but a small proportion comes from replication of the existing pool.[80]

Alveolar macrophages can directly phagocytose bacteria; however, the polysaccharide capsule of many bacteria is a significant impediment. For these pathogens, opsonization (by immunoglobulin, complement, and other opsonins discussed earlier) is required for effective phagocytosis.[81] Like neutrophils, macrophages use a variety of microbicidal molecules to kill pathogens, including nitric oxide[81] and NADPH-dependent production of ROS. Macrophages also play an important role in reducing inflammatory damage by phagocytosing apoptotic neutrophils and other cellular debris, and by secreting antiinflammatory cytokines such as IL-10 and TGF-β, as described earlier.

Dendritic Cells

Dendritic cells play a pivotal role in linking the innate and adaptive immune systems. They can be divided into myeloid and plasmacytoid groups, both of which mature into conventional dendritic cells. Although dendritic cells of myeloid origin migrate through the lymphatics and into lymph nodes, where they act primarily as antigen-presenting cells,[82] plasmacytoid dendritic cells migrate through small blood vessels primarily surveying for pathogens.[83] Macrophages seem to control the number of dendritic cells in the lung, keeping them suppressed unless there is acute infection.[84] Although alveolar macrophages have a half-life measured in weeks to months, dendritic cells have a fast turnover with a half-life of less than 2 days.[85] The primary function of dendritic cells in the lung seems to be as antigen-presenting cells. Dendritic cells that have captured foreign material mature, leave the lung, and enter lymphoid tissues where they activate naive T cells.[86] Although myeloid dendritic cells express a broad array of TLRs,[87] plasmacytoid dendritic cells express only TLR-7 and TLR-9 and are the most potent known producers of IFNs,[88] suggesting that they are key cells in the innate response to viral infection.

Natural Killer Cells

Natural killer (NK) cells are lymphocytes that are capable of killing infected cells without the need for antigen specificity (eg, as with cytotoxic lymphocytes). NK cells can also activate macrophages to enhance intracellular killing of phagocytosed pathogens. Key components of NK cell activity are perforin, a protein that perforates target cell membranes, and granzymes, which initiate apoptosis and hence death of the infected cell.[89] Infected cells typically reduce expression of class I HLA molecules on their surface, which is thought to be the signal for NK cells to target them.

ADAPTIVE IMMUNITY
Specific Humoral Immunity

The adaptive immune response is required when innate mechanisms fail to contain invading organisms. Key among the adaptive responses is the development of pathogen-specific immunoglobulins (antibodies). Primary disorders of antibody production, a number of which are recognized (Table 2), are all associated with bronchiectasis.

Secretory IgA helps protect the mucosal surface from a variety of pathogens, but is vulnerable to IgA-specific proteases released by common pathogens such as Streptococcus pneumoniae and Haemophilus influenzae.[2] Most IgA is produced locally by subepithelial plasma cells. The proportion of IgA subclasses is different between the lung and blood, with IgA2 contributing a higher proportion in the lung (around 30% compared with 10%–20% in blood). IgA2 is more resistant to IgA-specific proteases produced by many bacteria.[66] The importance of IgA in airway defense is unclear given that IgA deficiency is usually asymptomatic, so presumably it is only critical when other defects in immune response are present.[90]

IgG-mediated opsonization of bacteria to facilitate phagocytosis is highly effective at removing pathogens. The importance of IgG in helping maintain the integrity of the airway is shown by the high risk of bronchiectasis in patients with marked deficiencies of IgG, although selective subclass deficiencies are probably not sufficient to cause disease on their own.[72,73,91]

Antibodies may not always have a protective effect. IgG2 antibodies in particular may impair phagocytosis.[92] These deleterious IgG2 antibodies seem to be more common in patients with cystic fibrosis and pseudomonas infection,[92,93] and in patients with human immunodeficiency virus infection.[94]

Specific Cellular Immunity

Effective mucosal immunity requires activation of both T-lymphocytes and B-lymphocytes. As discussed earlier, the end result of much of the activity of the TLR system is the presentation of antigen to, and activation of, naive T cells in lung lymphoid tissue. Although B-cell activation leads to the production of antigen-specific immunoglobulin, the primary effector arm of T-cell activation is

Table 2
Primary disorders of antibody production

Syndrome	Deficiency	Useful References
Common variable immune deficiency	Low IgG, IgA, ± low IgM	101–103
X-linked agammaglobulinemia	Low IgG, IgA, and IgM	104,105
IgG subclass deficiencies	1 or more IgG1-4 low	106
Specific antibody deficiency	Normal IgG and subclasses but impaired response to vaccines	107,108
Selective IgA deficiency	Low IgA	90
Selective IgM deficiency	Low IgM	109
Hyper-IgM syndrome	High IgM, low IgG and IgA	110

the production of cytotoxic T-lymphocytes, which are characterized by the expression of CD8. CD8+ cytotoxic T-lymphocytes recognize specific epitopes on infected cells, and then target them for elimination using a similar arsenal to NK cells.[95] There is also recent research that suggests that CD8+ lymphocytes may have direct antimicrobial activity against an array of pathogens.[96]

As well as activating CD8+ cytotoxic T-lymphocytes, dendritic and other antigen-presenting cells activate CD4+ T-lymphocytes (known as T-helper lymphocytes). Although they have no cytotoxic or phagocytic activity, CD4+ T-lymphocytes secrete cytokines that significantly enhance the development of other adaptive immune functions including CD8+ cytotoxic T-lymphocytes. CD4+ T-lymphocytes have traditionally been divided into 2 classes based on their cytokine secretion pattern: Th1, with a predominance of IFN γ, which favors the development of cellular immunity, and Th2 with a predominance of IL-4, which favors the development of antibody or humoral immunity. A third subset, T-regulatory (T-reg) lymphocytes are characterized by the expression of CD25 (IL-2R α) and play a key role in downregulating the immune response by a variety of mechanisms including the secretion of IL-9, IL-10, TGF-β, and cytotoxic T-lymphocyte antigen 4.[97]

However, it has recently been recognized that CD4+ T-lymphocyte differentiation is more complex, with substantial attention given to the Th17 pathway.[98] Th17 T cells are characterized by their secretion of IL-17A, IL-17F, and IL-22, seem to play a key role in defense against extracellular pathogens, and have been implicated in the development of several autoimmune and allergic disorders.[98]

Adaptive Immunity and Immune Memory

An important end result of activating the adaptive immune system is the preservation of the immune memory of the pathogen so that, if reinfection occurs, subsequent immune responses will be faster and disease might be less severe. Although most CD8+ and CD4+ lymphocytes die with the resolution of infection, some remain as memory cells. Memory B-cells are also preserved.

SUMMARY

The immune system is complex, with multiple redundancies and overlapping mechanisms. The evolution of such a complex system is probably driven by the ingenuity of pathogens in developing ways to overcome immune barriers. Although there have been steady advances in all areas, it is in the innate immune system that there ahs

been a particular expansion of knowledge. The key role that small proteins and peptides such as defensins, cathelicidins, and collectins play are major new insights into how humans protect themselves against pathogens. How many of these newly understood systems have faults that lead to, or at least contribute to, the development of bronchiectasis will be a fruitful area of research in the next decade, particularly because they may be amenable to intervention with inhaled therapies, including stem cell approaches.

REFERENCES

1. Cole P, Wilson R. Host-microbial interrelationships in respiratory infection. Chest 1989;95:217S–21S.
2. Wanner A, Salathe M, O'Riordan TG. Mucociliary clearance in the airways. Am J Respir Crit Care Med 1996;154(6 Pt 1):1868–902.
3. Ware SM, Aygun MG, Hildebrandt F. Spectrum of clinical diseases caused by disorders of primary cilia. Proc Am Thorac Soc 2011;8(5):444–50.
4. Houtmeyers E, Gosselink R, Gayan-Ramirez G, et al. Regulation of mucociliary clearance in health and disease. Eur Respir J 1999;13(5):1177–88.
5. Gadsby DC, Vergani P, Csanady L. The ABC protein turned chloride channel whose failure causes cystic fibrosis. Nature 2006;440(7083):477–83.
6. Lopez-Vidriero MT. Mucus as a natural barrier. Respiration 1989;55(Suppl 1):28–32.
7. Moresco EM, LaVine D, Beutler B. Toll-like receptors. Curr Biol 2011;21(13):R488–93.
8. Caramalho I, Lopes-Carvalho T, Ostler D, et al. Regulatory T cells selectively express toll-like receptors and are activated by lipopolysaccharide. J Exp Med 2003;197(4):403–11.
9. Sha Q, Truong-Tran AQ, Plitt JR, et al. Activation of airway epithelial cells by toll-like receptor agonists. Am J Respir Cell Mol Biol 2004;31(3):358–64.
10. Simpson JL, Grissell TV, Douwes J, et al. Innate immune activation in neutrophilic asthma and bronchiectasis. Thorax 2007;62(3):211–8.
11. Chen R, Lim JH, Jono H, et al. Nontypeable *Haemophilus influenzae* lipoprotein P6 induces MUC5AC mucin transcription via TLR2-TAK1-dependent p38 MAPK-AP1 and IKKbeta-IkappaBalpha-NF-kappaB signaling pathways. Biochem Biophys Res Commun 2004;324(3):1087–94.
12. Koga T, Kuwahara I, Lillehoj EP, et al. TNF-alpha induces MUC1 gene transcription in lung epithelial cells: its signaling pathway and biological implication. Am J Physiol Lung Cell Mol Physiol 2007; 293(3):L693–701.
13. Kohri K, Ueki IF, Shim JJ, et al. *Pseudomonas aeruginosa* induces MUC5AC production via epidermal growth factor receptor. Eur Respir J 2002;20(5): 1263–70.

14. Lu W, Hisatsune A, Koga T, et al. Cutting edge: enhanced pulmonary clearance of *Pseudomonas aeruginosa* by Muc1 knockout mice. J Immunol 2006;176(7):3890–4.

15. Chamaillard M, Hashimoto M, Horie Y, et al. An essential role for NOD1 in host recognition of bacterial peptidoglycan containing diaminopimelic acid. Nat Immunol 2003;4(7):702–7.

16. Girardin SE, Boneca IG, Carneiro LA, et al. Nod1 detects a unique muropeptide from gram-negative bacterial peptidoglycan. Science 2003;300(5625): 1584–7.

17. Girardin SE, Boneca IG, Viala J, et al. Nod2 is a general sensor of peptidoglycan through muramyl dipeptide (MDP) detection. J Biol Chem 2003; 278(11):8869–72.

18. Hasegawa M, Fujimoto Y, Lucas PC, et al. A critical role of RICK/RIP2 polyubiquitination in Nod-induced NF-kappaB activation. EMBO J 2008;27(2):373–83.

19. Gomez MI, Lee A, Reddy B, et al. *Staphylococcus aureus* protein A induces airway epithelial inflammatory responses by activating TNFR1. Nat Med 2004;10(8):842–8.

20. Skerrett SJ, Liggitt HD, Hajjar AM, et al. Cutting edge: myeloid differentiation factor 88 is essential for pulmonary host defense against *Pseudomonas aeruginosa* but not *Staphylococcus aureus*. J Immunol 2004;172(6):3377–81.

21. Taylor PR, Tsoni SV, Willment JA, et al. Dectin-1 is required for beta-glucan recognition and control of fungal infection. Nat Immunol 2007;8(1):31–8.

22. Drickamer K. Two distinct classes of carbohydrate-recognition domains in animal lectins. J Biol Chem 1988;263(20):9557–60.

23. Lee HM, Yuk JM, Shin DM, et al. Dectin-1 is inducible and plays an essential role for mycobacteria-induced innate immune responses in airway epithelial cells. J Clin Immunol 2009;29(6):795–805.

24. Werner JL, Gessner MA, Lilly LM, et al. Neutrophils produce interleukin 17A (IL-17A) in a dectin-1- and IL-23-dependent manner during invasive fungal infection. Infect Immun 2011;79(10):3966–77.

25. Wu K, Yuan J, Lasky LA. Characterization of a novel member of the macrophage mannose receptor type C lectin family. J Biol Chem 1996;271(35): 21323–30.

26. Voglis S, Quinn K, Tullis E, et al. Human neutrophil peptides and phagocytic deficiency in bronchiectatic lungs. Am J Respir Crit Care Med 2009; 180(2):159–66.

27. Ganz T. Extracellular release of antimicrobial defensins by human polymorphonuclear leukocytes. Infect Immun 1987;55(3):568–71.

28. Diamond DL, Kimball JR, Krisanaprakornkit S, et al. Detection of beta-defensins secreted by human oral epithelial cells. J Immunol Methods 2001; 256(1-2):65–76.

29. Santaolalla R, Fukata M, Abreu MT. Innate immunity in the small intestine. Curr Opin Gastroenterol 2011;27(2):125–31.

30. King AE, Critchley HO, Kelly RW. Innate immune defences in the human endometrium. Reprod Biol Endocrinol 2003;1:116.

31. Schutte BC, Mitros JP, Bartlett JA, et al. Discovery of five conserved beta-defensin gene clusters using a computational search strategy. Proc Natl Acad Sci U S A 2002;99(4):2129–33.

32. Duits LA, Ravensbergen B, Rademaker M, et al. Expression of beta-defensin 1 and 2 mRNA by human monocytes, macrophages and dendritic cells. Immunology 2002;106(4):517–25.

33. Bals R, Wilson JM. Cathelicidins–a family of multifunctional antimicrobial peptides. Cell Mol Life Sci 2003;60(4):711–20.

34. Tjabringa GS, Rabe KF, Hiemstra PS. The human cathelicidin LL-37: a multifunctional peptide involved in infection and inflammation in the lung. Pulm Pharmacol Ther 2005;18(5):321–7.

35. Pompilio A, Scocchi M, Pomponio S, et al. Antibacterial and anti-biofilm effects of cathelicidin peptides against pathogens isolated from cystic fibrosis patients. Peptides 2011;32(9):1807–14.

36. Crouch E, Hartshorn K, Ofek I. Collectins and pulmonary innate immunity. Immunol Rev 2000;173:52–65.

37. Wright JR. Immunoregulatory functions of surfactant proteins. Nat Rev Immunol 2005;5(1):58–68.

38. McCormack FX. New concepts in collectin-mediated host defense at the air-liquid interface of the lung. Respirology 2006;11(Suppl):S7–10.

39. McIntosh JC, Mervin-Blake S, Conner E, et al. Surfactant protein A protects growing cells and reduces TNF-alpha activity from LPS-stimulated macrophages. Am J Physiol 1996;271(2 Pt 1):L310–9.

40. Borron P, McIntosh JC, Korfhagen TR, et al. Surfactant-associated protein A inhibits LPS-induced cytokine and nitric oxide production in vivo. Am J Physiol Lung Cell Mol Physiol 2000;278(4):L840–7.

41. Reidy MF, Wright JR. Surfactant protein A enhances apoptotic cell uptake and TGF-beta1 release by inflammatory alveolar macrophages. Am J Physiol Lung Cell Mol Physiol 2003;285(4):L854–61.

42. Weiss J, Elsbach P, Olsson I, et al. Purification and characterization of a potent bactericidal and membrane active protein from the granules of human polymorphonuclear leukocytes. J Biol Chem 1978; 253(8):2664–72.

43. Calafat J, Janssen H, Tool A, et al. The bactericidal/permeability-increasing protein (BPI) is present in specific granules of human eosinophils. Blood 1998;91(12):4770–5.

44. Canny G, Levy O, Furuta GT, et al. Lipid mediator-induced expression of bactericidal/permeability-increasing protein (BPI) in human mucosal epithelia. Proc Natl Acad Sci U S A 2002;99(6):3902–7.

45. Gazzano-Santoro H, Meszaros K, Birr C, et al. Competition between rBPI23, a recombinant fragment of bactericidal/permeability-increasing protein, and lipopolysaccharide (LPS)-binding protein for binding to LPS and gram-negative bacteria. Infect Immun 1994;62(4):1185–91.

46. Aichele D, Schnare M, Saake M, et al. Expression and antimicrobial function of bactericidal permeability-increasing protein in cystic fibrosis patients. Infect Immun 2006;74(8):4708–14.

47. Weiss J, Elsbach P, Shu C, et al. Human bactericidal/permeability-increasing protein and a recombinant NH2-terminal fragment cause killing of serum-resistant gram-negative bacteria in whole blood and inhibit tumor necrosis factor release induced by the bacteria. J Clin Invest 1992;90(3):1122–30.

48. Carroll MC. The complement system in regulation of adaptive immunity. Nat Immunol 2004;5(10):981–6.

49. Botto M, Kirschfink M, Macor P, et al. Complement in human diseases: lessons from complement deficiencies. Mol Immunol 2009;46(14):2774–83.

50. Keating SE, Baran M, Bowie AG. Cytosolic DNA sensors regulating type I interferon induction. Trends Immunol 2011;32(12):574–81.

51. Bartlett NW, Buttigieg K, Kotenko SV, et al. Murine interferon lambdas (type III interferons) exhibit potent antiviral activity in vivo in a poxvirus infection model. J Gen Virol 2005;86(Pt 6):1589–96.

52. Zhang Z, Hinrichs DJ, Lu H, et al. After interleukin-12p40, are interleukin-23 and interleukin-17 the next therapeutic targets for inflammatory bowel disease? Int Immunopharmacol 2007;7(4):409–16.

53. Kolls JK, Linden A. Interleukin-17 family members and inflammation. Immunity 2004;21(4):467–76.

54. Happel KI, Dubin PJ, Zheng M, et al. Divergent roles of IL-23 and IL-12 in host defense against Klebsiella pneumoniae. J Exp Med 2005;202(6):761–9.

55. Dubin PJ, Kolls JK. IL-23 mediates inflammatory responses to mucoid Pseudomonas aeruginosa lung infection in mice. Am J Physiol Lung Cell Mol Physiol 2007;292(2):L519–28.

56. Reynolds JM, Angkasekwinai P, Dong C. IL-17 family member cytokines: regulation and function in innate immunity. Cytokine Growth Factor Rev 2010;21(6):413–23.

57. Lukacs NW, Hogaboam C, Campbell E, et al. Chemokines: function, regulation and alteration of inflammatory responses. Chem Immunol 1999;72:102–20.

58. Mahalingam S, Karupiah G. Chemokines and chemokine receptors in infectious diseases. Immunol Cell Biol 1999;77(6):469–75.

59. Hill AT, Campbell EJ, Hill SL, et al. Association between airway bacterial load and markers of airway inflammation in patients with stable chronic bronchitis. Am J Med 2000;109(4):288–95.

60. Smart SJ, Casale TB. Interleukin-8-induced transcellular neutrophil migration is facilitated by endothelial and pulmonary epithelial cells. Am J Respir Cell Mol Biol 1993;9(5):489–95.

61. Harada A, Sekido N, Akahoshi T, et al. Essential involvement of interleukin-8 (IL-8) in acute inflammation. J Leukoc Biol 1994;56(5):559–64.

62. Mikami M, Llewellyn-Jones CG, Bayley D, et al. The chemotactic activity of sputum from patients with bronchiectasis. Am J Respir Crit Care Med 1998;157(3 Pt 1):723–8.

63. Cowburn AS, Condliffe AM, Farahi N, et al. Advances in neutrophil biology: clinical implications. Chest 2008;134(3):606–12.

64. Hager M, Cowland JB, Borregaard N. Neutrophil granules in health and disease. J Intern Med 2010;268(1):25–34.

65. Ooi CE, Weiss J, Elsbach P, et al. 25-kDa NH2-terminal fragment carries all the antibacterial activities of the human neutrophil 60-kDa bactericidal/permeability-increasing protein. J Biol Chem 1987;262(31):14891–4.

66. Burnett D, Crocker J, Stockley RA. Cells containing IgA subclasses in bronchi of subjects with and without chronic obstructive lung disease. J Clin Pathol 1987;40(10):1217–20.

67. Scribner DJ, Fahrney D. Neutrophil receptors for IgG and complement: their roles in the attachment and ingestion phases of phagocytosis. J Immunol 1976;116(4):892–7.

68. Fevang B, Mollnes TE, Holm AM, et al. Common variable immunodeficiency and the complement system; low mannose-binding lectin levels are associated with bronchiectasis. Clin Exp Immunol 2005;142(3):576–84.

69. Laarman AJ, Bardoel BW, Ruyken M, et al. Pseudomonas aeruginosa alkaline protease blocks complement activation via the classical and lectin pathways. J Immunol 2012;188(1):386–93.

70. Tung JP, Fraser JF, Wood P, et al. Respiratory burst function of ovine neutrophils. BMC Immunol 2009;10:25.

71. de Oliveira-Junior EB, Bustamante J, Newburger PE, et al. The human NADPH oxidase: primary and secondary defects impairing the respiratory burst function and the microbicidal ability of phagocytes. Scand J Immunol 2011;73(5):420–7.

72. Pasteur MC, Helliwell SM, Houghton SJ, et al. An investigation into causative factors in patients with bronchiectasis. Am J Respir Crit Care Med 2000;162(4 Pt 1):1277–84.

73. King PT, Hutchinson P, Holmes PW, et al. Assessing immune function in adult bronchiectasis. Clin Exp Immunol 2006;144(3):440–6.

74. Brinkmann V, Reichard U, Goosmann C, et al. Neutrophil extracellular traps kill bacteria. Science 2004;303(5663):1532–5.

75. Fuchs TA, Abed U, Goosmann C, et al. Novel cell death program leads to neutrophil extracellular traps. J Cell Biol 2007;176(2):231–41.

76. Yost CC, Cody MJ, Harris ES, et al. Impaired neutrophil extracellular trap (NET) formation: a novel innate immune deficiency of human neonates. Blood 2009; 113(25):6419–27.

77. Vermaelen K, Pauwels R. Pulmonary dendritic cells. Am J Respir Crit Care Med 2005;172(5): 530–51.

78. Stumbles PA, Upham JW, Holt PG. Airway dendritic cells: co-ordinators of immunological homeostasis and immunity in the respiratory tract. APMIS 2003;111(7–8):741–55.

79. van oud Alblas AB, van Furth R. Origin, kinetics, and characteristics of pulmonary macrophages in the normal steady state. J Exp Med 1979;149(6): 1504–18.

80. Blusse van oud Alblas A, van der Linden-Schrever B, van Furth R. Origin and kinetics of pulmonary macrophages during an inflammatory reaction induced by intravenous administration of heat-killed bacillus Calmette-Guerin. J Exp Med 1981;154(2):235–52.

81. Jonsson S, Musher DM, Chapman A, et al. Phagocytosis and killing of common bacterial pathogens of the lung by human alveolar macrophages. J Infect Dis 1985;152(1):4–13.

82. Zuniga EI, McGavern DB, Pruneda-Paz JL, et al. Bone marrow plasmacytoid dendritic cells can differentiate into myeloid dendritic cells upon virus infection. Nat Immunol 2004;5(12): 1227–34.

83. Liu YJ. IPC: professional type 1 interferon-producing cells and plasmacytoid dendritic cell precursors. Annu Rev Immunol 2005;23:275–306.

84. Jakubzick C, Tacke F, Llodra J, et al. Modulation of dendritic cell trafficking to and from the airways. J Immunol 2006;176(6):3578–84.

85. McWilliam AS, Napoli S, Marsh AM, et al. Dendritic cells are recruited into the airway epithelium during the inflammatory response to a broad spectrum of stimuli. J Exp Med 1996;184(6):2429–32.

86. Kapsenberg ML. Dendritic-cell control of pathogen-driven T-cell polarization. Nat Rev Immunol 2003; 3(12):984–93.

87. Condon TV, Sawyer RT, Fenton MJ, et al. Lung dendritic cells at the innate-adaptive immune interface. J Leukoc Biol 2011;90(5):883–95.

88. Kadowaki N, Ho S, Antonenko S, et al. Subsets of human dendritic cell precursors express different toll-like receptors and respond to different microbial antigens. J Exp Med 2001;194(6): 863–9.

89. Moretta A, Marcenaro E, Parolini S, et al. NK cells at the interface between innate and adaptive immunity. Cell Death Differ 2008;15(2):226–33.

90. Latiff AH, Kerr MA. The clinical significance of immunoglobulin A deficiency. Ann Clin Biochem 2007;44(Pt 2):131–9.

91. Stead A, Douglas JG, Broadfoot CJ, et al. Humoral immunity and bronchiectasis. Clin Exp Immunol 2002;130(2):325–30.

92. Hornick DB, Fick RB Jr. The immunoglobulin G subclass composition of immune complexes in cystic fibrosis. Implications for the pathogenesis of the Pseudomonas lung lesion. J Clin Invest 1990;86(4):1285–92.

93. Guttman RM, Waisbren BA. Bacterial blocking activity of specific IgG in chronic Pseudomonas aeruginosa infection. Clin Exp Immunol 1975; 19(1):121–30.

94. MacLennan CA, Gilchrist JJ, Gordon MA, et al. Dysregulated humoral immunity to nontyphoidal Salmonella in HIV-infected African adults. Science 2010;328(5977):508–12.

95. Bleackley RC. A molecular view of cytotoxic T lymphocyte induced killing. Biochem Cell Biol 2005;83(6):747–51.

96. Oykhman P, Mody CH. Direct microbicidal activity of cytotoxic T-lymphocytes. J Biomed Biotechnol 2010;2010:249482.

97. Shevach EM. Regulatory T cells in autoimmunity. Annu Rev Immunol 2000;18:423–49.

98. Hirota K, Martin B, Veldhoen M. Development, regulation and functional capacities of Th17 cells. Semin Immunopathol 2010;32(1):3–16.

99. Zhang D, Zhang G, Hayden MS, et al. A toll-like receptor that prevents infection by uropathogenic bacteria. Science 2004;303(5663):1522–6.

100. Yarovinsky F, Zhang D, Andersen JF, et al. TLR11 activation of dendritic cells by a protozoan profilin-like protein. Science 2005;308(5728):1626–9.

101. Quinti I, Soresina A, Spadaro G, et al. Long-term follow-up and outcome of a large cohort of patients with common variable immunodeficiency. J Clin Immunol 2007;27(3):308–16.

102. Thickett KM, Kumararatne DS, Banerjee AK, et al. Common variable immune deficiency: respiratory manifestations, pulmonary function and high-resolution CT scan findings. QJM 2002;95(10): 655–62.

103. Castigli E, Geha RS. Molecular basis of common variable immunodeficiency. J Allergy Clin Immunol 2006;117(4):740–6 [quiz: 747].

104. Ochs HD, Smith CI. X-linked agammaglobulinemia. A clinical and molecular analysis. Medicine 1996; 75(6):287–99.

105. Winkelstein JA, Marino MC, Lederman HM, et al. X-linked agammaglobulinemia: report on a United States registry of 201 patients. Medicine 2006; 85(4):193–202.

106. Herrod HG. Clinical significance of IgG subclasses. Curr Opin Pediatr 1993;5(6):696–9.

107. Ambrosino DM, Umetsu DT, Siber GR, et al. Selective defect in the antibody response to *Haemophilus influenzae* type b in children with recurrent infections and normal serum IgG subclass levels. J Allergy Clin Immunol 1988;81(6):1175–9.

108. Epstein MM, Gruskay F. Selective deficiency in pneumococcal antibody response in children with recurrent infections. Ann Allergy Asthma Immunol 1995;75(2):125–31.

109. Goldstein MF, Goldstein AL, Dunsky EH, et al. Selective IgM immunodeficiency: retrospective analysis of 36 adult patients with review of the literature. Ann Allergy Asthma Immunol 2006;97(6):717–30.

110. Winkelstein JA, Marino MC, Ochs H, et al. The X-linked hyper-IgM syndrome: clinical and immunologic features of 79 patients. Medicine 2003;82(6):373–84.

Pathogenesis of Bronchiectasis

Bart C. Moulton, MD, Alan F. Barker, MD*

KEYWORDS

- Bronchiectasis • Sputum • Pathogenesis • Airway epithelium

KEY POINTS

- The pathogenesis of bronchiectasis varies by case, but generally involves a cycle of inflammation and altered immune response to infection.
- Combination of high-resolution computed tomographic imaging and sampling of the airway biology, via sputum, bronchoalveolar lavage, biopsies, or exhaled breath condensates, may target mechanisms that can be interrupted without impairing the healing stages of infection and inflammation.
- Treatment at early stages may allow for appropriate cellular and chemokine responses, reducing airway damage and harboring of virulent organisms.

In 1821, René Théophile Hyacinthe Laënnec described bronchiectasis as an "affection of the bronchia is always produced by chronic catarrh, or by some other disease attended by long, violent, and often repeated fits of coughing."[1] In 1950, Lynne Reid[2] correlated bronchographic images with pathologic specimens and defined bronchiectasis as a permanent dilation of bronchi. Systematic data for the incidence or prevalence of bronchiectasis are not available; however, it is rare in developed countries.[3] Estimates for the United States show 100,000 affected individuals, qualifying bronchiectasis as a rare disease (<200,000 affected individuals).[4] Smaller studies in isolated populations of low socioeconomic status, such as Alaskan and Australian natives, suggest a prevalence of 1% to 2%.[5,6] Although neither symptoms nor definitions have changed since the initial descriptions, numerous advancements have occurred in the pathogenesis. This review describes the changes and advancement in the pathogenesis of bronchiectasis, including mechanisms of injury and host factors.

PATHOLOGIC FEATURES OF BRONCHIECTASIS

In 1898, Ewart classified bronchiectasis into 3 forms based on the grossly dilated appearance of the large airways: (1) regular or cylindrical, (2) fusiform, and (3) globular or sacculated with a bead-like modification of the affected large airway.[7] Because of Reid's classification, bronchiectasis is grouped based on the appearance of the airways, even today. Cylindrical bronchiectasis has uniform dilation of the affected bronchi (**Fig. 1**). Varicose bronchiectasis, because of the resemblance to varicose veins, has focal areas of constriction between areas of dilation (**Fig. 2**). Cystic or saccular bronchiectasis is the most damaged form, characterized by dilated bronchi that end in cysts and grapelike clusters (**Fig. 3**).[2] The current gold standard for imaging the airways and classifying bronchiectasis is high-resolution computed tomographic (HRCT) imaging.[8,9] The pathologic terminology has been maintained and adopted when describing computed tomographic (CT) images of the chest (**Table 1**).

Because most patients are not diagnosed until an advanced stage, the gross pathology is mainly available from surgical or autopsied specimens. With the decline of surgery for bronchiectasis and autopsies over the past several decades, descriptions of the pathologic conditions of the airway mainly come from reports that were available 5 or more decades ago. The lumina contain purulent mucus and necrotic debris reflecting

Pulmonary and Critical Care Medicine, Oregon Health and Science University, 3181 Southwest Sam Jackson Park Road, UHN67, Portland, OR 97239, USA
* Corresponding author.
E-mail address: barkera@ohsu.edu

Clin Chest Med 33 (2012) 211–217
doi:10.1016/j.ccm.2012.02.004
0272-5231/12/$ – see front matter © 2012 Elsevier Inc. All rights reserved.

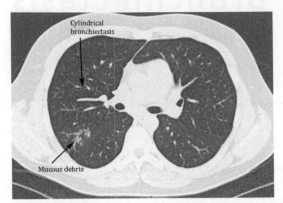

Fig. 1. Computed tomography (CT) image showing cylindrical bronchiectasis and lack of clearance of mucous debris.

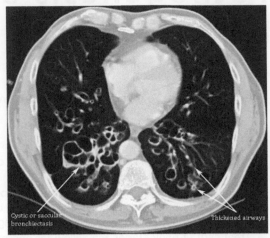

Fig. 3. CT image showing both thickened and dilated airways along with cystic bronchiectasis (grapelike clusters).

impaired clearance of microbial organisms and phagocytic cells. The results of physicochemical studies of sputum from Native American children from Alaska with bronchiectasis showed sputum that was less elastic and viscous, yet had higher transportability than banked sputum of patients with cystic fibrosis and chronic bronchitis.[10] Airway walls are thickened, due to transmural inflammation. Normal mucosal and muscular layers fail to heal because of repeated infectious insult and may be replaced by a fibrotic scar. In the more proximal airways, structural cartilage is lost or replaced by the scar. With the loss or destruction of supportive mural structure, airways may be dilated out to the periphery of the lung, and bronchi and bronchioles may be tortuous or even angulated by the surrounding scar. Proximally, lymph node enlargement occurs, sometimes narrowing a lobar bronchus as in the middle lobe syndrome. Because of recurrent infection and inflammation, neovascular bronchial arterioles

are enlarged below the mucosal surface. Erosion of the mucosa during infection contributes to the brisk bleeding sometimes seen. These changes are obviously indications of a far-advanced disease, destruction, necrosis, and attempts at repair.

Chest CT scans may provide earlier indications of susceptible or damaged airways. Patients with common variable immunodeficiency (CVID) are susceptible to recurrent bacterial infection and bronchiectasis. Inspiratory and expiratory HRCT scans were performed on 54 children aged 6 to 18 years with CVID in a stable state. The most common abnormality was expiratory air trapping (mosaic attenuation) seen in 71% to 80% of the study participants, and was the only abnormality in 9% to 15% of the study participants. The presence of air trapping in the expiratory HRCT scan results suggests that the inflammatory changes in the small airway are the cause, and raises the possibility of a reversal of these changes.[11]

Histologically, polymorphonuclear (PMN) transmural inflammation is accompanied in later stages by microabscesses of airways filled with necrotic debris, including bacteria or other infectious pathogens. Usual wavelike cilia are disrupted, fractured, or lost. Distal bronchioles may be obstructed by inflammatory debris or infected mucus. The inflammation may extend beyond airways into lung parenchyma yielding an appearance of pneumonia. Mural neovascular bronchial arterioles are recognized by their thick walls when compared with normal pulmonary capillaries. In 1952, Whitwell[12] coined the term follicular bronchiectasis. Follicular bronchiectasis has excessive formation of lymphoid tissue, and there is formation of follicles and nodes within walls of diseased bronchi.

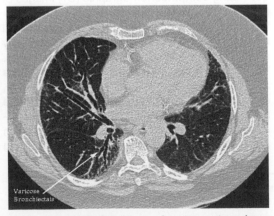

Fig. 2. High-resolution CT scan showing varicose bronchiectasis (dilated airways with fibrosis causing irregular and tortuous airways).

Table 1	
Pathologic conditions of bronchiectasis and their imaging correlates	
Pathologic Condition (Type)	**Chest CT Imaging**
Dilated airways (cylindrical)	Enlarged airways that do not taper to periphery Airway >1.5 times corresponding vessel (signet ring)
Thickened airways	Thick peripheral airways (1–3 mm), tram lines
Airways with mucus or necrotic debris	Irregular peripheral nodules in airways Tree-in-bud **(Fig. 4)**
Airways dilated and tortuous with constrictions (varicose)	Airways seen longitudinally are irregular in outline
Cysts or saccules off airways (cystic or saccular)	Clusters of cysts at terminal airways (grapelike clusters)
Airways narrowed or partially obstructed	Mosaic attenuation or air trapping

PATHOGENESIS

The underlying mechanism of bronchiectasis is described as a vicious cycle of transmural recurrent infection and subsequent inflammation.[13] Inflammation and infection cause damage primarily to the bronchi and bronchioles. Damaged airways are susceptible to infection with usually colonizing but severely damaging bacterial and fungal microbes, such as *Pseudomonas aeruginosa*, *Aspergillus fumigatus*, and nontuberculous mycobacteria. Impaired mucociliary clearance leads to the release of phagocytic enzymes and chemokines that erode mucosal barriers and create crevices and microabscesses that harbor potentially pathogenic organisms. Damaged airways are then more susceptible to infection, resulting in further damage. Airway damage from inflammation is mediated through both leukocytes and respiratory epithelial cells. Innate immune responses include release of neutrophil elastase (NE) and reactive oxygen species, major histocompatibility complex (MHC) genes involved in cell recognition, and activation of complement pathway. Acquired immune responses include antibody production in response to infectious antigens via B cells, T cells, and other antigen-presenting cells.

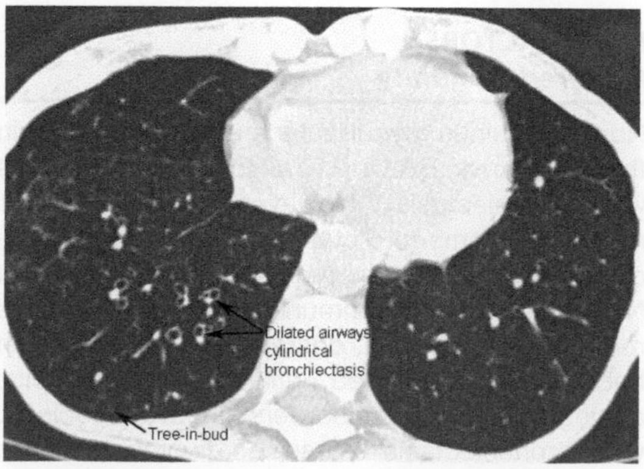

Airway Epithelium and Transport

The respiratory mucosa is quite resistant to infection. In addition to barrier resistance from tight junctions, secretion of bacterial toxic mucins, an efficient distal to proximal ciliary transport, and active transport of sodium and chloride for smooth aqueous protection, airway epithelium provides innate immunity through production of antibacterial peptides.[14–16] Mucociliary clearance is normally effective in moving particles at a rate of 1 to 2 cm/min.[17] Primary ciliary dyskinesia is the classic example of dysfunctional cilia leading to impaired clearance. Cystic fibrosis and Young syndrome result in mucus with abnormal properties, which prevents adequate clearance of microbes, thus increasing the risk of colonization and subsequent infection.[18,19] Sputum from patients with bronchiectasis containing excessive leukocyte elastase has been shown to reduce the beat frequency of cilia in vitro.[20,21] Individuals with cystic fibrosis also have abnormalities of mucosal transport, which involves a dysfunctional chloride channel. The nasal potential difference test analyzes the transport function of sodium and chloride transport across the airway epithelium. An abnormal nasal potential difference with a magnitude between that of normal and cystic fibrosis values was identified in patients with bronchiectasis and a single CFTR mutation, which suggests that the presence of a single CFTR mutation may play a role in the development of

Fig. 4. CT image showing tree-in-bud pattern of inflammation.

bronchiectasis.[22] In addition to physical barriers, the airway epithelium is involved in protective inflammation. Infection induces the airway epithelium to release inflammatory cytokines including macrophage inflammatory protein-2, interleukin (IL)-8, and tumor necrosis factor α (TNF-α). The presence of deleterious bacteria increases the expression of intercellular adhesion molecule 1 (ICAM-1).[23] ICAM-1 is a cell surface glycoprotein which, when activated by the cytokines TNF-α and IL-1, regulates neutrophil adhesion and macrophage transendothelial migration.[24] With increased ICAM-1, there is an increase in migration across endothelium into tissues. Although this process has the potential to recruit leukocytes to an area of infection with subsequent resolution, it causes further damage, which contributes to perpetuation of the vicious cycle.[13] Indications of the heightened inflammatory state in bronchiectasis are the elevated systemic markers including C-reactive protein and erythrocyte sedimentation rate.[25]

Macrophages

Macrophages are the first line of defense by leukocytes against bacterial invasion. The results of bronchial biopsies confirm a higher density in the lamina propria of bronchiectatic airways compared with normal airways. Patients with bronchiectasis who have frequent production of sputum have a significantly higher density of macrophages in the airway compared with patients with bronchiectasis who do not have regular production of sputum. No association between the density of neutrophils and the production of sputum is seen in bronchiectasis. TNF-α, produced by macrophages, is increased in bronchiectatic airways and is the main chemoattractant for neutrophils.[26,27]

Neutrophils

In normal individuals, more than 95% of cells in airway secretions are macrophages.[28] Neutrophils are the most dominant cells present in sputum, bronchoalveolar lavage (BAL), and bronchial mucosal biopsies of patients with bronchiectasis.[28,29] Bronchiectatic airways also have increased neutrophil infiltration of the lamina propria.[26] Neutrophils are recruited to airways in response to infection by the bacterial chemokines IL-1β, IL-8, IL-17, leukotriene B4, and TNF-α.[30–32] Once in airways, activated neutrophils release NE, cathepsin G, and proteinase 3. NE causes epithelial damage, reduced ciliary beating, mucous gland hyperplasia, and increased secretion of mucus.[33] This damage and mucociliary stagnation then allows further colonization of bacteria and neutrophil recruitment. Excessive NE also has

been shown to alter the structure of immunoglobulin and compromise mechanisms of complement defense, thus decreasing susceptibility of bacteria to phagocytosis by neutrophils.[33] Despite the presence of increased numbers of neutrophils in the airways of patients with bronchiectasis, the neutrophils may be ineffective. In a study of stable patients with bronchiectasis, high levels of human neutrophil peptides (HNP, also called α-defensins) in sputum were noted. HNP normally have an antimicrobial effect, but also impair neutrophil phagocytosis leading to loss of antimicrobicidal activity. Addition of α1-antitrypsin to sputum neutrophil cell cultures attenuated HNP activity and improved phagocytic activity.[34]

Lymphocytes

The number of lymphocytes is increased in bronchiectatic airways. The fact that bronchiectasis is associated with chronic lymphocytic leukemia and with the rare transporter antigen presentation (TAP) deficiency syndrome confirms a role for lymphocytes.[35] Studies are conflicting as to whether CD4+ or CD8+ T cells predominate.[29,36–38] Familial bronchiectasis has been noted in individuals with TAP syndrome. These individuals have a downregulation of major histocompatibility complex (MHC) class I molecules on T cells.[35] MHC class I molecules function in the body, recognizing foreign cells and peptides by presenting antigens to CD8+ cells, which generally have a cytotoxic function.[39] With the down-regulation of MHC class I in TAP deficiency syndrome, antigen cell recognition is decreased, thereby impairing immune response, which allows for further colonization and infection with bacteria. Homozygotes of human leukocyte antigen C group 1, a subclass of MHC class I, also have increased susceptibility to bronchiectasis. Thus, impaired antigen presentation and cytotoxic T cells may be another contributory source of the beginning of the vicious cycle.[40]

HOST FACTORS
Impaired Immunity

Nontuberculous mycobacteria (NTM) are found in the sputum or BAL of 10% to 20% of patients with bronchiectasis.[41] However, host immunologic response seems to dictate development of bronchiectasis rather than the pathogenic nature of NTM.[42] This host immune response may be related to MHC class, decreased opsonization of bacteria, or increased inflammatory response against self. Immune disorders that are associated with bronchiectasis are varied, which indicates that there is not a single defect. Rheumatoid arthritis, Sjögren syndrome, relapsing polychondritis, and inflammatory bowel disease are autoimmune conditions associated with bronchiectasis.[19] Also, immunodeficiency syndromes involving lower levels of IgG, IgM, IgA; combined variable immunodeficiency; or administration of immune-suppressing medications that inhibit lymphocytes have associations with bronchiectasis.[19,43] Thus, although impaired immune regulation is important in the genesis of bronchiectasis, a single defect or mechanism is unlikely.

Bacteria and Bacterial Products

The two most frequently isolated pathogens in the sputum of patients with bronchiectasis are *Haemophilus influenzae* and *P aeruginosa*. *P aeruginosa* is a ubiquitous gram-negative rod-shaped bacterium that rarely infects a normal host. In patients with bronchiectasis, a dysfunctional or damaged mucosal barrier and the pressure of repeated and broad-spectrum antibiotics are risk factors for *P aeruginosa* infection. Bacterial characteristics responsible for chronic and virulent pseudomonas infection include the motile and sticky structure of the bacteria, exotoxin and endotoxin virulence products of *P aeruginosa*, cell-to-cell signaling communications that inhibit antibiotic penetration, and genetic variability.

The cell wall of *P aeruginosa* contains a flagellum that allows facile mobility and also stimulates release of the proinflammatory chemokine, IL-8, on attachment to an epithelial surface. The cell wall also exhibits several pili that enhance adherence to the lipid membrane of epithelial cells and in addition stimulate the release of toll-like receptors, promoting internalization of *P aeruginosa*. Flagella and pili serve as primers for recruitment of phagocytic cells including PMNs.

After adherence and cellular entry of *P aeruginosa*, a variety of potent extracellular products are released. Alginate, a mucopolysaccharide, is a gelatinous product of *P aeruginosa* that enhances adherence of *P aeruginosa* to the epithelial cells. Alginate accounts for the glistening mucoidity and rounding up seen in cultures of *P aeruginosa*. Mucoid *P aeruginosa* is classically seen in cystic fibrosis but is also recognized in patients with non–cystic fibrosis bronchiectasis. Pyocyanin, a potent exotoxin produced by *P aeruginosa*, gives the blue-green color to sputum of patients infected with *P aeruginosa* but, most importantly, disrupts the epithelial cell wall, impairs ciliary function, and interferes with antioxidant defense. Proteases from *P aeruginosa* cleave and disable CXCR1, a chemokine receptor, leading to reduced neutrophil recruitment and failure of bacterial killing.[44] The glycoprotein α_1-antitrypsin is known to inhibit neutrophilic proteases, including NE found in lung.[45] α_1-Antitrypsin deficiency is associated with bronchiectasis.[46] Some studies have suggested that this relationship is due to the increase in chronic obstructive pulmonary disease (COPD) from α_1-antitrypsin deficiency or perhaps uninhibited NE damage to elastin-rich bronchi and bronchioles.[47] However, in a few patients with bronchiectasis and homozygous α_1-antitrypsin deficiency, there is minimal emphysema on chest CT imaging, indicating that there is more than just increased COPD involved in bronchiectasis associated with α_1-antitrypsin deficiency.[46] Lipopolysaccharide is a key endotoxin released from the *P aeruginosa* cell wall, accounting for many of the systemic manifestations of infection including fever, blood pressure alterations, and tissue necrosis, as seen with other gram-negative organisms.

P aeruginosa has developed genetic coordination via cell signaling or quorum sensing that allows the production of chemicals called lactones, which are the basis of biofilms, structured communities that coat epithelial surfaces and medical equipment, allowing bacterial persistence and exotoxin and endotoxin accumulation via reduced penetration of phagocytic cells and antibiotics. Biofilms are formed independently of alginate but serve similar functions. Biofilms may also induce and trap cytokines responsible for ongoing inflammation. Macrolides inhibit gene products responsible for quorum sensing and biofilm production.[48]

Impaired Repair

As first described by Reid,[2] bronchiectasis is a reduction in bronchial subdivision. Underlying this reduction is a delicate balance of inflammation for recruiting leukocytes to infected tissue and limiting the damage from the inflammation. When neutrophils are recruited, degradation of the nearby connective tissue occurs.[45] This damage occurs through NE released by the neutrophil and activated respiratory epithelium, presumably for antimicrobial effects of the NE.[49]

SUMMARY

The pathogenesis of bronchiectasis cannot be explained by a single cause. The current model is a vicious cycle of inflammation and altered response to infection. This cycle depends not only on the type and virulence of the pathogen but also on the host immune response. In this response, too much or too little can damage the airways or fail to clear the pathogen, thus increasing the probability of further infection. The past specimens for bronchiectasis including surgical and autopsied specimens are now rarely available, but also represent far-advanced stages of necrosis, destruction, and scar well beyond any possibility of repair or reversibility. The combination of sophisticated clinical tools, including HRCT imaging and sampling of the airway biology via sputum, BAL, biopsies, or exhaled breath condensates, may target mechanisms that can be interrupted without impairing the repair or healing stages of infection and inflammation. Treatment at early stages may allow for appropriate but not excessive cellular and chemokine responses. Earlier identification and treatment may reduce the airway damage and harboring of virulent organisms including *P aeruginosa* that perpetuate bronchiectasis.

REFERENCES

1. Laennec RT. A treatise on the disease[s] of the chest. New York: Published under the auspices of the Library of the New York Academy of Medicine by Hafner Pub. Co; 1962.
2. Reid LM. Reduction in bronchial subdivision in bronchiectasis. Thorax 1950;5(3):233–47.
3. Barker AF. Bronchiectasis. N Engl J Med 2002; 346(18):1383–93.
4. Weycker D, Edelsberg J, Oster G, et al. Prevalence and economic burden of bronchiectasis. Clin Pulm Med 2005;12(4):205–9.
5. Chang AB, Grimwood K, Mulholland EK, et al. Bronchiectasis in indigenous children in remote Australian communities. Med J Aust 2002;177(4):200–4.
6. Singleton R, Morris A, Redding G, et al. Bronchiectasis in Alaska native children: causes and clinical courses. Pediatr Pulmonol 2000;29(3):182–7.
7. Allbutt TC, Rolleston HD. A system of medicine. New York, London: Macmillan & Co; 1905.
8. Tasker AD, Flower CD. Imaging the airways. Hemoptysis, bronchiectasis, and small airways disease. Clin Chest Med 1999;20(4):761–73, viii.
9. Kang EY, Miller RR, Muller NL. Bronchiectasis: comparison of preoperative thin-section CT and pathologic findings in resected specimens. Radiology 1995;195(3):649–54.
10. Redding GJ, Kishioka C, Martinez P, et al. Physical and transport properties of sputum from children with idiopathic bronchiectasis. Chest 2008;134(6): 1129–34.
11. van de Ven AA, van Montfrans JM, Terheggen-Lagro SW, et al. A CT scan score for the assessment of lung disease in children with common variable immunodeficiency disorders. Chest 2010;138(2): 371–9.
12. Whitwell F. A study of the pathology and pathogenesis of bronchiectasis. Thorax 1952;7(3):213–39.
13. Cole PJ. Inflammation: a two-edged sword—the model of bronchiectasis. Eur J Respir Dis Suppl 1986;147:6–15.
14. Travis SM, Singh PK, Welsh MJ. Antimicrobial peptides and proteins in the innate defense of the airway surface. Curr Opin Immunol 2001;13(1): 89–95.
15. Lukinskiene L, Liu Y, Reynolds SD, et al. Antimicrobial activity of PLUNC protects against *Pseudomonas aeruginosa* infection. J Immunol 2011; 187(1):382–90.
16. Roche WR, Montefort S, Baker J, et al. Cell adhesion molecules and the bronchial epithelium. Am Rev Respir Dis 1993;148(6 Pt 2):S79–82.
17. Willoughby RA, Ecker GL, McKee SL, et al. Use of scintigraphy for the determination of mucociliary clearance rates in normal, sedated, diseased and exercised horses. Can J Vet Res 1991;55(4):315–20.
18. Goeminne PC, Dupont LJ. The sinusitis-infertility syndrome: Young's saint, old devil. Eur Respir J 2010;35(3):698.
19. Boyton RJ. Regulation of immunity in bronchiectasis. Med Mycol 2009;47(Suppl 1):S175–82.
20. Tegner H, Ohlsson K, Toremalm NG, et al. Effect of human leukocyte enzymes on tracheal mucosa and its mucociliary activity. Rhinology 1979;17(3):199–206.
21. Smallman LA, Hill SL, Stockley RA. Reduction of ciliary beat frequency in vitro by sputum from patients with bronchiectasis: a serine proteinase effect. Thorax 1984;39(9):663–7.
22. Bienvenu T, Sermet-Gaudelus I, Burgel PR, et al. Cystic fibrosis transmembrane conductance regulator channel dysfunction in non-cystic fibrosis bronchiectasis. Am J Respir Crit Care Med 2010;181(10): 1078–84.
23. Frick AG, Joseph TD, Pang L, et al. *Haemophilus influenzae* stimulates ICAM-1 expression on respiratory epithelial cells. J Immunol 2000;164(8):4185–96.
24. Yang L, Froio RM, Sciuto TE, et al. ICAM-1 regulates neutrophil adhesion and transcellular migration of TNF-alpha-activated vascular endothelium under flow. Blood 2005;106(2):584–92.
25. Wilson CB, Jones PW, O'Leary CJ, et al. Systemic markers of inflammation in stable bronchiectasis. Eur Respir J 1998;12(4):820–4.
26. Zheng L, Shum H, Tipoe GL, et al. Macrophages, neutrophils and tumour necrosis factor-alpha expression in bronchiectatic airways in vivo. Respir Med 2001;95(10):792–8.
27. Gaga M, Bentley AM, Humbert M, et al. Increases in CD4+ T lymphocytes, macrophages, neutrophils and interleukin 8 positive cells in the airways of patients with bronchiectasis. Thorax 1998;53(8): 685–91.
28. Loukides S, Bouros D, Papatheodorou G, et al. Exhaled H(2)O(2) in steady-state bronchiectasis: relationship with cellular composition in induced

sputum, spirometry, and extent and severity of disease. Chest 2002;121(1):81–7.

29. Eller J, Lapa e Silva JR, Poulter LW, et al. Cells and cytokines in chronic bronchial infection. Ann N Y Acad Sci 1994;725:331–45.

30. Roussel L, Houle F, Chan C, et al. IL-17 promotes p38 MAPK-dependent endothelial activation enhancing neutrophil recruitment to sites of inflammation. J Immunol 2010;184(8):4531–7.

31. Salva PS, Doyle NA, Graham L, et al. TNF-alpha, IL-8, soluble ICAM-1, and neutrophils in sputum of cystic fibrosis patients. Pediatr Pulmonol 1996; 21(1):11–9.

32. Beeh KM, Kornmann O, Buhl R, et al. Neutrophil chemotactic activity of sputum from patients with COPD: role of interleukin 8 and leukotriene B4. Chest 2003;123(4):1240–7.

33. Stockley RA. Neutrophils and protease/antiprotease imbalance. Am J Respir Crit Care Med 1999; 160(5 Pt 2):S49–52.

34. Voglis S, Quinn K, Tullis E, et al. Human neutrophil peptides and phagocytic deficiency in bronchiectatic lungs. Am J Respir Crit Care Med 2009; 180(2):159–66.

35. Gadola SD, Moins-Teisserenc HT, Trowsdale J, et al. TAP deficiency syndrome. Clin Exp Immunol 2000; 121(2):173–8.

36. Stockley RA. The role of proteinases in the pathogenesis of chronic bronchitis. Am J Respir Crit Care Med 1994;150(6 Pt 2):S109–13.

37. Sepper R, Konttinen YT, Ingman T, et al. Presence, activities, and molecular forms of cathepsin G, elastase, alpha 1-antitrypsin, and alpha 1-antichymotrypsin in bronchiectasis. J Clin Immunol 1995; 15(1):27–34.

38. Silva JR, Jones JA, Cole PJ, et al. The immunological component of the cellular inflammatory infiltrate in bronchiectasis. Thorax 1989;44(8):668–73.

39. Bjorkman PJ, Saper MA, Samraoui B, et al. The foreign antigen binding site and T cell recognition regions of class I histocompatibility antigens. Nature 1987;329(6139):512–8.

40. Boyton RJ, Smith J, Ward R, et al. HLA-C and killer cell immunoglobulin-like receptor genes in idiopathic bronchiectasis. Am J Respir Crit Care Med 2006;173(3):327–33.

41. Wickremasinghe M, Ozerovitch LJ, Davies G, et al. Non-tuberculous mycobacteria in patients with bronchiectasis. Thorax 2005;60(12):1045–51.

42. Tatano Y, Yasumoto K, Shimizu T, et al. Comparative study for the virulence of *Mycobacterium avium* isolates from patients with nodular-bronchiectasis- and cavitary-type diseases. Eur J Clin Microbiol Infect Dis 2010;29(7):801–6.

43. Rosen FS, Cooper MD, Wedgwood RJ. The primary immunodeficiencies. N Engl J Med 1995;333(7): 431–40.

44. Hartl D, Latzin P, Hordijk P, et al. Cleavage of CXCR1 on neutrophils disables bacterial killing in cystic fibrosis lung disease. Nat Med 2007;13(12):1423–30.

45. Llewellyn-Jones CG, Lomas DA, Stockley RA. Potential role of recombinant secretory leucoprotease inhibitor in the prevention of neutrophil mediated matrix degradation. Thorax 1994;49(6):567–72.

46. Parr DG, Guest PG, Reynolds JH, et al. Prevalence and impact of bronchiectasis in alpha1-antitrypsin deficiency. Am J Respir Crit Care Med 2007; 176(12):1215–21.

47. Cuvelier A, Muir JF, Hellot MF, et al. Distribution of alpha(1)-antitrypsin alleles in patients with bronchiectasis. Chest 2000;117(2):415–9.

48. Sadikot RT, Blackwell TS, Christman JW, et al. Pathogen-host interactions in *Pseudomonas aeruginosa* pneumonia. Am J Respir Crit Care Med 2005; 171(11):1209–23.

49. Zuyderduyn S, Ninaber DK, Schrumpf JA, et al. IL-4 and IL-13 exposure during mucociliary differentiation of bronchial epithelial cells increases antimicrobial activity and expression of antimicrobial peptides. Respir Res 2011;12:59.

The Initial Evaluation of Adults with Bronchiectasis

Mark L. Metersky, MD

KEYWORDS

• Bronchiectasis • Diagnosis • Immunodeficiency • Genetics • Microbiology • Radiology

KEY POINTS

• A systematic approach should be used to investigate the cause of bronchiectasis in newly diagnosed patients; however, testing should be guided by patient characteristics.

• In approximately 50% of patients, a specific cause of bronchiectasis is not determined; however, in a substantial percentage of patients, the finding of an underlying cause results in a change in therapy.

• In all newly diagnosed patients with bronchiectasis, sputum should be cultured for bacteria and mycobacteria, and fungal cultures could be considered in selected cases.

Bronchiectasis is an extremely heterogeneous disease in terms of the underlying causes, the demographic characteristics of affected patients, and the severity of disease.[1–3] Because some of these causes may respond to specific therapies or may increase the risk of certain complications, a systematic etiologic evaluation of a patient diagnosed with bronchiectasis is important. **Tables 1** and **2** list most of the recognized causes of bronchiectasis and a recommended scheme for diagnostic testing. Characteristic manifestations related to the underlying cause of disease may offer important clues to the underlying etiology and allow a targeted evaluation. Thus, there is not one panel of tests that is recommended for all patients. In this article the initial evaluation of an adult patient with bronchiectasis is reviewed.

Various authors[2,4] and expert panels[5,6] have published lists of diagnostic tests that should be performed on patients with bronchiectasis of unknown cause, with most lists including a group of tests that the authors believe should be performed on all patients and a second list of tests that should be performed if there are factors suggesting an increased likelihood of a specific diagnosis. It is noteworthy that essentially every one of the published lists is different. Many of the tests are recommended on the basis of little or no evidence that they lead to a specific diagnosis in a cost-effective manner[7] or that they lead to changes in treatment or patient outcomes. A good rule of thumb is that the longer the list of tests recommended for all patients, the more one should be skeptical. Doing all possible tests on all patients results in significant inconvenience and often direct cost for the patient and the healthcare system.

Several factors may alter the diagnostic yield of certain tests or the relative importance of any results that are obtained. These may include the age of the patient, age of onset, and severity of disease. Because the clinical presentation may suggest a specific cause, it often results in less inconvenience for the patient and less cost to initially perform testing only for the suspected cause and perform subsequent diagnostic testing if the initial testing is nonrevealing. How far away the patient lives from the treating physician may influence the testing scheme. For a patient who has flown several thousand miles to a specialized center, all potentially relevant tests may be ordered during the first visit, whereas for a patient who lives 10 minutes away, it is more cost-effective to order the most inexpensive

Division of Pulmonary and Critical Care Medicine, University of Connecticut School of Medicine, 263 Farmington Avenue, Farmington, CT 06030–1321, USA
E-mail address: Metersky@nso.uchc.edu

Clin Chest Med 33 (2012) 219–231
doi:10.1016/j.ccm.2012.03.004
0272-5231/12/$ – see front matter © 2012 Elsevier Inc. All rights reserved.

chestmed.theclinics.com

Table 1
Reported etiologies of bronchiectasis pooled from three cohort studies[a] and other reported etiologies

Etiologies Among Three Large Cohorts	Percent of Patients (n = 418 patients)[b]
Idiopathic	48
Postinfectious	25
Immunodeficiency (various)	8
Allergic bronchopulmonary aspergillosis	7
Primary ciliary dyskinesia	5
Young syndrome	3
Rheumatoid arthritis	2
Ulcerative colitis	2
Aspiration or gastroesophageal reflux	2
Yellow nail syndrome	1
Nontuberculous mycobacterial infection[c]	1
Cystic fibrosis	1
Diffuse panbronchiolitis	1
Congenital	<1
Other Reported Etiologies	
Acquired immunodeficiency	
Lymphoma	
HIV-related	
Organ or bone marrow transplant	
Autoimmune	
Relapsing polychondritis	
Ankylosing spondylitis	
Systemic lupus erythematosis	
Chronic obstructive pulmonary disease	
Congenital or genetic	
α_1-Antitrypsin deficiency	
Job syndrome (hyper immunoglobulin E syndrome)	
Marfan syndrome	
Mounier-Kuhn syndrome (tracheobronchomegaly)	
Williams-Campbell syndrome	
Endobronchial obstruction	
Neoplasm	
Foreign body	
Extrinsic compression by lymph nodes	
Inhalational exposure	
Smoke	
Ammonia	
Chlorine	
Traction	
Pulmonary fibrosis	
Sarcoidosis	

[a] Patients pooled from references.[7,9,10]
[b] Percentages add up to more than 100% because one study reported more than one etiology or association for some patients.
[c] Recent reports suggest that the current frequency of bronchiectasis caused by nontuberculous mycobacterial infection in the United States is significantly higher than 1%.

Table 2
Suggested testing for the initial evaluation of a newly diagnosed patient with bronchiectasis

Testing	Factors Increasing Likelihood of a Specific Diagnosis	Etiology
Suggested for all patients		
Pulmonary function testing with bronchodilator responsiveness ± arterial blood gas analysis		
Posteroanterior and lateral chest radiograph		
High-resolution CT scan of the chest		
Sputum for bacterial, mycobacterial, and fungal cultures		
Complete blood count with differential		
Quantitative immunoglobulins (IgG, IgA, IgM)	Concomitant sinus disease, recurrent infections	Common variable immunodeficiency
IgE level	Asthma, central bronchiectasis, prominent mucus plugging	Allergic bronchopulmonary aspergillosis
	Eczema, staphylococcal infections, retained primary teeth	Job syndrome
Suggested for most patients without a specific identified etiology		
α_1-Antitrypsin level	Emphysema	
Sweat chloride, nasal potential difference, or CF mutation screen	Concomitant sinus disease, younger age, upper-lobe disease	Cystic fibrosis
Suggested for selected patients without a specific identified etiology		
Aspergillus-specific IgG, IgE, aspergillus skin testing	Central bronchiectasis, asthma	Allergic bronchopulmonary aspergillosis
Bronchoscopy	Unilateral focal disease	Bronchial obstruction
Bronchoscopy with mycobacterial cultures	"Tree-in-bud" on high-resolution CT, nodules, cavities, scoliosis, pectus	Nontuberculous mycobacteria
Ciliary biopsy, ciliary functional testing, nasal nitric oxide	Childhood onset, sinus or ear infections, situs inversus Fertility problems	Primary ciliary dyskinesia
Swallow evaluation or esophageal pH measurement	*M avium* disease	Gastroesophageal reflux disease or aspiration
IgG subclass levels, response to immunization, tests for qualitative immune defects	Childhood onset, recurrent infections, dysmorphic features	Congenital immunodeficiency
Serologies for autoimmune disease	Arthritis, sicca syndrome	Rheumatoid arthritis, Sjögren syndrome

tests first and then order the more expensive or invasive tests only if needed. Resource availability and type of healthcare insurance may also be important factors. For example, in resource-poor countries, a diagnosis of α_1-antitrypsin deficiency or common variable immunodeficiency may not alter treatment considerations greatly, because replacement therapy may not be a realistic consideration. Even in wealthy countries, variable coverage may limit the ability to obtain certain tests or treatments.

Perhaps most importantly, the goals of testing for each patient should be considered before embarking on a battery of tests. Patients should also be made aware that in approximately 50% of patients, no specific cause is found, despite extensive evaluation.[8–11] Nonetheless, if a cause can be determined with reasonable cost and without undue inconvenience, patients generally would like an explanation of why they have bronchiectasis, even if the answer may not affect treatment decisions. For some diagnoses, knowing the cause may be important for genetic counseling if the patient is still in their childbearing years or has potentially affected children who can be advised to seek care early if they develop suggestive symptoms. In other patients, considering the goals of testing can minimize cost and inconvenience. For example, the author has forgone cystic fibrosis (CF) transmembrane conductance regulator (CFTR) DNA sequencing (cost >$1000) in more than one elderly patient despite a sweat chloride result greater than 40 and a nonrevealing CFTR mutation screening result, because the patients had very mild disease, good quality of life (QOL), and indicated that they would not want any specific therapy for CF.

WHY DETERMINE AN ETIOLOGY?

Several observational cohort studies of adults with bronchiectasis have been published in which the rate of determination of a specific cause was reported.[7–10] A specific cause was determined in between 26%[7] and 74%[10] in these series. **Table 1** shows the rate of idiopathic bronchiectasis and specific etiologies in results pooled from three of these studies (the Nicotra and coworkers[9] study was not included because specific numbers were not given for several of the etiologies). Varying rates can be explained by factors including differences in patient populations, referrals to certain centers for specific areas of expertise, and differences in the testing protocols between the centers. It is also noteworthy that these studies, only one of which is from the United States, demonstrate very low rates of bronchiectasis caused by nontuberculous mycobacterial (NTM) infection. This finding is contrary to the experience of centers in the United States.[12] Although a specific cause can only be determined in about 50% of patients, studies demonstrate that a significant segment of the causes result in changes in therapy. In the Pasteur and coworkers study,[10] 15% of patients received specific therapy based on the underlying diagnosis (allergic bronchopulmonary aspergillosis [ABPA], CF, gastroesophageal reflux, and common variable immunodeficiency). In the Shoemark cohort,[11] 37% of patients received a diagnosis that was thought to affect future management. Based on the results of these and other studies, a systematic effort to determine the etiology of patients with bronchiectasis is recommended by the British and the Spanish bronchiectasis guidelines and by other experts.[5,6,9,13] Even in the case of etiologies that do not require specific therapy, some lead to genetic testing and counseling of offspring. Furthermore, patients with bronchiectasis usually desire an explanation of why they have the disease, and seem to appreciate that explanation even if therapy is not altered.

HISTORY AND PHYSICAL EXAMINATION

Bronchiectasis is no different from most other conditions in that an appropriately targeted history and physical examination can provide important information. Key factors to elucidate include the age of symptom onset and the character of symptoms. The amount and character of sputum production can provide information regarding severity of disease and potential causes. For example, in a patient with scant sputum production despite prominent systemic symptoms, such as fever, sweats, and weight loss, infection with *Mycobacterium avium* complex should be considered. A history of childhood illnesses, such as pertussis or measles, is generally obtained, although the accuracy of designating one of these infections as the cause of bronchiectasis is suspect, given the frequency of these childhood infections in patients who were children before vaccines were commonly used. One should specifically query for symptoms suggesting comorbidities commonly associated with bronchiectasis. These include autoimmune diseases, such as rheumatoid arthritis and Sjögren syndrome. Gastrointestinal symptoms can suggest ulcerative colitis, a well-known cause of bronchiectasis. A history of pancreatitis or suggestive of pancreatic insufficiency may indicate CF, although most patients with adult-onset CF are pancreatic sufficient. Fertility problems suggest the possibility of primary ciliary dyskinesia (PCD), CF, or Young syndrome. A history of paranasal sinus disease is often seen in association with a systemic immune defect or a defect involving the entire respiratory tract, such as PCD or CF.

The physical examination can also provide useful information regarding cause and severity of illness. The character of spontaneous cough should be observed. It is not unusual to have a patient (usually female) who habitually swallows her sputum, and therefore denies sputum production,[14] but has an obvious "wet" cough. Examination can also provide clues to nutritional status. Sinus disease or nasal polyps may be evident. Thoracic skeletal abnormalities, such as pectus excavatum and scoliosis, and tall stature are more common in female patients with bronchiectasis caused by M avium and other NTM infections than in the general population.[15] The lung examination can reveal bronchiectasis-related findings, such as wheezing, rhonchi, and crackles. Prominent wheezing is unusual in idiopathic bronchiectasis and may suggest concomitant asthma and a diagnosis of ABPA. Evidence of pulmonary hypertension or right-heart failure may represent the sequela of severe disease, whereas mitral valve prolapse is more common in patients with bronchiectasis caused by NTM infection.[15] Examination of the nailbeds can reveal clubbing, also indicative of more severe disease, or yellow-colored nails, suggesting yellow nail syndrome.

IMAGING

A comprehensive review of the use of radiologic studies for the evaluation of bronchiectasis is beyond the scope of this article, but an excellent review is available elsewhere in this issue. Plain chest radiographs are usually abnormal in patients with bronchiectasis, but in approximately 50% the finding of "tramlines" or other abnormalities specific for bronchiectasis is not evident.[3,16] Common scenarios are that bronchiectasis is an unexpected finding when CT scanning is performed to more accurately evaluate a nonresolving abnormality initially thought to be pneumonia or when a CT is performed for unrelated reasons. A near universal finding in such scenarios is that in retrospect, the patient had suggestive symptoms for a long period preceding the diagnosis. High-resolution chest CT (HRCT) scans have largely replaced bronchography for the diagnosis of bronchiectasis. A recent study[17] evaluated the use of 3-T MRI in patients with bronchiectasis and found it to be highly accurate for many findings associated with bronchiectasis, although the authors acknowledged that the poorer spatial resolution of MRI limits the ability to visualize smaller airways and nodules. In situations where radiation exposure is problematic (ie, pregnancy), MRI seems to be a reasonable alternative.

The HRCT criteria for the finding of bronchiectasis include an airway internal diameter larger than the accompanying vessel pulmonary artery (the signet ring sign); the lack of tapering of the bronchus; and a bronchus visible within a centimeter of the pleural surface. In addition to identifying the presence of bronchiectasis, HRCT can also define the severity, based on the presence of (in order of increasing severity) cylindrical, varicose, and saccular disease. The severity of bronchiectasis can also be assessed on the basis of the extent of disease and in terms of the number of lobes involved, and a radiographic severity scoring system developed for use in CF[18] has been used to assess patients with non-CF bronchiectasis. Disease severity based on this radiographic score correlates with physiologic impairment and the severity of symptoms as assessed by the St. George's Respiratory Questionnaire, although in one report, the correlation with this questionnaire was only seen in patients with more severe disease.[19] It is also important to note that occasionally, after acute infection, there may be bronchial dilatation that resolves spontaneously (**Fig. 1**), so the diagnosis of bronchiectasis should be made with caution in a patient with recent symptoms suggesting acute infection who did not clearly have chronic symptoms previously.

Several radiographic findings associated with bronchiectasis are thought to provide clues to the cause of bronchiectasis. Predominantly upper-lobe disease (**Fig. 2**) is suggestive of CF. Central bronchiectasis, particularly in the presence of prominent mucus plugging, is suggestive of ABPA. Prominent nodularity in a tree-in-bud pattern or with cavitation is suggestive of NTM infection, as is the presence of predominantly middle lobe and lingular disease. Pectus excavatum may be more obvious on the CT scan than on physical examination, especially in women (**Fig. 3**). Patients with unilateral focal bronchiectasis are more likely to have disease related to focal airway obstruction, potentially caused by an endobronchial foreign body or neoplasm, both of which have treatment implications. An enlarged tracheal diameter (diameter >25 mm in men and >23 mm in women) is virtually diagnostic of tracheobronchomegaly or Mounier-Kuhn syndrome.[20]

Several studies have systematically evaluated the accuracy of determining the cause of bronchiectasis based on HRCT results, based largely on the previously mentioned patterns.[21–23] Cartier and colleagues[22] found that bilateral upper-lobe disease was more common in patients with CF and ABPA. Reiff and colleagues[23] found that

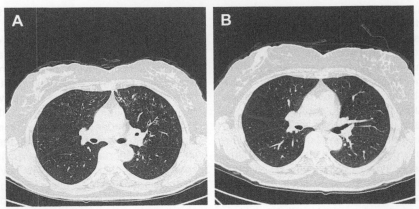

Fig. 1. CT image of a 69-year-old woman who presented with 3 months of cough and sputum after an acute lower respiratory tract infection (A) and a subsequent CT image demonstrating resolution of the bronchial dilatation 1 year later (B).

predominantly lower-lobe disease was associated with syndromes of impaired mucociliary clearance and ABPA was more commonly associated with central bronchiectasis, but these associations were not sensitive or specific enough to be usefully applied to individual patients. Lee and colleagues[21] agreed that the cause of bronchiectasis could not reliably be determined from HRCT patterns of disease. However, it seems reasonable to theorize that the presence of certain patterns of disease could help direct a subsequent etiologic evaluation to the more likely causes first, to increase cost effectiveness.

ETIOLOGIC TESTING
Immunodeficiency

All experts agree that quantitative immunoglobulins (IgG, IgA, and IgM) should be performed in every patient with bronchiectasis of unknown origin, because common variable immunodeficiency

is one of the most treatable underlying causes and one of the more common. In one series, bronchiectasis was seen in a patient with isolated IgM deficiency,[10] an immune defect often associated with impaired IgG response to antigen challenge. Whether or not to measure levels of IgG subclasses is somewhat controversial. In one study of predominantly adult patients with idiopathic bronchiectasis, 48% were found to have a low level of at least one subclass, most commonly IgG2, and these patients had impaired antibody responses to vaccine antigens compared with those without deficiency.[24] Martinez-Garcia[25] found that 12.5% of patients with idiopathic bronchiectasis had a low IgG subclass, also with IgG2 being the most commonly deficient subtype. However, several other investigators have found only rare patients with IgG subclass deficiency and no correlation between IgG subclass deficiency and humoral immune response to vaccine antigens.[9,26,27] That two of the studies demonstrating low IgG2 levels were from different groups

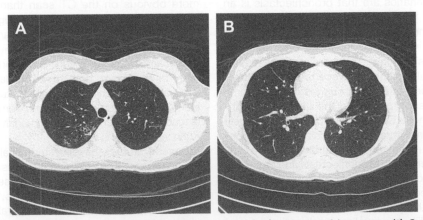

Fig. 2. CT slices through the upper lobes (A) and lower lobes (B) of a 26-year-old woman with 3 years of cough and sputum who was found to have cystic fibrosis.

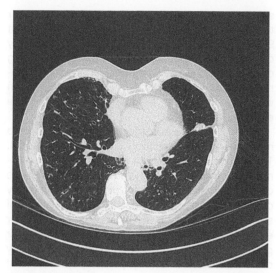

Fig. 3. Pectus excavatum in a 58-year-old woman with bronchiectasis caused by pulmonary *Mycobacterium avium* complex infection.

in Spain suggests the possibility of a relationship between ethnicity and IgG subclass deficiency. Elevated IgE levels can suggest bronchiectasis caused by either ABPA or hyperimmunoglobuline-mia E syndrome (HIES or Job syndrome), and therefore are performed routinely in some centers, although not recommended by the British Thoracic Society (BTS) guidelines.[5]

The performance of immunologic testing beyond immunoglobulin levels is recommended by some experts. The BTS guidelines recommend screening for humoral response to specific antigens, such as tetanus toxoid and capsular polysaccharides of *Streptococcus pneumoniae* and *Hemophilus influenza* type b.[5] Some specialized centers frequently search for other quantitative and qualitative immune defects, such as T- and B-cell number

and function; neutrophil function, including the oxidative burst; and innate immunity, including complement.[28] The yield of doing so in adults is thought to be low[9] and many experts do not recommend routine screening beyond immunoglobulin levels. In certain circumstances, it may be reasonable to do so, such as in the setting of congenital defects that suggest an immunodeficiency syndrome, unusually severe or frequent infections involving organs other than the lungs, or the occurrence of opportunistic infections.[5]

Genetic Disorders

The BTS guidelines recommend testing for α_1-antitrypsin deficiency only if there is concomitant emphysema.[5] However, a cohort study of patients with known α_1-antitrypsin deficiency demonstrated that there is a clinically distinct subset of patients with α_1-antitrypsin deficiency who have little or no evidence of emphysema, yet have radiographically and clinically severe bronchiectasis.[29] The author has diagnosed Pi ZZ α_1-antitrypsin deficiency in two older women, neither of whom had clinically significant emphysema (**Fig. 4**). Because α_1-antitrypsin deficiency is a diagnosis for which specific therapy is often provided (although there have been no studies that have tested for a benefit in α_1-antitrypsin deficiency–associated bronchiectasis), and because the testing is inexpensive, in contrast to the BTS guidelines,[5] the author recommends testing for α_1-antitrypsin deficiency in all patients with adult-onset bronchiectasis in whom no other cause is identified.

It is well recognized that patients with CF caused by the CFTR mutations that result in less severe functional abnormalities often present in adulthood with disease that is clinically similar to non-CF bronchiectasis.[30] Because the typical severe disease

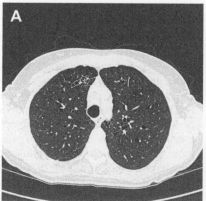
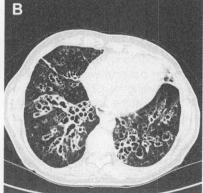

Fig. 4. (*A, B*) Representative CT slices of a 69-year-old woman with severe bronchiectasis caused by α_1-antitrypsin deficiency (ZZ), yet minimal evidence of emphysema.

and extrapulmonary manifestations are usually lacking, it is not possible to reliably identify adults with CF without specific testing. Even though the treatment of CF and non-CF bronchiectasis is similar, there are several reasons why it is quite important to identify patients with CF. First, genetic counseling of offspring often is indicated. Also, in many patients, treatment is altered. For example, DNase is an important component of CF treatment, but is contraindicated in non-CF bronchiectasis.[31] Finally, medications used for non-CF bronchiectasis are frequently not reimbursed by payers because they are not approved by the Food and Drug Administration (there are no medications that are approved by the Food and Drug Administration for use in bronchiectasis). Because many of these same medications are approved for use in CF or are proved to be beneficial in CF, a diagnosis often allows easier and less costly access for patients. These medications include hypertonic saline; inhaled antibiotics; and even chronic, low-dose macrolide therapy.

It is also increasingly apparent that the difference between CF and non-CF bronchiectasis is becoming more indistinct, complicating recommendations for screening protocols. Bienvenu and colleagues[32] recently studied a cohort of 122 idiopathic patients with bronchiectasis as defined by a normal sweat chloride (<60 mmol/L) and found that 22 (18%) had one CFTR mutation and 15 (12%) had two CFTR mutations. Furthermore, there was a continuum of airway CFTR dysfunction as measured by nasal epithelial potential difference, corresponding to the number of CFTR mutations, and the degree of dysfunction correlated with the phenotype of bronchiectasis as assessed by colonization with Pseudomonas sp and Staphylococcus aureus. The appropriateness of relying on a normal sweat chloride to rule out CF was therefore challenged by the authors, who suggested that a CF mutation screen test might be a more appropriate initial screening test.

The BTS guidelines[5] recommend testing for CF in all patients less than age 40 and in patients greater than the age of 40 who have suggestive features, such as predominantly upper-lobe disease or sinus disease. Pancreatic insufficiency can also be seen but is less common in patients with adult-onset CF. The appropriate testing for CF is not agreed on uniformly. Whereas some centers routinely screen all patients, the BTS guidelines[5] recommend screening those patients in whom CF is thought to be more likely based on clinical factors, such as age less than 40, upper lobe–predominant disease, sinus disease, malabsorption, or infertility. They recommend two determinations of sweat chloride and CFTR mutation analysis in those patients for whom screening is performed. The CFTR mutation

screening tests that are widely available screen for the most common mutations that result in about 90% of cases. If the screen is negative, or if only one mutation is detected, CFTR gene sequencing can be performed by several commercial laboratories, although frequently this requires a discussion with the insurance company because of the expense.

Based on these considerations, it is difficult to recommend one specific CF screening protocol. The author's practice is to do a single sweat chloride test on all patients who have no obvious cause of their bronchiectasis and to do further testing only on those patients in whom there is a higher index of suspicion or a sweat chloride of greater than or equal to 40 mmol/L. The BTS[5] protocol or other protocols may be chosen based on the availability of the various tests and the patient population, but a systematic approach is recommended.

PCD is an infrequent cause of bronchiectasis diagnosed in adulthood, but a few cases are seen in most published series.[7–10] In patients who do not give a history of chronic respiratory symptoms since childhood, the disease is rare enough that it is reasonable to forgo testing, especially because there is no specific therapy. In adults who have had symptoms since childhood, PCD should be considered. The saccharin test, which measures the time until the patient tastes saccharin after it is placed on the inferior nasal turbinate, is inexpensive and in theory could be performed in any center; however, it is very patient- and operator-dependent and can give misleading results.

Patients with PCD generally have very low nasal nitric oxide levels, offering an inexpensive screening tool for those centers that possess the necessary equipment. Although the absolute levels vary depending on the methodology and the report, patients with PCD rarely have nasal nitric oxide levels greater than 100 ppb.[33,34] In one study, a cut-off value of 105 ppb or lower had 94% sensitivity and 89% specificity for PCD.[33] Normal individuals and patients with other types of airway disease usually have nasal nitric oxide levels an order of magnitude higher than patients with PCD, but there is some overlap in patients with other types of airway disease, particularly CF.[34] Therefore, confirmation of the diagnosis of PCD through direct observation of ciliary structure or function is required. Ciliary biopsy with transmission electron microscopy reliably detects most ciliary structural defects leading to ciliary dyskinesia, although 3% of patients with PCD have no detectable ultrastructural abnormalities.[35] Some other defects are difficult to reliably detect with electron microscopy unless computer-assisted techniques are used.[35] Because of these issues, if there is a high clinical suspicion, only direct visualization of ciliary function can definitively exclude the diagnosis. This is generally only done in highly specialized centers, sometimes creating logistic difficulties in getting the viable samples to the center. It is also important to realize that ultrastructural defects and ciliary functional abnormalities can be seen in the setting of acute and chronic airway inflammation, so testing should be done with patients in their most stable state.[36]

Other, more rare genetic defects can result in bronchiectasis. Job syndrome (HIES) is caused by mutations in the gene encoding signal transducer and activator of transcription 3, a protein integral to signal transduction for multiple cytokines.[37] Patients characteristically have very high IgE levels; a history of eczema (which may remit in adulthood); and a history of staphylococcal infections including boils and pneumonia or lung abscesses. Failure of several primary teeth to spontaneously fall out, with a resulting requirement for extraction, is almost pathognomonic for HIES in the right clinical setting. Testing for signal transducer and activator of transcription 3 mutations is not commercially available but can be obtained by contacting the National Institutes of Health. Chronic antifungal therapy with posiconazole is recommended for affected patients to prevent invasive aspergillosis, a common cause of mortality from HIES.[38]

Miscellaneous Testing

There are several other testing modalities that should be considered in selected patients. Because autoimmune diseases, such as Sjögren syndrome or rheumatoid arthritis, can cause bronchiectasis, appropriate serologies should be obtained in any patient with suggestive features elicited by history or physical examination. Although some experts recommend such serologies[4] for all patients with bronchiectasis of undetermined cause, this does not seem to be a cost-effective approach because most patients have a prior diagnosis of the underlying disease before bronchiectasis is diagnosed.

Chronic aspiration caused by gastroesophageal reflux, other esophageal disease, and abnormal swallowing caused by laryngeal disease or neurologic disease can be a cause of bronchiectasis in patients without other risk factors. Gastroesophageal reflux has also been associated with bronchiectasis caused by *M avium* complex infection.[39,40] Thus, in selected patients, a swallow evaluation or esophageal pH monitoring may provide a cause and an opportunity to intervene.

Stable patients with bronchiectasis have elevated levels of inflammatory markers, such as C-reactive protein and erythrocyte sedimentation rate,[41] and these markers increase during exacerbations.[42] Murray and colleagues[42] also investigated the usefulness of following inflammatory markers, such as the erythrocyte sedimentation rate or C-reactive protein, so that follow-up measurements can be used to assess the patients' response to therapy. Although there were significant differences between levels before and after treatment of exacerbations, there is no evidence that using these markers yields any more information than assessing the response using easily available clinical markers, such as cough, fever, and weight gain. In another study, procalcitonin levels did not reliably differentiate between stable patients and those admitted to the hospital with an exacerbation of bronchiectasis, and therefore cannot be recommended.[43] These markers are not recommended for routine use in patients with bronchiectasis.

Because of the lack of biomarkers or other tests that reliably determine severity of disease or predict outcome, there has been significant interest in using QOL instruments to monitor patients with bronchiectasis. QOL instruments, such the Leicester Cough Questionnaire,[44] the St. Georges Respiratory Questionnaire,[45] and the recently developed bronchiectasis-specific QOL-B,[46] have been studied. They allow physicians to obtain an objective and reliable assessment of the patients' status and uncover some symptoms or concerns that would usually not be elucidated. Physicians seeing many patients with bronchiectasis could consider incorporating routine assessments of QOL into their practice.

PULMONARY FUNCTION TESTING

Pulmonary function testing, including spirometry with bronchodilator response testing, lung volumes, and diffusion capacity for carbon monoxide, is routinely recommended as part of the initial evaluation of patients. Severe impairment identifies patients with a worsened prognosis.[47] Because the intensity of therapy that a patient will accept is often determined in part by the treatment burden for the patient, identification of more severe disease may help convince the patient of the importance of adhering to recommended treatment. The finding of a bronchodilator response will likely identify patients who are more likely to receive benefit from inhaled bronchodilators and inhaled corticosteroids.[48] Arterial blood gas determination may be done for selected patients who have more severe disease in whom clinically significant hypoxemia or hypercarbia may indicate the need for long-term oxygen therapy or nocturnal noninvasive ventilatory support.

MICROBIOLOGIC TESTING

Because patients with bronchiectasis have a much larger variety of pathogens than patients with chronic obstructive pulmonary disease, microbiologic surveillance plays a more important role. All patients should have sputum cultured for bacterial pathogens when initially diagnosed. Approximately 30% of patients are chronically colonized with[9] and exacerbate because of *Pseudomonas aeruginosa*, and thus identifying the presence of this pathogen is important in directing therapy for future exacerbations. Furthermore, patients with chronic *Pseudomonas* infection have worsened long-term prognosis.[9] Other potentially resistant gram-negative bacilli are also cultured, although less frequently. More recently, methicillin-resistant *S aureus* has emerged as a problematic pathogen in some patients with bronchiectasis.

Because NTM infection is commonly seen in association with bronchiectasis (as a cause and complication), the initial evaluation should involve at least one sputum cultured for mycobacteria. If *M avium* complex is isolated and treatment is being considered, the isolate should be tested for sensitivity to macrolides, because the results predict response to therapy and ultimate prognosis.[49] Many laboratories do not routinely perform such testing, so the clinician usually must remember to specifically request it when *M avium* is isolated. Similarly, for several other NTM, sensitivities are important to guide therapy. Because patients with bronchiectasis caused by NTM may produce little sputum, in patients with characteristic CT findings or other reasons for a high suspicion if the initial sputum is negative or the patient is unable to produce an adequate sample, additional samples or even bronchoalveolar lavage and biopsy should be obtained. Not all patients who grow NTM require specific therapy because many are merely colonized, but even colonization with NTM is an important finding. First, colonization identifies a patient in whom NTM infection should be considered in the case of clinical worsening. Furthermore, chronic low-dose macrolide therapy, commonly used for its immunomodulatory effect, should be avoided in patients with NTM disease or colonization because it creates the risk for inducing macrolide resistance, markedly decreasing the chances of cure.[50] NTM and bronchiectasis is discussed in more detail elsewhere in this issue.

The sputum of patients with bronchiectasis often grows one or more fungi, including yeasts and molds, reflecting the impaired local airway host defenses. Usually, unless profound systemic immunosuppression occurs, these potentially opportunistic organisms are not clinically important. Because the growth of *Aspergillus* sp is associated with ABPA, some authors suggest performing a fungal culture as part of the initial evaluation. The other potentially important finding that can be obtained from a fungal culture is *Nocardia* sp, which is usually not detected using standard bacterial techniques. Although isolation of *Nocardia* sp often represents colonization, *Nocardia* sp can be pathogenic in patients with bronchiectasis who are not otherwise immunocompromised.[51] The author has treated a patient with *Nocardia* and *Pseudomonas* in her sputum whose fever and copious sputum did not respond to antipseudomonal therapy, but responded promptly to treatment with oral trimethoprim-sulfamethoxazole, despite the lack of evidence of infiltration on chest CT scan.

BRONCHOSCOPY

Most patients with bronchiectasis do not require bronchoscopy at the time of diagnosis. However, in a patient with unilateral focal bronchiectasis, a bronchoscopy should be performed to rule out an obstructing lesion, such as an aspirated foreign body, or obstruction from an endobronchial lesion, such as a carcinoid tumor, or extrinsic compression, such as can be caused by enlarged lymph nodes. Most patients with bronchiectasis can produce a sputum sample for microbiologic testing, avoiding the need for bronchoscopy for this purpose. One common exception is seen in patients with bronchiectasis caused by NTM, many of whom have scant sputum production despite significant disease. When NTM-related bronchiectasis is suspected, and the patient is unable to produce an adequate sputum sample, bronchoscopy should be performed, because the yield is three times greater than with sputum.[52]

WHAT CAUSES IDIOPATHIC BRONCHIECTASIS?

Some patients with idiopathic bronchiectasis undoubtedly suffered a childhood respiratory infection that resulted in irreversible damage, even if that infection is not recalled or appreciated by the patient. However, recent research has shed some light on some potential underlying genetic factors that seem to increase the risk of bronchiectasis. A total of 18% of patients with bronchiectasis and a sweat chloride of less than 60 mmol/L possess a single mutation of the CFTR, and although not fulfilling the diagnostic criteria for CF, have abnormalities in CFTR function as assessed by nasal potential difference. Fajac and colleagues[53] recently described abnormal sodium transport associated with mutations in the epithelial sodium channel ENaC in patients with idiopathic bronchiectasis. There is also an accumulating line of thinking that patients with idiopathic bronchiectasis may suffer from a "double hit" or "multiple hits" of genetic presdispositions, none of which in isolation is likely to cause bronchiectasis.[54] This could explain why some but not all patients with a single CFTR mutation develop bronchiectasis, and why bronchiectasis is sometimes seen in patients with isolated IgG subclass deficiency or a single α_1-antitrypsin mutation. Another example is seen in patients with common variable immunodeficiency, in whom coexisting deficiency of mannose binding lectin (a component of the innate immune system important in complement activation) increases the risk of developing bronchiectasis.[55]

SUMMARY

Bronchiectasis is caused by a myriad of underlying conditions or environmental insults to the bronchial tree. Despite a detailed evaluation, the cause remains undetermined in approximately 50% of cases. Nonetheless, it is important to use a systematic approach to the diagnostic evaluation of a patient with newly diagnosed bronchiectasis, because a substantial proportion of patients have a specific underlying diagnosis with implications for prognosis or treatment. Although there is no uniformly agreed on approach, there is broad consensus that all patients should be tested for quantitative immunoglobulin deficiency. Many experts believe that specific testing for α_1-antitrypsin deficiency and CF is indicated for most patients with bronchiectasis of unknown cause. Bronchoscopy should be performed on most patients with unilateral focal disease to exclude the possibility of an obstructing endobronchial lesion. Other tests, such as ciliary ultrastructure and function, aspergillus serologies, further testing for immunodeficiency, or an evaluation for possible aspiration, should be considered in selected patients. All patients should have baseline imaging including a chest radiograph and HRCT and a culture of respiratory secretions, including bacterial, mycobacterial, and sometimes fungal.

REFERENCES

1. O'Donnell AE. Bronchiectasis. Chest 2008;134(4): 815–23.
2. Barker AF. Bronchiectasis. N Engl J Med 2002; 346(18):1383–93.
3. Feldman C. Bronchiectasis: new approaches to diagnosis and management. Clin Chest Med 2011; 32(3):535–46.
4. Wilson R. Bronchiectasis. In: Niederman M, editor. Respiratory infections. 2nd edition. Philadelphia: Lippincott, Williams and Wilkins; 2001. p. 347–59.
5. Pasteur MC, Bilton D, Hill AT. British Thoracic Society guideline for non-CF bronchiectasis. Thorax 2010; 65(Suppl 1):i1–58.
6. Vendrell M, de Gracia J, Olveira C, et al. Diagnosis and treatment of bronchiectasis. Spanish Society of Pneumology and Thoracic Surgery. Arch Bronconeumol 2008;44(11):629–40.
7. Quast TM, Self AR, Browning RF. Diagnostic evaluation of bronchiectasis. Dis Mon 2008;54(8):527–39.
8. King PT, Holdsworth SR, Freezer NJ, et al. Characterisation of the onset and presenting clinical features of adult bronchiectasis. Respir Med 2006; 100(12):2183–9.
9. Nicotra MB, Rivera M, Dale AM, et al. Clinical, pathophysiologic, and microbiologic characterization of bronchiectasis in an aging cohort. Chest 1995; 108(4):955–61.
10. Pasteur MC, Helliwell SM, Houghton SJ, et al. An investigation into causative factors in patients with bronchiectasis. Am J Respir Crit Care Med 2000; 162(4 Pt 1):1277–84.
11. Shoemark A, Ozerovitch L, Wilson R. Aetiology in adult patients with bronchiectasis. Respir Med 2007;101(6):1163–70.
12. O'Donnell A, Prevots D, Olivier K, et al. The bronchiectasis research registry: clinical, microbiologic, and treatment characteristics. Eur Respir J 2010; 36:A4034.
13. Couderc LJ, Catherinot E, Rivaud E, et al. Are investigations for underlying causes needed for the management of an adult patient with bronchiectasis? Rev Pneumol Clin 2011;67(4):267–74.
14. Reich JM, Johnson RE. Mycobacterium avium complex pulmonary disease presenting as an isolated lingular or middle lobe pattern. The Lady Windermere syndrome. Chest 1992;101(6):1605–9.
15. Kim RD, Greenberg DE, Ehrmantraut ME, et al. Pulmonary nontuberculous mycobacterial disease: prospective study of a distinct preexisting syndrome. Am J Respir Crit Care Med 2008; 178(10):1066–74.
16. Goeminne P, Dupont L. Non-cystic fibrosis bronchiectasis: diagnosis and management in 21st century. Postgrad Med J 2010;86(1018):493–501.
17. Montella S, Santamaria F, Salvatore M, et al. Assessment of chest high-field magnetic resonance imaging in children and young adults with noncystic fibrosis chronic lung disease: comparison to high-resolution computed tomography and correlation

with pulmonary function. Invest Radiol 2009;44(9): 532–8.

18. Bhalla M, Turcios N, Aponte V, et al. Cystic fibrosis: scoring system with thin-section CT. Radiology 1991;179(3):783–8.

19. Eshed I, Minski I, Katz R, et al. Bronchiectasis: correlation of high-resolution CT findings with health-related quality of life. Clin Radiol 2007;62(2):152–9.

20. Noori F, Abduljawad S, Suffin DM, et al. Mounier-Kuhn syndrome: a case report. Lung 2010;188(4):353–4.

21. Lee PH, Carr DH, Rubens MB, et al. Accuracy of CT in predicting the cause of bronchiectasis. Clin Radiol 1995;50(12):839–41.

22. Cartier Y, Kavanagh PV, Johkoh T, et al. Bronchiectasis: accuracy of high-resolution CT in the differentiation of specific diseases. AJR Am J Roentgenol 1999;173(1):47–52.

23. Reiff DB, Wells AU, Carr DH, et al. CT findings in bronchiectasis: limited value in distinguishing between idiopathic and specific types. AJR Am J Roentgenol 1995;165(2):261–7.

24. De Gracia J, Rodrigo MJ, Morell F, et al. IgG subclass deficiencies associated with bronchiectasis. Am J Respir Crit Care Med 1996;153(2):650–5.

25. Martinez-Garcia MA, Perpina-Tordera M, Roman-Sanchez P, et al. Inhaled steroids improve quality of life in patients with steady-state bronchiectasis. Respir Med 2006;100(9):1623–32.

26. Stead A, Douglas JG, Broadfoot CJ, et al. Humoral immunity and bronchiectasis. Clin Exp Immunol 2002;130(2):325–30.

27. Hill SL, Mitchell JL, Burnett D, et al. IgG subclasses in the serum and sputum from patients with bronchiectasis. Thorax 1998;53(6):463–8.

28. King PT, Hutchinson P, Holmes PW, et al. Assessing immune function in adult bronchiectasis. Clin Exp Immunol 2006;144(3):440–6.

29. Parr DG, Guest PG, Reynolds JH, et al. Prevalence and impact of bronchiectasis in alpha1-antitrypsin deficiency. Am J Respir Crit Care Med 2007; 176(12):1215–21.

30. Nick JA, Rodman DM. Manifestations of cystic fibrosis diagnosed in adulthood. Curr Opin Pulm Med 2005;11(6):513–8.

31. O'Donnell AE, Barker AF, Ilowite JS, et al. Treatment of idiopathic bronchiectasis with aerosolized recombinant human DNase I. rhDNase Study Group. Chest 1998;113(5):1329–34.

32. Bienvenu T, Sermet-Gaudelus I, Burgel PR, et al. conductance regulator channel dysfunction in non-cystic fibrosis bronchiectasis. Am J Respir Crit Care Med 2010;181(10):1078–84.

33. Marthin JK, Nielsen KG. Choice of nasal nitric oxide technique as first-line test for primary ciliary dyskinesia. Eur Respir J 2011;37(3):559–65.

34. Corbelli R, Bringolf-Isler B, Amacher A, et al. Nasal nitric oxide measurements to screen children for primary ciliary dyskinesia. Chest 2004;126(4): 1054–9.

35. Storm van's Gravesande K, Omran H. Primary ciliary dyskinesia: clinical presentation, diagnosis and genetics. Ann Med 2005;37(6):439–49.

36. Cowan MJ, Gladwin MT, Shelhamer JH. Disorders of ciliary motility. Am J Med Sci 2001;321(1):3–10.

37. Paulson ML, Freeman AF, Holland SM. Hyper IgE syndrome: an update on clinical aspects and the role of signal transducer and activator of transcription 3. Curr Opin Allergy Clin Immunol 2008;8(6): 527–33.

38. Vinh DC, Sugui JA, Hsu AP, et al. Invasive fungal disease in autosomal-dominant hyper-IgE syndrome. J Allergy Clin Immunol 2010;125(6):1389–90.

39. Thomson RM, Armstrong JG, Looke DF. Gastroesophageal reflux disease, acid suppression, and Mycobacterium avium complex pulmonary disease. Chest 2007;131(4):1166–72.

40. Koh WJ, Lee JH, Kwon YS, et al. Prevalence of gastroesophageal reflux disease in patients with nontuberculous mycobacterial lung disease. Chest 2007;131(6):1825–30.

41. Wilson CB, Jones PW, O'Leary CJ, et al. Systemic markers of inflammation in stable bronchiectasis. Eur Respir J 1998;12(4):820–4.

42. Murray MP, Turnbull K, Macquarrie S, et al. Assessing response to treatment of exacerbations of bronchiectasis in adults. Eur Respir J 2009; 33(2):312–8.

43. Loebinger MR, Shoemark A, Berry M, et al. Procalcitonin in stable and unstable patients with bronchiectasis. Chron Respir Dis 2008;5(3):155–60.

44. Murray MP, Turnbull K, MacQuarrie S, et al. Validation of the Leicester Cough Questionnaire in non-cystic fibrosis bronchiectasis. Eur Respir J 2009; 34(1):125–31.

45. Wilson CB, Jones PW, O'Leary CJ, et al. Validation of the St. George's Respiratory Questionnaire in bronchiectasis. Am J Respir Crit Care Med 1997; 156(2 Pt 1):536–41.

46. Quittner AL, Salathe M, Gotfried M, et al. National validation of a patient-reported outcome measure for bronchiectasis: psychometric results on the QOL-B. Am J Respir Crit Care Med 2010;181:A5793.

47. Loebinger MR, Wells AU, Hansell DM, et al. Mortality in bronchiectasis: a long-term study assessing the factors influencing survival. Eur Respir J 2009; 34(4):843–9.

48. van Haren EH, Lammers JW, Festen J, et al. The effects of the inhaled corticosteroid budesonide on lung function and bronchial hyperresponsiveness in adult patients with cystic fibrosis. Respir Med 1995;89(3):209–14.

49. Griffith DE, Brown-Elliott BA, Langsjoen B, et al. Clinical and molecular analysis of macrolide resistance in Mycobacterium avium complex lung

disease. Am J Respir Crit Care Med 2006;174(8): 928–34.

50. Griffith DE, Aksamit T, Brown-Elliott BA, et al. An official ATS/IDSA statement: diagnosis, treatment, and prevention of nontuberculous mycobacterial diseases. Am J Respir Crit Care Med 2007;175(4): 367–416.

51. Ferrer A, Llorenc V, Codina G, et al. Nocardiosis and bronchiectasis. An uncommon association? Enferm Infecc Microbiol Clin 2005;23(2):62–6.

52. Tanaka E, Amitani R, Niimi A, et al. Yield of computed tomography and bronchoscopy for the diagnosis of *Mycobacterium avium* complex

pulmonary disease. Am J Respir Crit Care Med 1997;155(6):2041–6.

53. Fajac I, Viel M, Sublemontier S, et al. Could a defective epithelial sodium channel lead to bronchiectasis. Respir Res 2008;9:46.

54. Boucher RC. Bronchiectasis: a continuum of ion transport dysfunction or multiple hits? Am J Respir Crit Care Med 2010;181(10):1017–9.

55. Fevang B, Mollnes TE, Holm AM, et al. Common variable immunodeficiency and the complement system; low mannose-binding lectin levels are associated with bronchiectasis. Clin Exp Immunol 2005; 142(3):576–84.

Imaging of Bronchiectasis

John Bonavita, MD*, David P. Naidich, MD

KEYWORDS

- Bronchiectasis • Imaging • Airways • Computed tomography

KEY POINTS

- It is essential for clinicians to be familiar with methods for obtaining computed tomography (CT) images in patients with known or suspected bronchiectasis to ensure optimal diagnostic accuracy as well as to minimize radiation exposure.
- Clinicians should be familiar with the commonest direct and indirect findings in patients with bronchiectasis as well as potential pitfalls in diagnosis.
- Although direct visual assessment of the airways remains the mainstay of routine clinical practice, physicians should be aware of the numerous quantitative and automated CT methods that are now available to evaluate airway diseases.

Bronchiectasis is defined as localized, irreversible destruction of the walls of cartilage-containing airways with resultant dilatation.[1,2] Previously thought to be declining in incidence, bronchiectasis is now a commonly established diagnosis, largely a reflection of the impact of high-resolution CT (HRCT) scanning. From the time of its first introduction, HRCT has consistently proved to be the most sensitive and specific noninvasive method for diagnosing bronchiectasis, with implications for a role of CT to limit progression when the diagnosis is established early in its course, especially in children.[3] In addition, the detail afforded by 1-mm images of the peripheral airways has proved superior to virtually every other method for assessing the extent and severity of disease. Furthermore, in select cases, the pattern of disease on HRCT may prove sufficiently distinctive to limit differential diagnosis to only a few entities.[4,5] As discussed later, in this era of widespread availability of multidetector CT scanners, including those providing dual energy capability, newer methods for reconstructing images are now being investigated, opening potentially unique automated, quantitative methods for evaluating the peripheral airways.

This article focuses on a detailed consideration of techniques of image acquisition and reconstruction, followed by a review of diagnostic CT criteria, both direct and indirect, requisite to establish a diagnosis of bronchiectasis, including potential limitations and pitfalls. Newer methods for assessing the extent and severity of disease, as well as potential future quantitative methods, are discussed and illustrated. Given the availability of numerous review articles describing both clinical and imaging findings from specific causes,[1,6,7] a review of the wide range of causes of bronchiectasis remains outside the scope of the present review, although brief mention is made of CT findings that indicate specific causes, when appropriate.

MULTIDETECTOR CT IMAGING TECHNIQUE

Diagnostic accuracy requires meticulous imaging technique. Multidetector CT scanners enable routine visualization of airways as small as 2 mm in diameter throughout the thorax.[5] As a result, most current protocols emphasize volumetric data acquisition with scans obtained through the thorax in a single breath hold. Current commercially available scanners enable a complete data set to be acquired in a few seconds or less (with current scanners capable of even subsecond data acquisition),

Department of Radiology, New York University-Langone Medical Center, 550 First Avenue, IRM 232B, New York, NY 10022, USA
* Corresponding author.
E-mail address: John.bonavita@nyumc.org

Clin Chest Med 33 (2012) 233–248
doi:10.1016/j.ccm.2012.02.007
0272-5231/12/$ – see front matter © 2012 Elsevier Inc. All rights reserved.

minimizing respiratory and cardiac motion. More importantly, volumetric acquisition allows isotropic image reconstruction, resulting in images with equivalent spatial resolution regardless of the plane of reconstruction. The result of these improvements is the availability of nearly endless methods for either prospectively or retrospectively reconstructing scan data. Decisions that most importantly affect image quality include (1) choice of collimators, which defines the limit of spatial resolution; and, (2) choice of reconstruction algorithms defining both slice thickness and plane of reconstruction, in particular. Other major considerations include radiation dose and indications for the use of intravenous contrast administration.

The choice of which type of images to reconstruct typically involves consideration of the time needed to reconstruct images, including those requiring advanced reconstruction techniques such as multi-planar reconstruction, or maximum or minimum-intensity projection images (**Fig. 1**), as well as storage requirements necessary to archive potentially

several hundred additional images by current picture archiving and communication systems (PACS). The choice of which images to reconstruct, archive, and send to PACS for viewing reflects a balance between the types of reconstruction formats needed for routine clinical assessment (in particular, slice thickness and three-dimensional [3D] orientation) versus the total number of images to be reconstructed and archived. In the era of volumetric acquisition of CT data, the number of scans reconstructed can be numbered in the hundreds. Current scanners include improved storage capability, rendering archiving requirements of less immediate concern. Allowing for considerable variation in routine clinical scan parameters used in daily clinical practice, it is recommended that the thinnest possible collimation should be used to acquire data, so that high-resolution images can be reconstructed without the need to separately acquire a second high-resolution data set. As a consequence, studies should now routinely include a combination of both

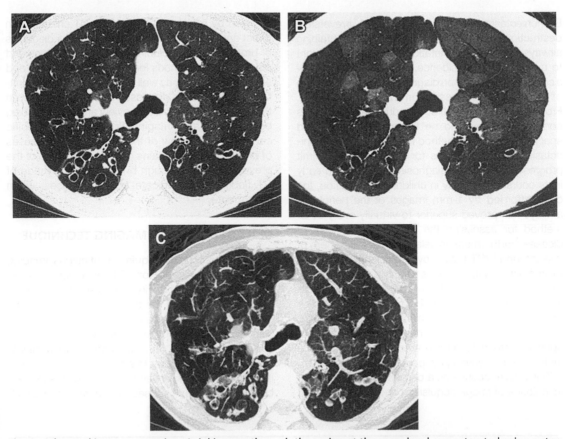

Fig. 1. Advanced image processing. Axial images through the carina at the same level reconstructed using a standard lung algorithm (*A*), minimum-intensity projection (MinIP) (*B*) and maximum intensity projection (MIP) images, respectively. Although routine reconstructions show the presence of bronchiectasis with associated mosaic lung attenuation, the MinIP image (*B*) enhances recognition of the extent of air trapping by effectively subtracting parenchymal vessels from the image, whereas the MIP (C) image shows to better advantage the distribution of parenchymal vessels.

thick (contiguous 5 mm) and thin (1–2 mm every 10 mm) images in every case, effectively making every study an HRCT examination. This protocol replaces the older concept of a separate high-resolution study, as initially recommended for evaluating diffuse lung disease,[8] with a role for performing traditional high-resolution studies with 1-mm images reconstructed every 10 mm, to reduce radiation exposure to patients in whom repeated follow-up studies are indicated, especially in younger individuals.

The most important indication for initial volumetric acquisition of data using thin collimation is the ability to prospectively and/or retrospectively reconstruct contiguous, high-resolution, 1-mm images through the thorax. The value of having access to contiguous 1-mm images for evaluating the peripheral airways cannot be overemphasized. Although 1-mm images reconstructed every 10 mm improve visualization of airway morphology compared with routine 5 mm thick images, the ability to sequential track airway anatomy using high-resolution images over several centimeters frequently proves invaluable, especially in more subtle cases (**Fig. 2**). In addition, availability of contiguous high-resolution images is essential for

more advanced visualization techniques, including 3D methods for depicting airway anatomy as well as minimum-intensity and maximum-intensity projection images (see **Fig. 1**). More problematic is the notion of routinely prospectively reconstructing contiguous 1-mm images for clinical evaluation on PACS, because this typically results in 100 to 200 additional images that need to be archived.

Other considerations besides choice of collimation and methods of reconstruction include the usefulness of acquiring additional expiratory images and issues related to radiation dose. In select cases, acquiring additional expiratory images can be helpful by allowing visualization of both focal and diffuse air trapping. Numerous studies have shown that air trapping frequently accompanies bronchiectasis, reflecting a combination of both large and small airway obstruction.[9–15] Typically performed selectively with only a few additional high-resolution images acquired (usually through the upper, mid, and lower lung zones, respectively), the need for routine acquisition is debatable. Although quantitative evaluation using visual scoring systems have been proposed, these suffer from considerable

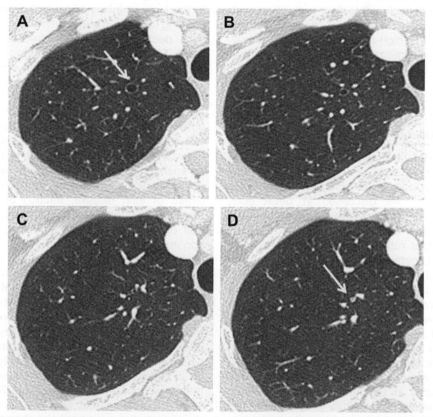

Fig. 2. Focal bronchial stricture. (*A–D*) Contiguous 1-mm high-resolution images through the right upper lobe show a dilated peripheral bronchus (*arrow* in *A*) that progressively narrows to a point of marked narrowing/ stenosis (*arrow* in *D*). Contiguous high-resolution imaging enables fine delineation of airway anatomy even in the lung periphery.

interobserver variation. True quantitative evaluation of the extent of air trapping may be performed but requires that contiguous 1-mm images be reconstructed, entailing considerable increase in radiation dose and often the need to access advanced image workstations.

Radiation exposure related to CT scanning also represents a recently highlighted concern. Although it is axiomatic that radiation exposure should be minimized whenever possible, low-dose CT techniques provide image quality sufficient for accurate diagnosis of most diseases affecting the airways and lung in all save the most obese individuals.[16,17] Although there is a slight increase in radiation exposure resulting from use of the thin collimation necessary for obtaining contiguous 1-mm high-resolution images as discussed earlier, diagnostic images can almost always be obtained using low-dose (80–100 mAs) exposure coupled with current dose modulation techniques used on modern multidetector scanners, partially offsetting concerns about excess radiation. As previously discussed, in cases in which excessive radiation exposure is of particular concern, one available solution is to initially perform volumetric data acquisition, with subsequent follow-up examinations performed with a dedicated high-resolution technique obtaining 1-mm axial images every 10 mm only, again using a low-dose imaging technique.

CT DIAGNOSIS: VISUAL INTERPRETATION
Bronchial Dilatation

Bronchial dilatation remains the most important CT finding to establish a diagnosis of bronchiectasis, and typically relies solely on simple visual identification.[18] As discussed in detail later, although several quantitative metrics have been proposed, most often including lumen diameter, bronchoarterial ratio, lumen area (LA) and wall thickness/diameter ratio (T/D ratio), none of these have proved of value in everyday clinical practice. Instead, visual assessment based on the finding of an airway with an internal diameter greater than the diameter of the adjacent pulmonary artery has served as the most common definition, an appearance referred to as a signet-ring sign (Fig. 3). The accuracy of this sign has been validated in early studies comparing CT with bronchography in patients with bronchiectasis. Although this sign is generally reliable, care must be taken not to misinterpret bronchial dilatation as bronchiectasis in the setting of underlying parenchymal consolidation (so-called reversible bronchiectasis) (Table 1).

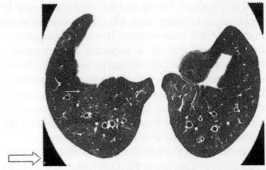

Fig. 3. Bronchiectasis. Axial 1-mm image through the lung bases shows classic appearance of airways greater in diameter than their accompanying pulmonary artery branches; the so-called signet-ring sign. Note that there is also accompanying mosaic lung attenuation (*arrow*) consistent with associated obstructive small airway disease. (*Reprinted from* Webb WR, Muller NL, Naidich DP. High resolution CT of the lung. Philadelphia: Lippincott Williams & Wilkins; 2009. p. 493; with permission, Fig. 16-1B, #3800.)

An appearance that superficially mimics bronchiectasis is most commonly seen in patients with diffuse lung fibrosis, in which case airway dilatation in the lung periphery is caused by peribronchial scarring rather than true localized irreversible bronchial destruction (so-called traction bronchiectasis) (Fig. 4). In patients with fibrotic idiopathic interstitial pneumonias, the extent and severity of traction bronchiectasis has proved to be an important predictor of disease mortality.[19–21] As reported by Edey and colleagues[19] in a study of 146 consecutive patients diagnosed with fibrotic interstitial pneumonias, of the variables analyzed, including the extent and severity of traction bronchiectasis, parenchymal reticulation, and microscopic and macroscopic honeycombing, as well as the overall extent of lung disease, traction bronchiectasis most strongly indicated higher mortality, regardless of the pattern of background parenchymal abnormalities (hazard ratio 1.04, confidence interval [CI] 1.03–1.06, $P = .001$).

Another variation in appearance that may also result in an erroneous impression of bronchiectasis is evaluation of thick, rather than thin, CT sections. Care should be exercised not to misinterpret physiologically dilated airways as bronchiectatic, as occurs, for example, in individuals who live at high altitudes,[22] in elderly patients,[18] or on images obtained through the lung bases in the prone position. In one study of HRCT findings in 85 subjects without cardiopulmonary disease divided into 3 groups based on their ages, significant correlation between bronchoarterial ratio and age was noted ($r = 0.768$, $P<.0001$), with bronchoarterial ratio greater than 1 being identified in

Table 1
Bronchiectasis: HRCT findings

Direct Signs	Indirect Signs

1. Bronchial dilatation
    Increased bronchoarterial ratio
    Contour abnormalities
	1. Bronchial wall thickening
	    Best assessed visually on images obtained
	        at right angles through vertically
	        oriented airways

2. Lack of airway tapering >2 cm distal to point of bifurcation	2. Mucoid impaction/fluid-filled airways
	    Tubular or Y-shaped structures; branching
	        or rounded opacities in cross section ±
	        air-fluid levels

3. Airway visibility within 1 cm of the costal pleura of fissures	3. Bronchiolitis
	    Clustered ill-defined centrilobular
	        nodules with a tree-in-bud
	        configuration

	4. Mosaic attenuation caused by air trapping
	    Best identified on expiratory HRCT
	        images

	5. Mosaic perfusion of the pulmonary
	    identified on contrast-enhanced dual energy
	    CT of the pulmonary parenchyma

	6. Bronchial artery hyperplasia

Modified from Naidich DP, Webb WR, Grenier PA, et al. Imaging of the airways. Philadelphia: Lippincott Williams & Wilkins; 2005. p. 109.

41% of individuals more than 65 years of age.[18] Although generally accurate, visual inspection may lead to overestimation of airway dilatation as a result of a subtle optical illusion in which the diameters of hollow circles appear larger than those of solid circles despite their identical size, a phenomenon that only occurs when airways are sectioned at right angles.

Normal airways diminish in caliber as they extend toward the lung periphery. In distinction, bronchiectatic airways fail to taper normally, a finding best appreciated toward the outer one-third of the lungs (**Fig. 5**). Although lack of tapering has been reported as the most sensitive sign of subtle cylindrical bronchiectasis,[23] some variation in lumen diameter normally occurs as airways extend toward the lung periphery. In one report evaluating serial changes in airway LA and wall thickness using semiautomated image processing in asymptomatic individuals, although lumen area typically decreased as airways extended toward the perimeter ($r = -0.765$, $P<.001$), in 101 (10.7%) of 943 bronchi, LA increased in size by a minimum of 10%.[24] In contrast, dilated, bronchiectatic airways may mimic the appearance of either cystic or cavitary lung disease, especially when presenting as an isolated finding. When severe, dilated cystic airways often appear clustered, especially in association with diminished lobar or sublobar volumes, potentially mimicking focal honeycombing (**Fig. 6**).

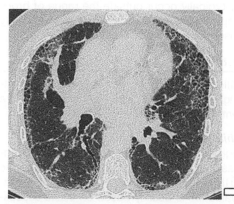

Fig. 4. Traction bronchiectasis. One-millimeter high-resolution image through the lower lobes shows evidence of end-stage lung disease with extensive subpleural reticulation and honeycombing in a patient with idiopathic pulmonary fibrosis. Note the presence of an irregular, dilated airway in the medial aspect of the superior segment of the right lower lobe (*arrow*) typical of traction bronchiectasis. The extent and severity of traction bronchiectasis is an important prognostic sign in patients with idiopathic interstitial pneumonias.

Mucoid Impaction

Nearly as important as identification of dilated air-filled bronchi for diagnosing bronchiectasis is the

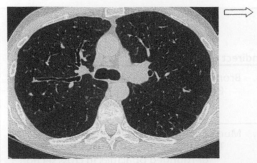

Fig. 5. Focal bronchiectasis. One-millimeter high-resolution image through the carina shows obvious lack of tapering of the right upper lobe posterior segmental bronchus (*arrow*), which indicates cylindrical bronchiectasis.

finding of mucoid impacted airways.[25] The appearance of fluid-filled airways depends on both their size and orientation relative to the CT scan plane. Larger fluid-filled airways result in abnormal lobular or branching structures when they lie in the same plane as the CT scan, or as well-defined nodular opacities when imaged in cross section (**Figs. 7 and 8**). Although the density of mucoid impacted airways may measure in the range of fluid, high-density secretions are more typically identified. In difficult cases, acquiring precontrast and postcontrast-enhanced CT images may be of value by documenting a lack of enhancement. Use of contrast may also be of value in cases in which

there is concern for the presence of a proximal obstructing lesion (see **Fig. 7**, **Fig. 9**). Rarely, retained secretions appear sufficiently dense to mimic calcification, a finding especially characteristic of allergic bronchopulmonary aspergillosis (ABPA) (**Fig. 10**). This possibility has recently led to a new method for classifying ABPA that is intended to improve prediction of outcomes based on CT findings. In a study of 234 patients with documented ABPA, Agarwal and colleagues[26] correlated CT findings, including the presence of high-density mucoid impacted airways, with clinical, spirometric, and serologic findings and showed that, on multivariate analysis, the finding correlating best with immunologic markers, and the strongest predictor of relapses was the presence of higzh-density mucoid impacted airways (odds ratio, 7.38; 95% CI, 3.21–17.0).

Most often, mucus-impacted airways are identified in association with other signs of bronchial inflammation, including evidence of infectious bronchiolitis, identifiable as clusters of poorly defined centrilobular nodules with a tree-in-bud configuration. Less commonly, foci of mucoid impaction may present as isolated abnormalities in the lung periphery. Although raising a suspicion of a proximal slow-growing endobronchial lesion (eg, peripheral carcinoid tumors), these cases usually prove to be isolated foci of chronic airway inflammation. In select cases, further confirmation may require the use of either a follow-up contrast-enhanced CT or a positron emission tomography CT examination for confirmation because these lesions typically occur outside the range of bronchoscopic evaluation and rarely can be definitively diagnosed on transthoracic needle biopsy.

Indirect Signs

In addition to direct signs, several important ancillary signs associated with bronchiectasis are frequently identified.

Bronchial wall thickening

Although frequently present in patients with bronchiectasis, bronchial wall thickening is a nonspecific finding that may be reversible (**Fig. 11**). Routine clinical evaluation is usually based on visual assessment, with quantitative measurements only rarely obtained in routine clinical practice.[27–30] As outlined in a recent comprehensive review article by Williamson and colleagues,[5] few/many/several measurements related to the bronchial wall have been proposed. These measurements include wall thickness, wall T/D ratio, segmental bronchial wall area, and wall area percent (WA%). As discussed later, similarly to quantitative methods for assessing bronchial dilatation, these measurements remain

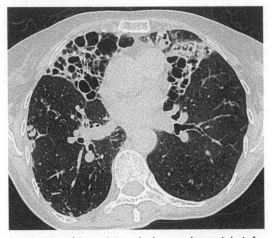

Fig. 6. Bronchiectasis/atypical mycobacterial infection. One-millimeter high-resolution image at the level of the right inferior pulmonary vein shows extensive cystic bronchiectasis throughout the middle lobe and lingula, with a so-called cluster of grapes appearance superficially mimicking extensive honeycombing. This distribution of disease is typical of atypical mycobacterial infection.

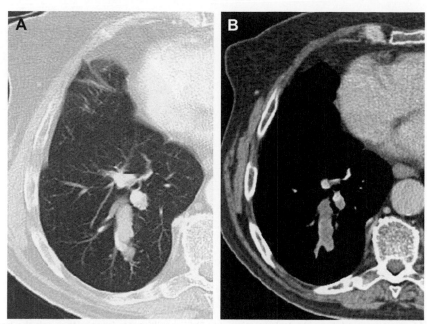

Fig. 7. Focal mucoid impaction. (*A, B*) Identical 5-mm images through the right lower lobe with lung (*A*) and mediastinal (*B*) windows, respectively, show a tubular, branching density extending posteriorly toward the lung periphery, consistent with focal mucoid impaction. Confirmation of the fluid-filled nature of this lesion is easily obtained by administration of intravenous contrast media, which has the additional value in select cases of excluding a proximal obstructing lesion. (*Reprinted from* Webb WR, Muller NL, Naidich DP. High resolution CT of the lung. Philadelphia: Lippincott Williams & Wilkins; 2009. p. 500; with permission, Fig. 16-16.)

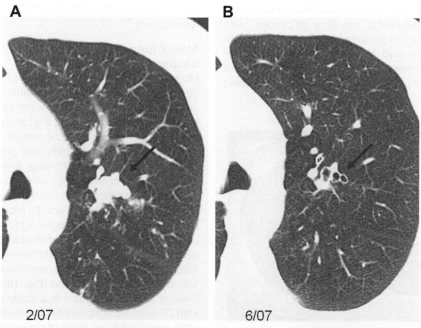

Fig. 8. Focal mucoid impaction. (*A, B*) One-millimeter high-resolution images through the left midlung obtained in the same patient 4 months apart. A focal lobular density is apparent in the midportion of the lung obscuring underlying hilar vessels and airways (*arrow* in *A*). At bronchoscopy, no endobronchial lesions were identified. Several months later, the airways appear normal in caliber; findings consistent with resolving focal mucoid impaction.

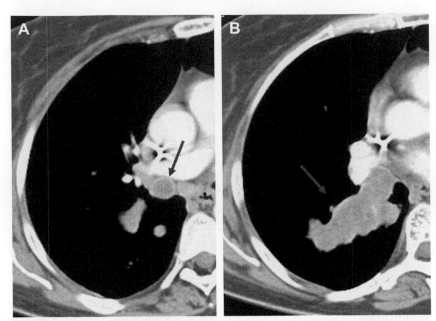

Fig. 9. Mucoid impaction: endobronchial obstruction. (*A, B*) Five-millimeter images through the bronchus intermedius (*arrow* in *A*) and proximal right lower lobe bronchus (*arrow* in *B*), respectively, following administration of intravenous contrast media show that there is obstruction of the bronchus intermedius resulting in extensive mucoid impaction through the superior segment. In this case, bronchoscopy showed an obstructing endobronchial lesion that subsequently proved to be metastatic colon cancer (compare with **Fig. 7**). (*Reprinted from Naidich DP, Webb RW, Müller NL, et al. Computed tomography and magnetic resonance of the thorax. Lippincott Williams & Wilkins; 2007. p. 520; with permission, Fig. 5-69.*)

difficult to use as part of routine clinical practice. Both quantitative and visual evaluation of wall thickness vary depending on slice thickness, with optimal evaluation performed with high-resolution 1-mm sections, and depending on the appropriate choice of window levels and widths, with optimal evaluation obtained with window levels centered

between −250 and −700 Hounsfield units (HU) and window widths between 1000 and 1400 HU, respectively.[31]

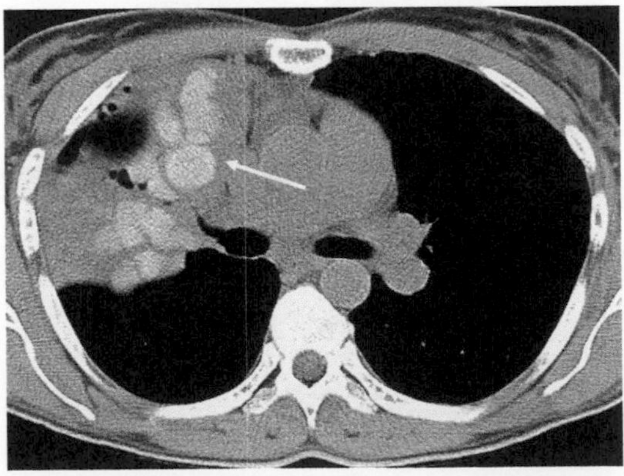

Mosaic lung attenuation/expiratory air trapping

Mosaic attenuation is a term used to denote heterogeneous lung density, often exhibiting a distinctly geographic distribution. This nonspecific finding typically results from one of the following 3 causes: (1) Foci of abnormally increased lung density caused by a variety of infiltrative and/or airspace filling diseases; (2) alternating low-density and high-density foci reflecting variations in lung perfusion, characteristically the result of chronic embolic pulmonary hypertension; and (3) foci of abnormally decreased lung density caused by focal air trapping in patients with underlying obstructive small airway disease (see **Figs. 1** and **3**). Differentiation between these causes is best accomplished on images acquired in deep expiration (**Fig. 12**). As noted by Hansell and colleagues[32] in a study of 70 patients with CT evidence of bronchiectasis, mosaic attenuation was visible on 20% of cases on images obtained in inspiration, whereas air trapping could be identified on 34% of images obtained in expiration. Air trapping could be identified in 17% of lobes in which no CT evidence of bronchiectasis was

Fig. 10. Mucoid impaction/ABPA. Five-millimeter noncontrast image shows extensive consolidation throughout the right upper lobe within which high-density material is noted filling the right upper lobe airways (*arrow*). This appearance is diagnostic of ABPA.

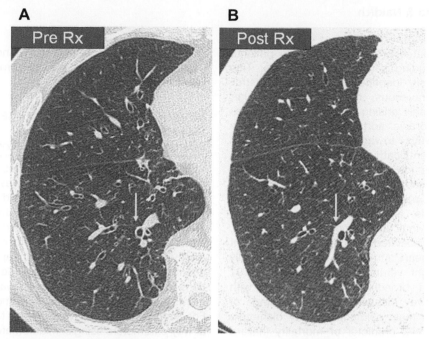

Fig. 11. Bronchial wall thickening. (*A, B*) One-millimeter high-resolution images through the right lower lobe obtained several weeks apart. Initially, there is evidence of diffuse bronchial wall thickening (*arrow* in *A*) associated with mild peripheral airway dilatation. Note that following antibiotic therapy, these reverted to a normal appearance. This case shows that bronchial wall thickening is a nonspecific, potentially reversible finding.

apparent, leaving these investigators to speculate that small airway inflammation may precede the development of inflammatory changes in larger airways.

Vascular abnormalities

In addition to morphologic changes within the airways and lungs, 2 other findings related to bronchiectasis are worth noting. The first is the

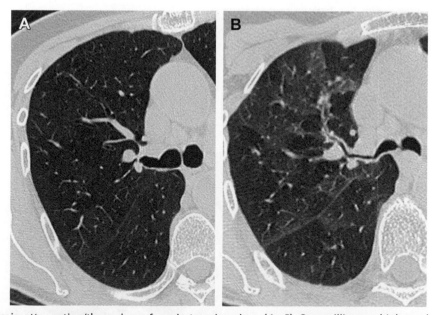

Fig. 12. Mosaic attenuation/the value of expiratory imaging. (*A, B*) One-millimeter high-resolution images through the carina and proximal right upper lobe bronchus (RULB) obtained in inspiration and expiration, respectively, show typical appearance of focal air trapping resulting in well-defined geographic areas of alternating increased and decreased lung density characteristic of obstructive small airway disease. Note that, although the peripheral airways appear normal both in inspiration and expiration, there is also marked narrowing of the carina and RULB consistent with tracheobronchomalacia.

finding of dilated bronchial arteries in patients with longstanding severe bronchiectasis. This finding is easily identified following administration of intravenous contrast as irregular, tortuous vessels arising from the proximal descending thoracic aorta extending along the central airways toward the pulmonary hila (**Fig. 13**). Identification of hypertrophied bronchial arteries may explain hemoptysis that is otherwise unaccounted for in select cases. Also seen in patients with longstanding severe bronchiectasis are dilated main pulmonary arteries that indicate pulmonary hypertension, frequently associated with findings consistent with right heart strain or failure, especially a dilated right ventricle. In one study of 91 patients with bronchiectasis, compared with standard airway measurement, the average of right and left main pulmonary artery diameters proved the best predictor of mortality (hazard ratio, 1.24; 95% CI, 1.13–1.35; P<.0001), independently of the extent or severity of bronchiectasis.[33] In addition, although mosaic attenuation is frequently seen in patients with extensive bronchiectasis, the result of associated obstructive small airway disease, accompanying alterations in lung perfusion may also be identified. As discussed later, dual energy CT scanners now enable direct visualization and potential quantification of abnormal patterns of lung vascularity (**Fig. 14**).

ADVANCED QUANTITATIVE IMAGE TECHNIQUES
Quantitative Evaluation of the Airways

To date, although several CT features for assessing airways have been proposed (as discussed earlier), and despite generally good correlation with routine physiologic measurements, limitations in spatial resolution as well as a lack of agreement regarding the optimal algorithm to measure the airway wall have restricted clinical application of quantitative airway measurements. Serious limitations for the use of quantitative airway measurements have been repeatedly documented.[6,34,35] For example, in one study attempting to quantitate airway parameters using semiautomated methods to evaluate airways dimensions on 2 mm thick sections in 52 individuals without evidence of cardiopulmonary disease, Matsuoka and colleagues[24] showed that WA% varied by more than 5% between 2 contiguous sections in 274 (29%) of 943 bronchi, whereas wall thickness/airway diameter ratio changed by more than 0.02 in 338 (35.8%) of these same airways.

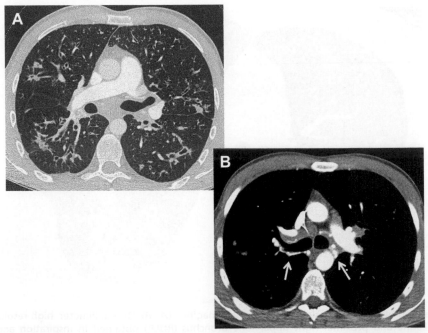

Fig. 13. Bronchiectasis/bronchial arterial hypertrophy. (*A*) One-millimeter high-resolution image through the midlung showing diffuse large and small airway inflammation in a patient with cystic fibrosis. (*B*) Contrast-enhanced 5-mm section through the carina in the same patient showing marked distension of the proximal bronchial arteries (*arrows* in *B*).

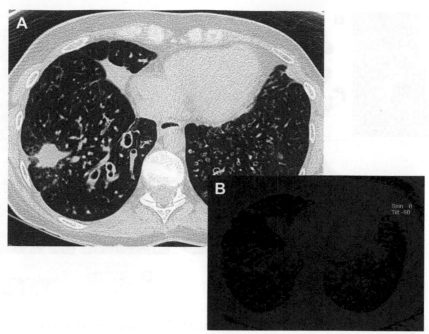

Fig. 14. Bronchiectasis/dual energy CT (DECT) imaging. (*A*) Routine 1-mm high-resolution image through the lung bases shows marked asymmetric bronchiectasis and focal mucoid impaction in the right lower lobe. (*B*) Color-coded map of iodine distribution obtained from a contrast-enhanced dual energy CT study showing marked variation in lung perfusion with a darker appearance throughout the right lower lobe caused by decreased iodine distribution relative to the left. This finding is consistent with asymmetric bronchiectasis resulting in reflex vasoconstriction. DECT represents a promising new method for quantitatively mapping vascular alterations in the lung from a variety of causes, including chronic airway inflammation.

To identify airways that are most appropriate for quantitative evaluation, Brillet and colleagues[36] proposed several validation criteria based on initial 3D segmentation of the airways, including restricting analysis to segmental and subsegmental airways only; evaluating only airways with lumen areas greater than 4 mm and greater than 7 mm in length; ensuring that the percentage of the airway length not directly touching an adjacent vessel be greater than 55% for validation of wall area; and a minimum of 10 contiguous cross-sectional images. Applying these criteria to sequential acquisitions in 10 asthmatic patients, complete segmentation of the airways was possible, allowing automated evaluation of both lumen area and wall thickness area in 78% and 98% of bronchi, respectively, with validation criteria met for 81% of segmental airways and 57% of subsegmental airways, respectively.[36] These same investigators subsequently showed that, despite rigorous application of these similar validation criteria, variability between successive multidetector CT examinations limits the reproducibility, and hence clinical applicability, of airway measurements.[35]

Although as a consequence of these limitations visual inspection remains the standard for clinical assessment of airway disorders, the potential for new methods for obtaining clinically useful automated quantitative airway evaluation remains to be evaluated. It was recently shown that it is possible to automatically segment the airway tree, following which color-coded maps of specific airway dimensions can be displayed (**Fig. 15**).

CT Grading: Extent and Severity of Disease

As a logical extension of the morphologic detail provided by CT for evaluating the airways and lung parenchyma, a variety of different CT-based methods for assessing the extent and severity of disease have been proposed. Although of only limited value in distinguishing the various causes of bronchiectasis,[28] assessing disease extent and severity is important, especially in patients for whom sequential CT studies are to be used to evaluate response to therapy and progression of disease.[29,37–41] These various attempts at grading have focused on combining several features to create a global estimate of the extent and severity of disease. They have emphasized a few or all of the following: generations of bronchial divisions (including the number of lobes involved); peribronchial thickening; mucoid impaction (both

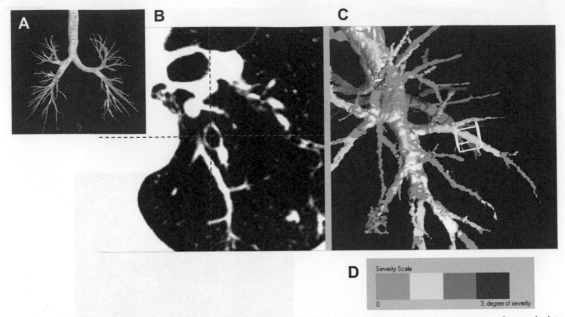

Fig. 15. Automated 3D evaluation of airway dilatation. (*A*) 3D segmentation of the airway tree, color coded to show abnormal regions of airway dilatation defined by an abnormal bronchoarterial ratio. This automated image is derived from a routine CT study using 1-mm collimation to provide contiguous 1-mm high-resolution images throughout the thorax in a single breath hold. Similar automated images showing a feature of the airway wall of dimensions can similarly be derived from routine volumetrically acquired CT images. (*B*) Coned-down view derived from *A* showing to better advantage a detailed view of the left lower lobe airways, color coded to display airways with abnormal bronchoarterial ratios. (*C*) Coned-down view of a branch of the superior segmental airway (identifiable by red crosshairs) specifically selected from the corresponding 3D image identified by the white box in *B*. Use of 3D segmentation allows individual airways to be sectioned at right angles for more precise quantitative evaluation. (*D*) Color guide indicating severity of disease.

large and small airway, the latter identified as resulting in a tree-in-bud pattern), signs of obstructive airway disease including CT evidence of emphysema; and mosaic attenuation (especially as documented on expiratory images).

Allowing for differences in emphasis, these various grading systems have in common the intent of the various approaches to establish a single metric meant as a convenient method for following disease progression.[29,37,42] In this regard, visual CT scoring systems have consistently shown good correlations with more traditional radiographic, clinical, and functional criteria.[43,44] Roberts and colleagues[43] showed that the extent and severity of airway dilatation and wall thickening in patients with bronchiectasis correlated with the severity of airflow obstruction, with focal air trapping on expiratory images showing the best correlation ($r = -0.55, P<.00005$). Visual scoring has also proved reproducible. As reported by Brody and colleagues,[41] in a study in which 3 radiologists scored 16 high-resolution CT scans in children with cystic fibrosis, with each study interpreted twice separated by at least 11 months, overall reproducibility of scoring was 95%, with the highest reproducibility noted for the presence of bronchiectasis and hyperinflation (95% and 88%, respectively).

However, despite these findings, the use of visual CT scoring has not translated to routine clinical practice. The need to evaluate a large number of images and potential variables has proved a tedious and time-consuming task that is impractical, especially without automation. Although methods that score airway abnormalities on a lobar basis are easier to use than those based on segmental scoring, even these have limited practicality and reproducibility.[45] Added to these problems is a reluctance to acquire additional expiratory images because of extra radiation exposure.

Given these limitations, attempts have been made to introduce both semiautomated and, in particular, automated evaluation of the extent and severity of disease in patients with bronchiectasis, albeit with varying success.[46–50] Recently, these ideas were expanded to generate both automated color-coded quantitative 3D airway maps independently depicting bronchial wall thickening, bronchial/arterial ratios, lack of airway tapering, and even foci of mucoid impaction (see **Fig. 15**).[51] Still further exploration of the possibility of an automated global scoring system to evaluate the extent and severity of disease in patients with bronchiectasis has recently been reported. In a preliminary retrospective study, Odry and colleagues[52] compared automated CT scoring using contiguous, high-resolution, 1-mm images in 23 patients with documented bronchiectasis caused by atypical mycobacterial infections of varying severity, with visual scoring by 2 independent experienced radiologists. Using evaluation of bronchial lumen/artery ratios, bronchial wall/artery ratios, as well as foci of mucoid impaction to create a single global score, these investigators found positive correlations between automated and reader's global scores ($r = 0.609$, $P = .01$), extent of bronchiectasis ($r = 0.69$, $P = .0004$), and severity of bronchiectasis ($r = 0.61$, $P = .01$). Although only a weak correlation between computer-generated and reader's scoring of bronchial wall thickening was initially shown ($r = -0.10$, $P = .40$), when wall thickness in 24 lobes showing the greatest disparity of interpretation were reevaluated by readers using electronic calipers through perpendicularly reconstructed bronchi, Spearman rank correlation improved to $r = 0.62$ ($P = .009$), leading to a revised global score of $r = 0.67$ ($P = .001$).[52] Although clearly requiring further validation, it is apparent that true routine, automated, quantitative global scoring of bronchiectasis is feasible and, if established, would represent an important milestone in the use of CT to assess patients with a wide variety of airway diseases.

Dual Energy CT

The recent introduction of commercially available dual energy CT (DECT) scanners promises to further expand the means available for evaluating airway and lung diseases. DECT enables the simultaneous acquisition of volumetric CT data at 2 different energy levels, allowing differentiation of materials by their unique chemical compositions.[53–55] This includes the specific ability to separately map the presence of iodine within tissues, and hence quantitatively measure contrast enhancement without the need to first acquire precontrast images. To date, most attention has focused on the use of DECT to evaluate patients with suspected pulmonary embolic disease.[53–55] In addition to highlighting the pulmonary arterial tree because of increased sensitivity to the presence of iodine within vessels, DECT

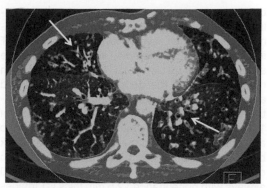

Fig. 16. Bronchial wall enhancement/DECT. Atypical mycobacterial infection. DECT image through the lower lung fields color coded to indicate the presence of iodine by the blue, and absence of iodine by red, following intravenous contrast enhancement. In this patient with documented *Mycobacterium avium-intracellulare* (MAI) infection primarily involving the middle lobe, the walls of these airways are colored blue, indicating enhancement (*arrow* on *right*) distinct from noninflamed, nonenhancing airways (*arrow* on *left*). Preliminary data suggest that DECT allows quantitative measurements of bronchial wall enhancement potentially serving as a CT biomarker of inflammation.

also simultaneously allows visualization of the distribution of iodine throughout the lung parenchyma (see **Fig. 14**). The ability to match alterations in vascular distribution with alterations in lung density caused by air trapping offers an additional way to evaluate the extent and severity of disease in patients with diffuse airway disorders. Although still experimental, it is also feasible to quantitate the extent of contrast enhancement within the bronchial wall (**Fig. 16**). On the assumption that an increase in vascularity results from airway inflammation, it is possible to infer that DECT measurements of bronchial wall enhancement serve as a biomarker for a wide variety of diseases that result in bronchiectasis, among other cases of airway inflammation or infection. This potential remains speculative, pending further clinical validation.

SUMMARY

Despite limitations, HRCT continues to be the gold standard for establishing the anatomic extent and severity of bronchiectasis. In addition, HRCT allows considerable insight into the physiologic consequences of bronchiectasis, as shown in particular by numerous studies correlating anatomic findings with physiologic parameters of airway obstruction. Although this article focuses on bronchiectasis, the use of HRCT to evaluate the airways in virtually all diseases affecting the airways has long been established. Although typically based on visual assessment, this includes several novel approaches to CT interpretation. For example, recent reports have shown that there is good correlation between measurements of the density of airway walls and airway obstruction in patients with chronic obstructive pulmonary disease (COPD).[56,57] In a study of 114 subjects with documented COPD, Yamashiro and colleagues[57] found that measuring mean peak bronchial wall attenuation in third, fourth, and fifth order bronchi originating from the right B1 and B10 airways with nonenhanced 2.5 mm thick CT images correlated significantly with FEV_1 as percentage of predicted value ($P<.0001$), exceeding correlations with measurements of lumen area and bronchial WA%. These findings suggest that measuring peak airway wall density may also prove of value for assessing the severity of bronchiectasis as well as potentially serving as a biomarker for measuring response to therapy. Although the use of mean bronchial wall density remains to be prospectively established for patients with COPD as well as bronchiectasis, along with the recently introduced methods for automated assessment previously mentioned, including color-coded 3D maps and dual energy measurements of airway wall enhancement, such novel approaches are evidence that the full potential of CT for evaluating airways disease has yet to be fully explored.

REFERENCES

1. Javidan-Nejad C, Bhalla S. Bronchiectasis. Thorac Surg Clin 2010;20:85–102.
2. Morechi MA, Fiel SB. An update on bronchiectasis. Curr Opin Pulm Med 1995;1:119–24.
3. Chang AB, Burnes CA, Everard ML. Diagnosing and preventing chronic suppurative lung disease (CSLD) and bronchiectasis. Paediatr Respir Rev 2011;12:97–103.
4. Boiselle PM, Dippolito G, Copeland J, et al. Multiplanar and 3D imaging of the central airways: comparison of image quality and radiation dose of single-detector row CT and multi-detector row CT at differing tube currents in dogs. Radiology 2003;228(1):107–11.
5. Williamson JP, James AL, Phillips MJ, et al. Quantifying tracheobronchial tree dimensions: methods, limitations and emerging techniques. Eur Respir J 2009;34:42–55.
6. Feldman C. Bronchiectasis: new approaches to diagnosis and management. Clin Chest Med 2011;32:535–46.
7. Zaid AA, Elnazir B, Greally P. A decade of non-cystic fibrosis bronchiectasis 1996-2006. Ir Med J 2010;103:77–9.
8. Naidich DP, Webb WR, Grenier PA, et al. Bronchiectasis. In: Imaging of the airways. Philadelphia: Lippincott Williams & Wilkins; 2005. p. 106–46.
9. Aziz ZA, Padley SP, Hansell DM. CT techniques for imaging the lung: recommendations for multislice and single slice computed tomography. Eur J Radiol 2004;52(2):119–36.
10. Bankier AA, Schaefer-Prokop C, De Maertelaer V, et al. Air trapping: comparison of standard-dose and simulated low-dose thin-section CT techniques. Radiology 2007;242(3):898–906.
11. Grenier PA, Beigelman-Aubry C, Fetita C, et al. Multidetector-row CT of the airways. Semin Roentgenol 2003;38(2):146–57.
12. Loeve M, Lequin MH, de Bruijne M, et al. Cystic fibrosis: are volumetric ultra-low-dose expiratory CT scans sufficient for monitoring related lung disease. Radiology 2009;253:223–9.
13. Nishino M, Hatabu H. Volumetric expiratory high-resolution CT of the lung. Eur J Radiol 2004;52(2):180–4.
14. Nishino M, Washko GR, Hatabu H. Volumetric expiratory HRCT of the lung: clinical applications. Radiol Clin North Am 2010;48:177–83.
15. Ozer C, Duce MN, Ulubaş B, et al. Inspiratory and expiratory HRCT findings in Behçet's disease and correlation with pulmonary function tests. Eur J Radiol 2005;56(1):43–7.
16. Boiselle PM, Ernst A. State-of-the-art imaging of the central airways. Respiration 2003;70(4):383–94.
17. Zhang J, Hasegawa I, Feller-Kopman D, et al. Dynamic expiratory volumetric CT imaging of the central airways: comparison of standard-dose and low-dose techniques. Acad Radiol 2003;10:719–24.
18. Matsuoka S, Uchiyama K, Shima H, et al. Bronchoarterial ratio and bronchial wall thickness on high-resolution CT in asymptomatic subjects: correlation with age and smoking. Am J Roentgenol 2003;180(2):513–8.
19. Edey AJ, Devaraj AA, Barker RP, et al. Fibrotic idiopathic interstitial pneumonias: HRCT findings that predict mortality. Eur Radiol 2011;21:1586–93.
20. Lloyd CR, Walsh SLF, Hansell DM. High-resolution CT of complications of idiopathic fibrotic lung disease. Br J Radiol 2011;84:581–92.
21. Fujimototo H, Taniguchu H, Johkoh T, et al. Acute exacerbation of idiopathic pulmonary fibrosis: high-resolution CT scores predict mortality. Eur Radiol 2012;22(1):83–92.
22. Lynch DA, Tschumper B, Cink TM, et al. Frequency of bronchial dilatation at high-resolution CT in asthmatics and control subjects. Radiology 1991;181(P):250.
23. Kang EY, Miller RR, Müller NL. Bronchiectasis: comparison of preoperative thin-section CT and pathologic findings in resected specimens. Radiology 1995;195:649–54.

24. Matsuoka S, Kurihara Y, Nakajima Y, et al. Serial change in airway lumen and wall thickness at thin-section CT in asymptomatic subjects. Radiology 2005;234(2):595–603.

25. Martinez S, Heyneman LE, McAdams HP, et al. Mucoid impactions: finger-in-glove sign and other CT and radiographic features. Radiographics 2008; 28:1369–82.

26. Agarwal R, Khan A, Gupta D, et al. An alternate method of classifying allergic bronchopulmonary aspergillosis based on high-attenuation mucus. PLoS One 2010;5:e15346.

27. Diederich S, Jurriaans E, Flower CD. Interobserver variation in the diagnosis of bronchiectasis on high-resolution computed tomography. Eur Radiol 1996;6(6):801–6.

28. Kim JS, Müller NL, Park CS, et al. Cylindrical bronchiectasis: diagnostic findings on thin-section CT. AJR Am J Roentgenol 1997;168:751–64.

29. Bhalla M, Turcios N, Aponte V, et al. Cystic fibrosis: scoring system with thin-section CT. Radiology 1991;179:783–8.

30. Remy-Jardin M, Amara A, Campistron P, et al. Diagnosis of bronchiectasis with multislice spiral CT: accuracy of 3-mm-thick structured sections. Eur Radiol 2003;13(5):1165–71.

31. Bankier AA, Fleischmann D, Mallek R, et al. Bronchial wall thickness: appropriate window settings for thin-section CT and radiologic-anatomic correlation. Radiology 1996;199(3):831–6.

32. Hansell DM, Wells AU, Rubens MB, et al. Bronchiectasis: functional significance of area of decreased attenuation at expiratory CT. Radiology 1994;193: 369–74.

33. Devaraj A, Wells AU, Meister MG, et al. Pulmonary hypertension in patients with bronchiectasis: prognostic significance of CT signs. AJR Am J Roentgenol 2011;196(6):1300–4.

34. Coxson HO. Quantitative computed tomography assessment of airway wall dimensions. Proc Am Thorac Soc 2008;5:940–5.

35. Brillet PY, Fetita CI, Capderou A, et al. Variability of bronchial measurements obtained by sequential CT using two computer-based methods. Eur Radiol 2009;19:1139–47.

36. Brillet PY, Fetita CI, Beigelman-Aubry C, et al. Quantification of bronchial dimensions at MDCT using dedicated software. Eur Radiol 2007;17(6):1483–9.

37. Ooi GC, Khong PL, Chan-Yeung M, et al. High-resolution CT quantification of bronchiectasis: clinical and functional correlation. Radiology 2002;225(3): 663–72.

38. Altin R, Savranlar A, Kart L, et al. Presence and HRCT quantification of bronchiectasis in coal workers. Eur J Radiol 2004;52(2):157–63.

39. de Jong PA, Nakano Y, Lequin MH, et al. Progressive damage on high resolution computed tomography despite stable lung function in cystic fibrosis. Eur Respir J 2004;23(1):93–7.

40. Edwards EA, Narang I, Li A, et al. HRCT lung abnormalities are not a surrogate for exercise limitation in bronchiectasis. Eur Respir J 2004;24(4):538–44.

41. Brody AS, Kosorok MR, Li Z, et al. Reproducibility of a scoring system for computed tomography scanning in cystic fibrosis. J Thorac Imaging 2006;21: 14–21.

42. Smith IE, Jurriaans E, Diederich S, et al. Chronic sputum production: correlations between clinical features and findings on high resolution computed tomographic scanning of the chest. Thorax 1996; 51(9):914–8.

43. Roberts HR, Wells AU, Milne DG, et al. Airflow obstruction in bronchiectasis: correlation between computed tomography features and pulmonary function tests. Thorax 2000;55:198–204.

44. Shah RM, Sexauer W, Ostrum BJ, et al. High-resolution CT in the acute exacerbation of cystic fibrosis: evaluation of acute findings, reversibility of those findings, and clinical correlation. AJR Am J Roentgenol 1997;169:375–80.

45. de Jong PA, Ottink MD, Robben SG, et al. Pulmonary disease assessment in cystic fibrosis: comparison of CT scoring systems and value of bronchial and arterial dimension measurements. Radiology 2004;2331:434–9.

46. Berger P, Perot V, Desbarats P, et al. Airway wall thickness in cigarette smokers: quantitative thin-section CT assessment. Radiology 2005;235:1055–64.

47. Prasad M, Sowmya A, Wilson P. Automatic detection of bronchial dilatation in HRCT lung images. J Digit Imaging 2008;21(Suppl 1):S148–63.

48. CARS 2004 - Computer Assisted Radiology and Surgery. Proceedings of the 18th International Congress and Exhibition International Congress Series 2004;1268:967–72.

49. Venkatraman R, Raman R, Raman B, et al. Fully automated system for three dimensional bronchial morphology using volumetric multidetector computed tomography of the chest. J Digit Imaging 2006;19: 132–9.

50. Odry BL, Kiraly AP, Godoy MC, et al. Automated airway evaluation system for multi-slice computed tomography using airway lumen diameter, airway wall thickness and bronchoarterial ratio. Conference Proceedings SPIE Medical Imaging 2006;6143:243–53.

51. Kiraly AP, Odry BL, Godoy MC, et al. Computer-aided diagnosis of the airways: beyond nodule detection. J Thorac Imaging 2008;23:105–13.

52. Odry BL, Kiraly AP, Godoy MC, et al. Automated CT scoring of airway diseases: preliminary results. Acad Radiol 2010;17(9):1136–45.

53. Godoy MC, Naidich DP, Marchiori E, et al. Basic principles and post-processing techniques of dual-energy CT: illustrated by selected congenital

abnormalities of the thorax. J Thorac Imaging 2009; 24:271–87.

54. Remy-Jardin M, Faivre JB, Pontana F. Thoracic applications of dual-energy CT. Radiol Clin North Am 2010;48:193–205.

55. Thieme SF, Becker CR, Hacker M, et al. Dual energy CT for the assessment of lung perfusion–correlation to scintigraphy. Eur J Radiol 2008;68:269–374.

56. Washoko GR, Dransfield MT, San Jose Estpat R, et al. Airway wall attenuation: a biomarker of airway disease in subjects with COPD. J Appl Physiol 2009;107:185–91.

57. Yamashiro T, Matsuoka S, Sna Jose Estepar R, et al. Quantitative assessment of bronchial wall attenuation with thin-section CT: an indicator of airflow obstruction in chronic obstructive pulmonary disease. AJR Am J Roentgenol 2010;195:363–9.

Genetic Causes of Bronchiectasis

Christine M. Gould, MD[a,b,*], Alexandra F. Freeman, MD[c],
Kenneth N. Olivier, MD, MPH[d]

KEYWORDS

- Bronchiectasis • Genetic • Impaired mucociliary clearance • Immunodeficiency
- Congenital anomalies of the airway

KEY POINTS

- Our understanding of the pathologic cycle leading to the development of bronchiectasis is enhanced by greater understanding of the genetic influences contributing to its development.
- This article discusses how allelic variations, gene modifiers, HLA associations, and the interplay of developmental, host, and environmental factors all contribute in lesser and greater degrees, depending on the specific disease, toward the development of bronchiectasis in a spectrum of disease processes.
- Genome-wide linkage analysis, family-based genetic linkage studies, and the testing of candidate genes may greatly advance our understanding of the complexity of the genetic basis of bronchiectasis.

Bronchiectasis is the permanent dilatation of bronchi with destruction of the elastic and muscular bronchial wall components primarily as a result of acute or chronic infection.[1] It remains a significant contributor to chronic lung disease in both the developed and developing world.[2] Although the exact prevalence of bronchiectasis worldwide is unknown, early and recurrent lower airway infections remain the primary causes in the developing world, whereas cystic fibrosis (CF) remains the most common cause in developed nations. With advances in sanitation, childhood immunization programs, and the wide availability of antimicrobial therapy, bronchiectasis secondary to recurrent and severe infection alone has declined, with an increasing proportion of patients being recognized as having underlying conditions predisposing to its development.[3] Multiple institutional studies have now examined the causes of non-CF bronchiectasis and highlight the rising importance of immunodeficiency, impairments in mucociliary clearance, and intrinsic airway anomalies as determinants of disease.[4–7] Ethnic variations in the incidence of bronchiectasis have also been reported, suggesting heritable susceptibility to disease.[8]

Understanding the genetic influences on the development of bronchiectasis remains complex because disease progression more likely involves a complicated interaction of multiple contributing factors, each playing a greater or lesser role in an affected individual (**Fig. 1**). However, insight

The authors have nothing to disclose.

[a] Division of Pulmonary & Sleep Medicine, Children's National Medical Center, 111 Michigan Avenue, Northwest, Washington, DC 20010, USA
[b] Department of Pediatrics, Walter Reed National Military Medical Center, 8901 Wisconsin Avenue, Bethesda, MD 20889, USA
[c] Laboratory of Clinical Infectious Diseases, National Institute of Allergy and Infectious Diseases, National Institutes of Health, 9000 Rockville Pike, Building 10, Room 12C116, Bethesda, MD 20892-1888, USA
[d] Laboratory of Clinical Infectious Diseases, National Institute of Allergy and Infectious Diseases, National Institutes of Health, 9000 Rockville Pike, Building 10, Room 11N234, Bethesda, MD 20892-1888, USA
* Corresponding author.
E-mail address: christine.gould@us.army.mil

Clin Chest Med 33 (2012) 249–263
doi:10.1016/j.ccm.2012.03.002
0272-5231/12/$ – see front matter Published by Elsevier Inc.

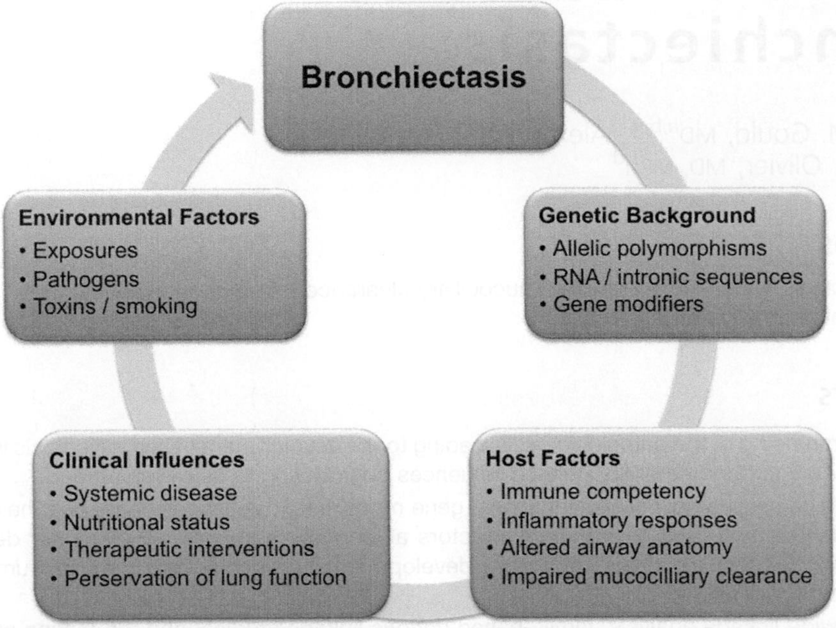

Fig. 1. Influences on the development of bronchiectasis.

into the genetic basis of syndromes associated with bronchiectasis provides insight into the pathogenesis of bronchiectasis, thus enhancing our ability to target effective therapy.[9] The genetic basis of syndromes associated with bronchiectasis is explored here (Table 1, online supplementary material).

ETIOLOGIC FACTORS
Congenital Defects of the Airways

Inherent defects within the airway structure itself or other anatomic defects leading to focal compression of the airway can result in bronchiectasis. Many such lesions are believed to have a familial component, although the specific gene defect(s) have yet to be identified and pathogenesis is more likely multifactorial in origin. Focal examination or radiographic findings in conjunction with a history of recurrent infection affecting a region of the lung should raise the clinical suspicion of bronchial obstruction, ectopy, stenosis, or malacia. Compressive lesions such as a vascular ring or sling or other space-occupying lesions such as bronchogenic cysts, congenital cystic adenomatoid malformations, or bronchopulmonary sequestrations may further alter bronchial anatomy. Regardless of the inciting lesion, bronchiectasis stems from altered mucociliary clearance either from the defect itself or by obstruction from impaired clearance of mucus through the narrowed segment. Inspissated secretions are prone to recurrent infection, with resultant inflammation and airway damage, leading to bronchiectasis.

Case reports of monozygotic twin and other familial occurrence of congenital airway lesions suggest that genetic influences are likely present though a unifying genetic hypothesis is currently lacking.[10–13] Defective regulation of fetal transcription factors, growth factors, and other signaling molecules are likely under complex genetic control and may contribute to the development of congenital airway defects.[14]

Familial Congenital Bronchiectasis (Williams-Campbell Syndrome)

Perhaps the most suggestive of the genetic influences on congenital airway anomalies is the rare syndrome of familial congenital bronchiectasis. This congenital disorder is characterized by diffuse tracheobronchomalacia caused by deficient or complete absence of cartilage within the bronchi. Williams and Campbell first described the disorder in 1960, when they reported on 5 children with symptoms of cough, wheezing, and recurrent pulmonary infections. Autopsy of 1 child showed deficiency of cartilage, with deficient or complete absence of cartilage within the bronchi.[15] Williams and colleagues[16] further described an additional 11 children with similar features of cartilaginous deficiencies leading to segmental and subsegmental bronchi dilatation and collapse. Subsequent case reports have further reported familial occurrence, yet the inheritance and genetic basis of this rare disease have yet to be described.[17,18]

This syndrome presents radiographically with cystic bronchiectasis distal to the third-generation bronchi with emphysematous dilatation distally (**Fig. 2**).[19] The ectatic bronchi show a characteristic ballooning on inspiration and collapse on expiration.[20] Pulmonary function testing may reflect gross hyperinflation, with severe airway obstruction, large residual volumes, poor static elastic recoil, and severely impaired expiratory flow rates.[20]

Tracheobronchomegaly (Mounier-Kuhn Syndrome)

Tracheobronchomegaly, also known as the Mounier-Kuhn syndrome, is a rare congenital anomaly of the trachea and main bronchi caused by atrophy or complete absence of elastic fibers and thinning of muscular components of the airway. First described by Mounier-Kuhn in 1932, this defect results in marked airway flaccidity and subsequent dynamic airway dilation during inspiration and collapse during expiration. The defect is generally described as occurring from the trachea to the fourth bronchial branch, with these hypercompliant airways developing large outpouchings of redundant musculomembranous tissue. The abnormal airway dynamics and pooling of secretions predispose to the development of chronic pulmonary suppuration, bronchiectasis, emphysema, and pulmonary fibrosis. The condition seems more common in men and is typically diagnosed in the third or fourth decades of life. The clinical presentation varies and may be mild to severe in nature. Pulmonary function testing may reveal an obstructive ventilatory defect with large residual volumes,

although normal function has been reported.[21,22] Radiographically, tracheobronchomegaly is defined by a transverse and sagittal diameter for the trachea and main stem bronchi that exceed the upper limits of the means plus 3 standard deviations (**Fig. 3**).[23] Endoscopically, the trachea and bronchi appear distended on inspiration and may completely collapse or occlude on expiration (see Video 1, online supplementary material).[24]

The genetic characterization of this syndrome has yet to be elucidated; however, there does seem to be some familial susceptibility to the disease, with associations with Ehlers-Danlos syndrome (EDS) in adults and cutis laxa in children.[25–27] Along with sporadic occurrences, an autosomal recessive inheritance pattern has also been postulated.[28]

IMPAIRED MUCOCILIARY CLEARANCE

Mucociliary clearance is an important defense mechanism in the respiratory tract, with disease resulting from alterations in any of its primary components of regulation of ion transport by airway epithelium, ciliary function, mucus secretion, and effective cough. Multiple disease states as well as environmental factors may lead to the impairment of mucociliary clearance, resulting in bacterial colonization and infection, with subsequent airway damage and bronchiectasis. Within this category of diseases, there are monogenic and multigenic diseases such as CF and the ciliopathies, which have provided great insight into the pathogenesis of bronchiectasis. In other diseases, the gene-environment interaction shows prominence, such as in Young syndrome, in which genetic susceptibility to a toxic environmental exposure may play a key role.

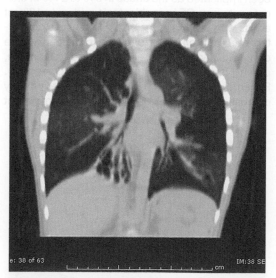

Fig. 2. Four-year-old with Williams-Campbell syndrome. Note distal dilatation of airways and evidence of air trapping.

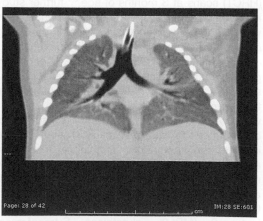

Fig. 3. 9-month-old with tracheobronchomegaly. 3.5-mm inner diameter endotracheal tube in place.

Cystic fibrosis

CF is the most common autosomal recessive disorder in Europe and North America and the most frequent known cause of bronchiectasis in the developed world. Disease incidence is approximately 1 in 3200 live births, with a carrier frequency for non-Hispanic Whites of approximately 1 in 25.[29] CF is a monogenic disease caused by mutations in the CF transmembrane conductance regulator (CFTR) gene that encodes an adenosine triphosphate-binding cassette protein that functions as a chloride ion channel and regulator of salt and water transport across the apical membrane of exocrine epithelial cells. The respiratory tract, exocrine pancreas, intestine, male genital tract, hepatobiliary system, and exocrine sweat glands are all affected to variable degrees, resulting in a complex multisystem disease.

Genetically, CF is classically diagnosed by the demonstration of 2 in trans clinically relevant CFTR gene mutations. More than 1800 mutations and polymorphisms of CFTR have been reported, with F508del being the most common disease-causing mutation.[30] Commercial genetic tests are widely available, and are effective in revealing an ever-increasing number of known disease-causing CFTR mutations. However, 1% to 5% of CF mutations remain unidentified after comprehensive gene analysis in patients with CF,[31] suggesting possible deep-intronic splicing mutations.[32,33]

Although it is well established that CF lung disease may lead to bronchiectasis, there are no specific allelic mutations of the CFTR that are directly linked with the presence or severity of bronchiectasis. However, there are noted associations with CFTR mutations that result in more severe lung disease. Given that up to 80% of children diagnosed with CF through newborn screening have abnormal high-resolution computed tomography (HRCT) scans at 3 months of age,[34] further study into bronchiectasis-associated allelic variations is warranted and may one day determine the timing of HRCT screening and therapeutic intervention.

In addition to CFTR genotype, secondary genetic factors, such as modifier gene expression, are now known to significantly influence the severity of CF lung disease and the development of bronchiectasis. Modifier genes contributing to disease manifestation include inflammatory and antiinflammatory mediators, antioxidants, mediators of airway reactivity, molecules involved in CFTR trafficking, and alternative ion channels.[35] The best-studied CF candidate modifiers include mannose-binding lectin 2 (MBL2), glutathione S-transferase, transforming growth factor β1 (TGF-β1), tumor necrosis factor α, β$_2$-adrenergic receptor, and HLA class II antigens.[36]

The modifier genes MBL2 and TGF-β1 seem to have significant contributory effects on CF lung disease. MBL plays a role in innate immunity with MBL deficiency resulting in a predilection to bacterial and viral infections. MBL-deficient CFTR genotypes are associated with lower lung function measures (FEV$_1$ [forced expiratory volume in the first second of expiration] and FVC [forced vital capacity]) as well as earlier acquisition of Pseudomonas aeruginosa.[37] On the other hand, TGF-β1 plays an important role in the regulation of inflammation and tissue remodeling.[38] In CFTR genotypes, the increased expression of TGF-β1 has been correlated with worse lung function.[39,40] In addition to mucociliary clearance impairment, MBL and TGF-β1 likely contribute to the pathologic cycle of CF bronchiectasis as a result of increased pathogen susceptibility and altered host response.

CF shows a wide phenotypic variability seen in terms of organ involvement, disease severity, and clinical progression even amongst familial cohorts (Figs. 4–6). The large number and class variation of CFTR gene mutations, the existence of modifier genes, environmental factors, such as viral and bacterial pathogens, as well as the timing and aggressiveness of medical intervention may account for this phenotypic variation.[41,42]

Primary Ciliary Dyskinesia

Primary ciliary dyskinesia (PCD) represents a rare and genetically heterogeneous disorder that has been implicated as the cause in 9% to 21% of children with non-CF bronchiectasis and up to 13% of adults with bronchiectasis.[43,44] Disease is characterized by structural or functional defects of motile cilia, resulting in impaired mucociliary clearance, organ lateralization, and sperm dysmotility. Patients may present with neonatal respiratory distress (75% of full-term infants), recurrent

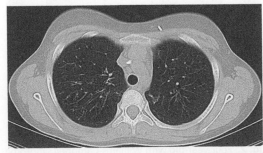

Fig. 4. 12-year-old with CF. Note upper lung zone involvement.

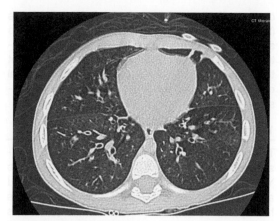

Fig. 5. 2-year-old with CF. Note early ectatic changes with maximal medical therapy.

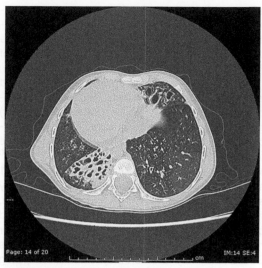

Fig. 7. 6-year-old with PCD and situs inversus totalis. Note mid to lower lung field involvement.

otosinopulmonary infections (may result in hearing loss), situs inversus (~50%) or heterotaxy (~6%), male infertility (~50%), and bronchiectasis in early childhood (**Fig. 7**).[37,42] Pulmonary function tests usually show progressive obstructive or mixed ventilatory defects, with significant deficits reported at an early age.[45,46]

The diagnosis of PCD is classically made by recognition of clinical phenotype and identification of ciliary ultrastructural defects by transmission electron microscopy. However, diagnostic challenges arise in PCD because of the variability of clinical phenotype, limited commercial genetic testing, and a spectrum of ciliary ultrastructural deficits to include normal variants seen in up to 28% of patients.[47] Video microscopy, arguably a more physiologic assay in terms of effective mucociliary clearance, may also be more useful diagnostically in the identification of aberrations in

ciliary beat frequency or waveform despite normal ultrastructure; however, the expertise to accurately interpret these assays is not widely available. In addition, nasal nitric oxide (NO) production has recently been found to be extremely low in PCD (10%–15% of normal), which may serve as a rapid, noninvasive, sensitive screening test for PCD, although its role in the diagnosis of PCD is yet to be fully defined.[48]

The genetic basis of PCD continues to be elucidated. PCD-causing mutations have been identified in 11 genes, encoding various axonemal components and accounting for up to 50% of all cases of PCD.[49] Most of these gene defects affect the structural integrity of the outer dynein arm (ODA) and show an autosomal recessive inheritance pattern, although there are reports of families showing autosomal dominant or X-linked inheritance.[50,51] ODA gene defects include dynein, axonemal, intermediate chain 1 (*DNAI1*) and 2 (*DNAI2*), heavy chain 5 (*DNAH5*) and 11 (*DNAH11*), and thioredoxin domain containing 3 (*TXNDC3*).[52–54] *DNAI1* mutations are reported to account for 14% of disease-causing mutations in patients with known ODA defects, whereas *DNAH5* mutations occur in up to 49%.[55,56] Defects in the *KTU* (chromosome 14 open reading frame 104) and *LRRC50* (located on chromosome 16q24) genes result both in inner dynein arm (IDA) and ODA anomalies.[49,57] Mutations in *RSPH9* and *RSPH4A* (radial spoke head 9 homolog and 4 homolog A) seem to cause central microtubular pair derangements.[58] Most recently, gene deficits in *CCDC39* and *CCDC40* have been associated with microtubule disorganization

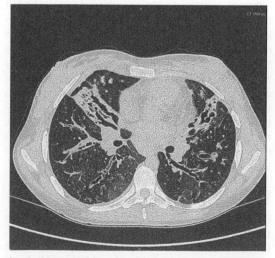

Fig. 6. 20-year-old with advanced CF lung disease.

and the PCD phenotype.[49] Up to 28% of diagnosed patients with PCD have no identified ultrastructural defects.[59] Mutations in *DNAH11* have been associated with the clinical phenotype of PCD and normal ciliary ultrastructure.[47]

The PCD phenotype has also been associated with other clinical syndromes. *RPGR* (retinitis pigmentosa guanosine triphosphatase regulator) gene mutations have been associated with complex dynein arm defects with postulated linkage to X-linked PCD in men with retinitis pigmentosa.[60] Mutations in *OFD1*, the oral-facial-digital type 1 syndrome gene, have been described in a family showing X-linked recessive mental retardation, macrocephaly, and PCD.[61] Further associated ciliopathies, such as autosomal dominant or recessive polycystic kidney disease as well as Bardet-Biedl syndrome, may have overlapping pulmonary signs and symptoms, even bronchiectasis, with PCD.[62,63]

The recognition of the PCD clinical phenotype, specialized ciliary structure and function testing, nasal NO measurement and commercial genetic testing may all be used to secure a diagnosis. In addition, referral to a specialized center and commercial genetic testing, which is now available for 11 PCD-associated mutations, may further aid in early detection of disease and maximized medical benefit in terms of preservation of lung function and the prevention of bronchiectasis.[37,45,64]

Middle Lobe Syndrome

The middle lobe syndrome (MLS) is an uncommon condition that is characterized by damage to the middle lobe, commonly resulting in bronchiectasis and often requiring surgical intervention. It is reported as accounting for ~1% of patients with non-CF pediatric bronchiectasis in a tertiary care center.[65] Although there is no consistent definition or definitive cause of the condition, it is generally believed to be caused by inadequate clearance of secretions as a result of intrinsic lung properties or from secondary obstruction resulting in atelectasis, inflammation, recurrent infection, and bronchiectasis. The pathophysiology of MLS involves suboptimal drainage of secretions because of the narrow diameter and acute take-off angle of the lobar bronchus or extrinsic obstruction by peribronchial lymph node swelling as well as inefficient collateral ventilation because of the relative anatomic isolation of the middle lobe.[66]

Clinically, patients with MLS most commonly present with recurrent infection, chronic productive cough, chest pain, and dyspnea.[67] Increased bronchial hyperreactivity is also seen.[68] Radiographically, atelectasis (21%–50%), consolidation or patchy infiltrates (16%–50%), and bronchiectasis (37%–39%) are common.[69,70] MLS occurs across age groups, with a female predominance.[70,71] Although the genetic basis of this syndrome has yet to be defined, there are multiple reports of familial occurrence[72–76] with at least 1 postulation of an autosomal recessive mode of inheritance.[77]

Young Syndrome

The clinical triad of bronchiectasis, chronic rhinosinusitis, and obstructive azoospermia defines Young syndrome. Inheritance has been reported as autosomal recessive, although the genetics have yet to be fully elucidated.[78] The impairments in mucociliary clearance are postulated to be secondary to abnormal mucous rheology as opposed to inherent ciliary dysfunction, although subtle structural defects have yet to be ruled out.[70,79] It is differentiated from CF by normal sweat gland and pancreatic function as well as azoospermia caused by blockage between the caput and body of the epididymis as opposed to aplasia of the vas deferens as seen in CF.[80] Sweat chloride testing, *CFTR* genetic analysis, nasal potential difference, or testicular ultrasonography help distinguish it from CF. Respiratory function is generally only mildly impaired, although bronchiectasis is a defining feature of the syndrome.

Given the clinical similarities of Young syndrome with CF, multiple studies have investigated the possibility of the syndrome as an allelic form of CF. These studies have failed to show a significant occurrence of *CFTR* gene mutations in Young syndrome.[71,81,82] However, *CFTR* mutations may be missed in the absence of thorough genetic analysis, making the unequivocal exclusion of the CF genotype not possible.[83]

The prevalence of Young syndrome is unknown, although is estimated to account for ~3% of adult bronchiectatic populations.[9,84] Disease prevalence does seem to be declining and is rare in men born after 1955.[77] The decline in incidence has been noted since the elimination of mercury from teething powders in the United Kingdom and Australia, leading some to postulate a link to toxic mercury exposure.[85,86] In addition to elimination of a possible toxic environmental influence, the decline in the prevalence of Young syndrome may also be a result of further advances and improvements in the diagnosis of CF and PCD.

DISORDERS OF HUMORAL IMMUNITY

Disorders of the humoral immune response are categorized by defective antibody production and account for approximately 70% of all primary immune deficiencies (PID)[87] and most

PID-associated bronchiectasis. The most common are X-linked agammaglobulinemia (XLA) and common variable immune deficiency (CVID).[4,82,88,89] Chronic or recurrent rhinosinopulmonary disease with encapsulated bacteria such as *Streptococcus pneumoniae* and *Haemophilus influenzae* predominate in humoral deficiencies,[90] with viral pathogens playing a lesser role because of the preservation of T-cell function. Aggressive diagnosis and treatment of pulmonary infections prevent lung damage; however, bronchiectasis often still develops. In addition to standard airway clearance techniques, higher trough IgG levels and prophylactic sputum culture-driven antimicrobial therapy may be warranted.[91]

In addition to the variable polymorphisms accounting for unique forms of immune dysfunction in PID, additional genetic influences in the form of HLA class II associations may further predispose to the development of bronchiectasis in PID by influencing specific pathogen susceptibility, overexuberant inflammatory responses, or reflecting an immune response gene effect in predisposition to autoimmunity.[92,93]

X-linked agammaglobulinemia

XLA is the most profound humoral immunodeficiency and is characterized by the near-to-complete or complete absence of circulating B lymphocytes and serum immunoglobulins. The disorder is caused by an early blockage of B-cell differentiation due to a mutation in the X chromosome gene encoding Bruton thyroxin kinase (*BTK*). A critical signaling transduction pathway for BTK is one initiated by the B-cell antigen receptor (BCR) complex with pre-BCR regulating proliferation, differentiation, and survival early in B-cell ontogeny so that autosomal recessive forms of agammaglobulemia have also been identified as a result of mutations in components of the pre-BCR protein complex (Mb1/Igα, μHC, λ-like) or signaling cascade (BLNK/SLP65).[94] The nature of gene defect may affect severity of clinical phenotype and mortality, as suggested by the observation that adults with XLA have a higher representation of splice-site mutations and a lower proportion of frameshift mutations than children with XLA.[86]

Clinically, patients generally present after the first 6 to 9 months of life because of early protection by maternal antibodies, although as many as 20% of diagnoses are delayed to the third or fourth year of life, likely becuase of the widespread use of antibiotics.[95] Pyogenic sinopulmonary infections begin after the waning of maternal antibody protection. Thymic size and structure are normal as a result of normal T-cell numbers and function, although tonsils, adenoids, and cervical lymph nodes may be small because of the lack of germinal centers in lymphoid tissue.

Common variable immune deficiency

CVID presents at a later age than XLA and is the most common form of primary hypogammaglobulinemia, occurring in approximately 1 in 10 to 25,000 individuals.[96,97] It represents a heterogeneous group of disorders defined by a marked reduction of at least 2 standard deviations below the mean for age of IgG and IgA or IgM associated with a defective antibody response to protein and polysaccharide antigens.[98] Clinically, patients present with recurrent pyogenic sinopulmonary infections in the second or third decades of life; this later presentation could account for the higher incidence of lung disease seen with CVID when compared with XLA.[99] Bronchiectasis and lymphoid interstitial pneumonitis may develop and there is also an increased risk of autoimmune disease and malignancy. The development of bronchiectasis is aided by unregulated inflammation intrinsic to the disease as well as a low number of IgM memory B cells and reduced IgM anti-pneumococcal polysaccharide antibodies seen in a subset of these patients noted to be at higher risk for recurrent encapsulated bacterial infections.[100]

CVID is a genetically and clinically heterogeneous disorder, with approximately 10% to 20% of individuals having an identified heritable cause.[95] The high degree of familial clustering, marked ethnic differences in population prevalence, familial association, and predominant inheritance patterns in multiple-case pedigrees strongly suggest a genetic predisposition. Familial linkage studies have now identified the presence of a susceptibility locus within the HLA region on chromosome 6.[101] Monogenic polymorphisms in *ICOS*, *CD19*, *TACI*, *BAFF-R*, and *MSH5* deficiencies all seem to be associated with CVID variants.[102]

HYPERIMMUNOGLOBULIN E SYNDROME

Autosomal dominant hyperimmunoglobulin E syndrome (HIES; Job syndrome) is a rare primary immunodeficiency characterized by markedly increased serum IgE concentrations, eczema, recurrent skin and lung infections, skeletal anomalies, coarse facial features, and defective eruption of permanent teeth. IgE levels are generally greater than 2 standard deviations above the mean but may be lower in affected infants and may wane in adult years.[103] Autosomal dominant HIES is caused by mutations of the signal transduction and activator of transcription 3 (*STAT3*) gene.[104] STAT3 enables TH17 lymphocyte differentiation and Th17-based cytokine signaling, which allows upregulation of antimicrobial peptides; therefore, defects in this pathway likely account for susceptibility to bacterial and candida infections along epithelial borders. It also has numerous roles in lung processes relevant to epithelial integrity after injury so that defective airway remodeling after infection likely contributes to pneumatocele formation and progression to bronchiectasis (**Fig. 8**), which then allows secondary infection with molds, nontuberculous mycobacteria, and *Pseudomonas aeruginosa*.

OTHER
Inherited Connective Tissue Disorders

The inherited connective tissue disorders comprise mainly monogenic defects that modulate connective tissue biosynthesis and autoimmune disorders with complex genetic causes. They potentially affect every portion of the pulmonary system, including the pleura, alveoli, interstitium, vasculature, lymphatic tissue, and airways. Lung disease, both functionally and radiographically, associated with these disorders may precede the clinical presentation of the collagen disease by several years.[105,106] In children, recognition of the inherited connective tissue disorders of Marfan syndrome (MFS) and Ehlers-Danlos syndrome (EDS) may prevent significant disease morbidity and mortality. Although the more common pulmonary manifestations of these disorders include interstitial lung disease and pulmonary hypertension; defects in airway integrity, circulating immune complexes, and other immunoregulatory deficiencies may all contribute to the ultimate development of bronchiectasis.

MFS is an autosomal dominant systemic disorder of connective tissue integrity caused by mutations in the fibrillin-1 gene (*FBN1*), resulting in defective fibrillin production, a major component

of extracellular microfibrils. There is a high degree of clinical variability in this disease, with cardinal features involving the ocular, skeletal, and cardiovascular systems. Pulmonary anomalies occur in 10% of affected individuals, with restrictive thoracic cage anomalies, bronchogenic cysts, bullae, blebs, spontaneous pneumothoraces, and emphysema being seen (**Fig. 9**).[107] The lung disease in MFS has been attributed to the loss of connective tissue integrity as a result of abnormal fibrillin; however, animal models have shown abnormal septation of distal alveoli, suggesting a role for developmental deficits.[108] These anatomic anomalies were corrected by blocking TGF-β, a powerful cytokine that modulates cell survival and phenotype signaling, revealing that the pathogenesis of lung disease in MFS is likely based on excessive TGF-β signaling.[109]

Diagnosis of MFS remains clinical and is based on family history and characteristic findings across organ systems. Genetic testing is also available, with ~70% to 93% of individuals with the classic phenotype of MFS showing sequence variants of *FBN1*.[98,110] Multiple *FBN1* mutations have been identified and associated with a wide variability in clinical phenotypes.[111] Further, mutations in a second fibrillin gene (*FBN2*), associated with congenital contractural arachnodactyly (Beal syndrome), have much phenotypic overlap with MFS.[112] Heterozygous mutations in the genes encoding TGF-β receptors I (*TGFBR1*) and II (*TGFBR2*) have also been linked to Marfan-associated disorders, such as Loeys-Dietz aortic aneurysm syndrome, MFS type 2, and familial thoracic aortic aneurysms and dissections.[113–116] The phenotypic overlap of these syndromes may be explained in part by the role of fibrillin-1 in regulating the bioavailability of TGFBR1.[117]

EDS is a heterogeneous tissue disorder characterized by articular hypermobility, skin extensibility, and abnormal wound healing. Diagnosis of EDS is by family history and classic

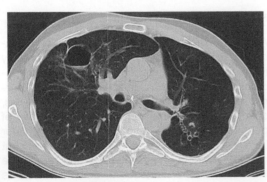

Fig. 8. 34-year-old with HIES.

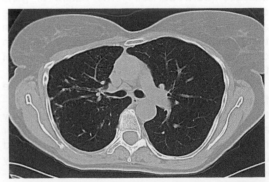

Fig. 9. 63-year-old with *FBN2* mutation (congenital contractural arachnodactyly).

phenotypic characteristics and confirmed by genetic testing. Pulmonary manifestations in EDS are most commonly seen in the vascular (type IV) and kyphoscoliotic (type VI) forms of EDS and generally believed to be caused by tissue fragility and altered respiratory mechanics. Hemoptysis and tracheobronchomegaly may be seen as well as bullae and pneumothoraces with or without generalized emphysema. Early diagnosis may be secured by family history and early manifestations of the diseases with neonatal hypotonia, joint laxity and thoracic scoliosis suggestive of the kyphoscoliotic form[118] of the disease and congenital hip dislocation, talipes equinovarus (club foot), easy bruising, and pneumothorax or pneumohemothorax suggestive of vascular EDS.[119] Bronchiectasis may be caused by impaired mucociliary clearance or anatomic derangements, as well as altered immune, inflammatory, or reparative responses.

Genetically, autosomal dominant inheritance of mutations in the *COL3A1* gene, encoding the α1-chain of type V collagen, result in the vascular form of EDS.[120] Alternatively, autosomal recessive inheritance of mutations in the *PLOD1* gene, encoding the enzyme procollagen-lysine, 2-oxo-glutarate 5 dioxygenase-1, which aids in the cross-linking of collagen, determine a kyphoscoliotic form of the syndrome.[121] Penetrance of both forms nears 100%, although the age of presentation may vary and incidence is unknown.

α_1-Antitrypsin Deficiency

α_1-Antitrypsin (AAT) deficiency is a genetic disorder that affects 1 in 2000 to 5000 individuals.[122] It is characterized by the development of chronic obstructive pulmonary disease (COPD) and liver disease. Inheritance is via an autosomal recessive pattern caused by mutations in the *SERPINA1* gene, leading to deficient or dysfunctional AAT. AAT is a codominantly expressed serpin (serine protease inhibitor) and is a major inhibitor of neutrophil elastase in the tissues and serum (protease-antiprotease hypothesis). The most common *SERPINA1* allele is the M type, with the MM genotype producing normal AAT level and function. S and Z alleles produce low to deficient levels of the gene product, respectively, so individuals with the ZZ allele types (PiZZ) are most severely AAT deficient. Diagnosis relies on the finding of low levels of AAT in serum or plasma and evidence of a deficient variant of the AAT protein by protease inhibitor typing or detection of homogeneous mutations of the *SERPINA1* gene. It is generally accepted that for an AAT allele to result in clinical disease, serum levels must by less than 35% of normal values.[123]

Pulmonary manifestations of AAT deficiency are heterogeneous, although they generally present as severe, early-onset panacinar emphysema, with a basilar predominance in the fourth or fifth decade of life.[124] It accounts for approximately 1% of COPD and patients are generally homozygous for non-M (null, S, or Z) variants.[125,126] Bronchiectasis, with or without concomitant emphysema, is seen in up to 40% of patients.[107,127,128]

The pathophysiology of the AAT deficiency lung disease seen has been attributed to the loss of protein function, allowing for unopposed neutrophil elastase activity. In addition, AAT itself has antiinflammatory effects and may inhibit immune responses to stimulate tissue repair and matrix production and have antibacterial properties.[126] In the AAT-deficient individual, cumulative pulmonary insults in the form of repeated lower airway infection or toxic environmental exposures, most notably smoking, result in progressive alveolar and airway damage. In support of this theory, intravenous AAT augmentation therapy seems to have clinical efficacy, with studies suggesting slower FEV1 declines, fewer lung infections, enhanced survival, reduced lung inflammation, and slower loss of lung density.[109,129] In addition to the loss of function effect, more recent evidence suggests that the misfolded AAT protein may further acquire a toxic gain of function, promoting exaggerated endoplasmic reticulum stress responses and inflammation within the lung.[130,131]

Several studies have also suggested a distinct phenotype of AAT deficiency in which severe bronchiectasis coexists with mild emphysema,[132–134] whereas others have suggested that bronchiectasis is a consequence of emphysema rather than as a primary effect of AAT deficiency.[132] Another hypothesis stemmed from the observation that the *11478G→A* polymorphism is associated with accelerated atherosclerosis.[135] In that atherosclerosis is associated with stiffening of arteries through degradation of elastin fibers in the arterial wall, this hypothesis might be analogous to the degradation of elastin in airways, resulting in emphysema and progressive airflow obstruction; however, population studies failed to show significant differences in the rate of lung function decline in patients with COPD with and without the AAT *SERPINA1 11478G→A* variant.[136]

Modifying genetic factors likely play an important role in the significant phenotypic variation of lung disease of individuals with AAT deficiency. Clinical differences in families with AAT deficiency cannot be solely explained by smoking or ascertainment bias and may be caused by variations within genes involved in inflammatory pathways.[137] AAT deficiency candidate gene studies have revealed significant associations with polymorphisms of the inflammatory cytokine tumor necrosis factor α with chronic bronchitis[137] and the antiinflammatory cytokine interleukin 10 with airflow obstruction.[138]

As in CF, the genetic basis of AAT deficiency is highly complex despite its monogenic origin. The wide variability in the development and severity of COPD and bronchiectasis in the most severely AAT-deficient individuals alludes to this complexity, in which a significant role of specific genotype-phenotype interactions, modifier gene influences, environmental exposures, and gene-environment interactions acting in concert determine disease manifestation.

Yellow Nail Syndrome

Yellow nail syndrome (YNS) is a rare condition clinically defined by the triad of yellow atrophic nails, lymphedema, and chronic pulmonary disease. Respiratory manifestations include pleural effusions, chronic sinusitis, recurrent pneumonias, and bronchiectasis (up to 44% of patients in 1 series).[139] The pathophysiology of the syndrome is uncertain although dysfunctional lymphatic drainage has been postulated,[124,126] with others suggesting a microvasculopathy with protein leak as the basis of disease.[140,141] The bronchiectasis of YNS is difficult to explain; ciliary dysmotility,[142] immunodeficiency,[139,143] and dysfunctional bronchial lymphatic drainage[139,144] have all been investigated without significant substantiation. Although familial reports suggest a genetic basis of disease as a dominantly inherited condition with variable expression, sporadic occurrence seems to dominate the literature.[139,145]

SUMMARY

Our understanding of the pathologic cycle leading to the development of bronchiectasis is enhanced by greater understanding of the influences contributing to its development. Genome-wide linkage analysis, family-based genetic linkage studies, and the testing of candidate genes have the ability to greatly advance our understanding of the complexity of the genetic basis of bronchiectasis. This article discusses how allelic variations, gene modifiers, HLA associations, and the interplay of developmental, host, and environmental factors all contribute in lesser and greater degrees, depending on the specific disease, toward the development of bronchiectasis in a spectrum of disease processes.

ACKNOWLEDGMENTS

We would like to acknowledge Dr Nabile M. Safdar of the Department of Diagnostic Imaging at Children's National Medical Center, Washington DC, for providing radiographic images and Ms Susan Keller, MLS, and Deborah Gilbert, MLS, of the Medical Library at Children's National Medical Center, Washington DC, for assistance with obtaining references.

SUPPLEMENTARY DATA

Supplementary data related to this article can be found online at doi:10.1016/j.ccm.2012.03.002.

REFERENCES

1. Barker A. Bronchiectasis. N Engl J Med 2002;346: 1383–93.
2. Callahan CW, Redding GJ. Bronchiectasis in children: orphan disease or persistent problem? Pediatr Pulmonol 2002;33:492–6.
3. Lewitson N. Bronchiectasis. In: Hilman B, editor. Pediatric respiratory disease. Philadelphia: WB Saunders; 1993. p. 222–9.
4. Eastham KM, Fall AJ, Mitchell L, et al. The need to redefine non-cystic fibrosis bronchiectasis in childhood. Thorax 2004;59:324–7.
5. Edwards EA, Asher MI, Byrnes CA. Paediatric bronchiectasis in the twenty-first century: experience of a tertiary children's hospital in New Zealand. J Paediatr Child Health 2003;39:111–7.
6. Kim HY, Kwon JW, Seo J, et al. Bronchiectasis in children: 10-year experience at a single institution. Allergy Asthma Immunol Res 2011;3(1):39–45.
7. Li AM, Sonnappa S, Lex C, et al. Non-CF bronchiectasis: does knowing the aetiology lead to changes in management? Eur Respir J 2005;26:8–14.
8. Twiss J, Metcalfe R, Edwards E, et al. New Zealand national incidence of bronchiectasis "too high" for a developed country. Arch Dis Child 2005;90: 737–40.
9. Pasteur M, Helliwell S, Houghton J, et al. An investigation into causative factors in patients with bronchiectasis. Am J Respir Crit Care Med 2000;162: 1277–84.
10. Brodlie M, Spencer DA. Bronchomalacia occurring in monozygotic twins–further information about its inheritance. Acta Paediatr 2009;98(9):1531–3.
11. Wong KS, Lien R, Lin TY. Congenital tracheobronchial stenosis in monozygotic twins. Eur J Pediatr 1998;157(12):1023–5.
12. Abuhamad AZ, Bass T, Katz ME, et al. Familial recurrence of pulmonary sequestration. Obstet Gynecol 1996;87(5):843–5.
13. Novak RM. Laryngotracheoesophageal cleft and unilateral pulmonary hypoplasia in twins. Pediatrics 1981;67(5):732–4.
14. Roth-Kleiner M, Post M. Genetic control of lung development. Biol Neonate 2003;84(1):83–8.

15. Williams H, Cambell P. Generalized bronchiectasis associated with deficiency of cartilage in the bronchial tree. Arch Dis Child 1960;35:182–91.

16. Williams HE, Landau LI, Phelan PD. Generalized bronchiectasis due to extensive deficiency of bronchial cartilage. Arch Dis Child 1972;47(253):423–8.

17. Wayne KS, Taussig LM. Probable familial congenital bronchiectasis due to cartilage deficiency (Williams-Campbell syndrome). Am Rev Respir Dis 1976;114(1):15–22.

18. Jones VF, Eid NS, Franco SM, et al. Familial congenital bronchiectasis: Williams-Campbell syndrome. Pediatr Pulmonol 1993;16(4):263–7.

19. Hartman TE, Primack SL, Lee KS, et al. CT of bronchial and bronchiolar diseases. Radiographics 1994;14(5):991–1003.

20. George J, Jain R, Tariq SM. CT bronchoscopy in the diagnosis of Williams-Campbell syndrome. Respirology 2006;11(1):117–9.

21. Blake MA, Clarke PD, Fenlon HM. Thoracic case of the day. Mounier-Kuhn syndrome (tracheobronchomegaly). J Thorac Imaging 1991;6(2):1–10.

22. Ghanei M, Peyman M, Aslani J, et al. Mounier-Kuhn syndrome: a rare cause of severe bronchial dilatation with normal pulmonary function test: a case report. Respir Med 2007;101(8):1836–9.

23. Shin MS, Jackson RM, Ho KJ. Tracheobronchomegaly (Mounier-Kuhn syndrome): CT diagnosis. AJR Am J Roentgenol 1988;150:777–9.

24. Schwartz M, Rossoff L. Tracheobronchomegaly. Chest 1994;106:1589–90.

25. Johnston RF, Green RA. Tracheobronchiomegaly. Report of five cases and demonstration of familial occurrence. Am Rev Respir Dis 1965;91:35–50.

26. Aaby GV, Blake HA. Tracheobronchiomegaly. Ann Thorac Surg 1966;2(1):64–70.

27. Woodring JH, Howard RS 2nd, Rehm SR. Congenital tracheobronchomegaly (Mounier-Kuhn syndrome): a report of 10 cases and review of the literature. J Thorac Imaging 1991;6(2):1–10.

28. Celik B, Bilgin S, Yuksel C. Mounier-Kuhn syndrome: a rare cause of bronchial dilation. Tex Heart Inst J 2011;38(2):194–6.

29. Rosenstein BJ, Cutting GR. The diagnosis of cystic fibrosis: a consensus statement. Cystic Fibrosis Foundation Consensus Panel. J Pediatr 1998; 132(4):589–95.

30. The cystic fibrosis mutation database. Available at: http://www.genet.sickkids.on.ca/cftr/. Accessed November 2011.

31. Castellani C, Cuppens H, Macek M Jr, et al. Consensus on the use and interpretation of cystic fibrosis mutation analysis in clinical practice. J Cyst Fibros 2008;7(3):179–96.

32. Dequeker E, Stuhrmann M, Morris MA, et al. Best practice guidelines for molecular genetic diagnosis of cystic fibrosis and CFTR-related disorders–updated European recommendations. Eur J Hum Genet 2009;17(1):51–65.

33. Costa C, Pruliere-Escabasse V, de Becdelievre A, et al. A recurrent deep-intronic splicing CF mutation emphasizes the importance of mRNA studies in clinical practice. J Cyst Fibros 2011;10(6):479–82.

34. Sly PD, Brennan S, Gangell C, et al, Australian Respiratory Early Surveillance Team for Cystic Fibrosis (AREST-CF). Lung disease at diagnosis in infants with cystic fibrosis detected by newborn screening. Am J Respir Crit Care Med 2009; 180(2):146–52.

35. Cutting GR. Modifier genes in Mendelian disorders: the example of cystic fibrosis. Ann N Y Acad Sci 2010;1214:57–69.

36. Merlo CA, Boyle MP. Modifier genes in cystic fibrosis lung disease. J Lab Clin Med 2003; 141(4):237–41.

37. Noone PG, Leigh MW, Sannuti A, et al. Primary ciliary dyskinesia: diagnostic and phenotypic features. Am J Respir Crit Care Med 2004;169(4):459–67.

38. Akhurst RJ. TGF beta signaling in health and disease. Nat Genet 2004;36(8):790–2.

39. Drumm ML, Konstan MW, Schluchter MD, et al. Gene Modifier Study Group. Genetic modifiers of lung disease in cystic fibrosis. N Engl J Med 2005;353(14):1443–53.

40. Bremer LA, Blackman SM, Vanscoy LL, et al. Interaction between a novel TGFB1 haplotype and CFTR genotype is associated with improved lung function in cystic fibrosis. Hum Mol Genet 2008; 17(14):2228–37.

41. Wolfenden LL, Schechter MS. Genetic and non-genetic determinants of outcomes in cystic fibrosis. Paediatr Respir Rev 2009;10(1):32–6.

42. Zariwala MA, Knowles MR, Leigh MW. Primary ciliary dyskinesia [Internet]. In: Pagon RA, Bird TD, Dolan CR, et al, editors. GeneReviews. Seattle (WA): University of Washington; 1993. January 24, 2007 [updated October 6, 2009].

43. Kapur N, Karadag B. Differences and similarities in non-cystic fibrosis bronchiectasis between developing and affluent countries. Paediatr Respir Rev 2011;12(2):91–6.

44. Verra F, Escudier E, Bignon J, et al. Inherited factors in diffuse bronchiectasis in the adult: a prospective study. Eur Respir J 1991;4(8):937–44.

45. Ellerman A, Bisgaard H. Longitudinal study of lung function in a cohort of primary ciliary dyskinesia. Eur Respir J 1997;10(10):2376–9.

46. Marthin JK, Petersen N, Skovgaard LT, et al. Lung function in patients with primary ciliary dyskinesia: a cross-sectional and 3-decade longitudinal study. Am J Respir Crit Care Med 2010;181(11):1262–8.

47. Zariwala MA, Omran H, Ferkol TW. The emerging genetics of primary ciliary dyskinesia. Proc Am Thorac Soc 2011;8:430–3.

48. Leigh MW, O'Callaghan C, Knowles MR. The challenges of diagnosing primary ciliary dyskinesia. Proc Am Thorac Soc 2011;8:434–7.

49. Loges NT, Olbrich H, Becker-Heck A, et al. Deletions and point mutations of LRRC50 cause primary ciliary dyskinesia due to dynein arm defects. Am J Hum Genet 2009;85(6):883–9.

50. Narayan D, Krishnan SN, Upender M, et al. Unusual inheritance of primary ciliary dyskinesia (Kartagener's syndrome). J Med Genet 1994;31(6):493–6.

51. Krawczyński MR, Witt M. Pcd and RP: X-linked inheritance of both disorders? Pediatr Pulmonol 2004;38(1):88–9.

52. Bartoloni L, Blouin JL, Pan Y, et al. Mutations in the DNAH11 (axonemal heavy chain dynein type 11) gene cause one form of situs inversus totalis and most likely primary ciliary dyskinesia. Proc Natl Acad Sci U S A 2002;99(16):10282–6.

53. Duriez B, Duquesnoy P, Escudier E, et al. A common variant in combination with a nonsense mutation in a member of the thioredoxin family causes primary ciliary dyskinesia. Proc Natl Acad Sci U S A 2007;104(9):3336–41.

54. Loges NT, Olbrich H, Fenske L, et al. DNAI2 mutations cause primary ciliary dyskinesia with defects in the outer dynein arm. Am J Hum Genet 2008; 83(5):547–58.

55. Zariwala MA, Leigh MW, Ceppa F, et al. Mutations of DNAI1 in primary ciliary dyskinesia: evidence of founder effect in a common mutation. Am J Respir Crit Care Med 2006;174(8):858–66.

56. Hornef N, Olbrich H, Horvath J, et al. DNAH5 mutations are a common cause of primary ciliary dyskinesia with outer dynein arm defects. Am J Respir Crit Care Med 2006;174(2):120–6.

57. Omran H, Kobayashi D, Olbrich H, et al. Ktu/PF13 is required for cytoplasmic pre-assembly of axonemal dyneins. Nature 2008;456(7222):611–6.

58. Castleman VH, Romio L, Chodhari R, et al. Mutations in radial spoke head protein genes RSPH9 and RSPH4A cause primary ciliary dyskinesia with central-microtubular-pair abnormalities. Am J Hum Genet 2009;84(2):197–209.

59. Jorissen M, Willems T, Van der Schueren B, et al. Ultrastructural expression of primary ciliary dyskinesia after ciliogenesis in culture. Acta Otorhinolaryngol Belg 2000;54:883–9.

60. Moore A, Escudier E, Roger G, et al. RPGR is mutated in patients with a complex X linked phenotype combining primary ciliary dyskinesia and retinitis pigmentosa. J Med Genet 2006; 43(4):326–33.

61. Budny B, Chen W, Omran H, et al. A novel X-linked recessive mental retardation syndrome comprising macrocephaly and ciliary dysfunction is allelic to oral-facial-digital type I syndrome. Hum Genet 2006;120(2):171–8.

62. Leigh MW. Primary ciliary dyskinesia. In: Chernick V, Boat TF, Wilmott RW, et al, editors. Disorders of the respiratory tract of children. Philadelphia: Saunders-Elsevier; 2006. p. 902–9.

63. Davis SD, Knowles M, Leigh M. Introduction: primary ciliary dyskinesia and overlapping syndromes. Proc Am Thorac Soc 2011;8:421–2.

64. Coren ME, Meeks M, Morrison I, et al. Primary ciliary dyskinesia: age at diagnosis and symptom history. Acta Paediatr 2002;91(6):667–9.

65. Banjar HH. A review of 151 cases of pediatric non-cystic fibrosis bronchiectasis in a tertiary care center. Ann Thorac Med 2007;2(1):3–8.

66. Inners CR, Terry PB, Traystman RJ, et al. Collateral ventilation and the middle lobe syndrome. Am Rev Respir Dis 1978;118(2):305–10.

67. Einarsson JT, Einarsson JG, Isaksson H, et al. Middle lobe syndrome: a nationwide study on clinicopathological features and surgical treatment. Clin Respir J 2009;3(2):77–81.

68. Priftis KN, Anthracopoulos MB, Mermiri D, et al. Bronchial hyperresponsiveness, atopy, and bronchoalveolar lavage eosinophils in persistent middle lobe syndrome. Pediatr Pulmonol 2006;41(9): 805–11.

69. Kwon KY, Myers JL, Swensen SJ, et al. Middle lobe syndrome: a clinicopathological study of 21 patients. Hum Pathol 1995;26(3):302–7.

70. Le Lannou D, Jezequel P, Blayau M, et al. Obstructive azoospermia with agenesis of vas deferens or with bronchiectasia (Young's syndrome): a genetic approach. Hum Reprod 1995;10(2): 338–41.

71. Friedman KJ, Teichtahl H, De Kretser DM, et al. Screening Young syndrome patients for CFTR mutations. Am J Respir Crit Care Med 1995; 152(4 Pt 1):1353–7.

72. Dees SC, Spock A. Right middle lobe syndrome in children. JAMA 1966;197(1):8–14.

73. Danielson GK, Hanson CW, Cooper EC. Middle lobe bronchiectasis. Report of an unusual familial occurrence. JAMA 1967;201(8):605–8.

74. Hoo JJ. Familial middle lobe bronchiectasis. Clin Genet 1979;15(1):85–8.

75. Livingston GL, Holinger LD, Luck SR. Right middle lobe syndrome in children. Int J Pediatr Otorhinolaryngol 1987;13(1):11–23.

76. Takahashi H, Kimura S, Nagai I, et al. A case of middle lobe syndrome occurring in two sisters. Jpn J Surg 1990;20(5):597–601.

77. Hendry WF, A'Hern RP, Cole PJ. Was Young's syndrome caused by exposure to mercury in childhood? BMJ 1993;307(6919):1579–82.

78. Handelsman DJ, Conway AJ, Boylan LM, et al. Young's syndrome. Obstructive azoospermia and chronic sinopulmonary infections. N Engl J Med 1984;310(1):3–9.

79. de longh R, Ing A, Rutland J. Mucociliary function, ciliary ultrastructure, and ciliary orientation in Young's syndrome. Thorax 1992;47(3):184–7.

80. Pryor JP. Cystic fibrosis and Young's syndrome. Lancet 1998;352(9133):1065 [author reply: 1065–6].

81. Dörk T, Dworniczak B, Aulehla-Scholz C, et al. Distinct spectrum of CFTR gene mutations in congenital absence of vas deferens. Hum Genet 1997;100(3–4):365–77.

82. Barker AF, Craig S, Bardana EJ Jr. Humoral immunity in bronchiectasis. Ann Allergy 1987;59(3):179–82.

83. Goeminne PC, Dupont LJ. The sinusitis-infertility syndrome: Young's saint, old devil. Eur Respir J 2010;35(3):698.

84. Shoemark A, Ozerovitch L, Wilson R. Aetiology in adult patients with bronchiectasis. Respir Med 2007;101(6):1163–70.

85. Arya AK, Beer HL, Benton J, et al. Does Young's syndrome exist? J Laryngol Otol 2009;123(5):477–81.

86. Broides A, Yang W, Conley ME. Genotype/phenotype correlations in X-linked agammaglobulinemia. Clin Immunol 2006;118(2–3):195–200.

87. Buckley RH. Pulmonary complications of primary immunodeficiencies. Paediatr Respir Rev 2004;5(Suppl A):S225–33.

88. Nikolaizik WH, Warner JO. Aetiology of chronic suppurative lung disease. Arch Dis Child 1994;70(2):141–2.

89. Cazzola G, Valletta EA, Ciaffoni S, et al. Neutrophil function and humoral immunity in children with recurrent infections of the lower respiratory tract and chronic bronchial suppuration. Ann Allergy 1989;63(3):213–8.

90. Conley ME, Dobbs AK, Farmer DM, et al. Primary B cell immunodeficiencies: comparisons and contrasts. Annu Rev Immunol 2009;27:199–227.

91. Freeman AF, Holland SM. Antimicrobial prophylaxis for primary immunodeficiencies. Curr Opin Allergy Clin Immunol 2009;9(6):525–30.

92. Boyton RJ, Smith J, Jones M, et al. Human leucocyte antigen class II association in idiopathic bronchiectasis, a disease of chronic lung infection, implicates a role for adaptive immunity. Clin Exp Immunol 2008;152(1):95–101.

93. Boyton RJ. Regulation of immunity in bronchiectasis. Med Mycol 2009;47(Suppl 1):S175–82.

94. Moreau T, Calmels B, Barlogis V, et al. Potential application of gene therapy to X-linked agammaglobulinemia. Curr Gene Ther 2007;7(4):284–94.

95. Scharenberg AM, Hannibal MC, Torgerson T, et al. Common variable immune deficiency overview [Internet]. In: Pagon RA, Bird TD, Dolan CR, et al, editors. GeneReviews. Seattle (WA): University of Washington; 1993. Updated July 5, 2006.

96. Notarangelo LD, Plebani A, Mazzolari E, et al. Genetic causes of bronchiectasis: primary immune deficiencies and the lung. Respiration 2007;74(3):264–75.

97. Dosanjh A. Chronic pediatric pulmonary disease and primary humoral antibody based immune disease. Respir Med 2011;105(4):511–4.

98. Loeys B, De Backer J, Van Acker P, et al. Comprehensive molecular screening of the FBN1 gene favors locus homogeneity of classical Marfan syndrome. Hum Mutat 2004;24(2):140–6.

99. Aghamohammadi A, Allahverdi A, Abolhassan H, et al. Comparison of pulmonary diseases in common variable immunodeficiency and X-linked agammaglobulinaemia. Respirology 2010;15(2):289–95.

100. Carsetti R, Rosado MM, Donnanno S, et al. The loss of IgM memory B cells correlates with clinical disease in common variable immunodeficiency. J Allergy Clin Immunol 2005;115(2):412–7.

101. Kralovicova J, Hammarström L, Plebani A, et al. Fine-scale mapping at IGAD1 and genome-wide genetic linkage analysis implicate HLA-DQ/DR as a major susceptibility locus in selective IgA deficiency and common variable immunodeficiency. J Immunol 2003;170(5):2765–75.

102. Deane S, Selmi C, Naguwa SM, et al. Common variable immunodeficiency: etiological and treatment issues. Int Arch Allergy Immunol 2009;150(4):311–24.

103. Freeman AF, Holland SM. The hyper-IgE syndromes. Immunol Allergy Clin North Am 2008;28(2):277–91, viii.

104. Holland SM, DeLeo FR, Elloumi HZ, et al. STAT3 mutations in the hyper-IgE syndrome. N Engl J Med 2007;357:1608–19.

105. Dinwiddle R, Sonnappa S. Systemic diseases of the lung. Paediatr Respir Rev 2005;6(3):181–9.

106. Lynch DA. Lung disease related to collagen vascular disease. J Thorac Imaging 2009;24(4):299–309.

107. Shin MS, Ho KJ. Bronchiectasis in patients with alpha 1-antitrypsin deficiency. A rare occurrence? Chest 1993;104(5):1384–6.

108. Neptune ER, Frischmeyer PA, Arking DE, et al. Dysregulation of TGF-beta activation contributes to pathogenesis in Marfan syndrome. Nat Genet 2003;33(3):407–11.

109. Stoller JK, Aboussouan LS. alpha1-Antitrypsin deficiency. 5: intravenous augmentation therapy: current understanding. Thorax 2004;59(8):708–12.

110. Dietz HC. Marfan syndrome [Internet]. In: Pagon RA, Bird TD, Dolan CR, et al, editors. GeneReviews. Seattle (WA): University of Washington, Seattle; 1993. April 18, 2001 [updated June 30, 2009].

111. Furtado LV, Wooderchak-Donahue W, Rope AF, et al. Characterization of large genomic deletions in the FBN1 gene using multiplex ligation-dependent probe amplification. BMC Med Genet 2011;12(1):119.

112. Callewaert BL, Loeys BL, Ficcadenti A, et al. Comprehensive clinical and molecular assessment

of 32 probands with congenital contractural arachnodactyly: report of 14 novel mutations and review of literature. Hum Mutat 2009;30(3):334–41.

113. Mizuguchi T, Collod-Beroud G, Akiyama T, et al. Heterozygous TGFBR2 mutations in Marfan's syndrome. Nat Genet 2004;36(8):855–60.

114. Loeys BL, Chen J, Neptune ER, et al. A syndrome of altered cardiovascular, craniofacial, neurocognitive and skeletal development caused by mutations in TGFBR1 and TGFBR2. Nat Genet 2005;37(3): 275–81.

115. Mizuguchi T, Matsumoto N. Recent progress in genetics of Marfan syndrome and Marfan-associated disorders. J Hum Genet 2007;52(1):1–12.

116. Stheneur C, Collod-Béroud G, Faivre L, et al. Identification of 23 TGFBR2 and 6 TGFBR1 gene mutations and genotype-phenotype investigations in 457 patients with Marfan syndrome type I and II, Loeys-Dietz syndrome and related disorders. Hum Mutat 2008;29(11):E284–95.

117. Chaudhry SS, Cain SA, Morgan A, et al. Fibrillin-1 regulates the bioavailability of TGFbeta1. J Cell Biol 2007;176:355–67.

118. Yeowell HN, Steinmann B. Ehlers-Danlos syndrome, kyphoscoliotic form [Internet]. In: Pagon RA, Bird TD, Dolan CR, et al, editors. GeneReviews. Seattle (WA): University of Washington; 1993. February 2, 2000 [updated February 19, 2008].

119. Pepin MG, Byers PH. Ehlers-Danlos syndrome type IV [Internet]. In: Pagon RA, Bird TD, Dolan CR, et al, editors. GeneReviews. Seattle (WA): University of Washington; 1993. September 2, 1999 [updated May 3, 2011].

120. Pepin M, Schwarze U, Superti-Furga A, et al. Clinical and genetic features of Ehlers-Danlos syndrome type IV, the vascular type. N Engl J Med 2000;342(10):673–80.

121. Yeowell HN, Walker LC, Farmer B, et al. Mutational analysis of the lysyl hydroxylase 1 gene (PLOD) in six unrelated patients with Ehlers-Danlos syndrome type VI: prenatal exclusion of this disorder in one family. Hum Mutat 2000;16(1):90.

122. Stoller JK, Aboussouan LS. Alpha1-antitrypsin deficiency. Lancet 2005;365(9478):2225–36.

123. Köhnlein T, Welte T. Alpha-1 antitrypsin deficiency: pathogenesis, clinical presentation, diagnosis, and treatment. Am J Med 2008;121(1):3–9.

124. Beer DJ, Pereira W Jr, Snider GL. Pleural effusion associated with primary lymphedema: a perspective on the yellow nail syndrome. Am Rev Respir Dis 1978;117(3):595–9.

125. Silverman EK, Sandhaus RA. Clinical practice. Alpha1-antitrypsin deficiency. N Engl J Med 2009; 360(26):2749–57.

126. Bull RH, Fenton DA, Mortimer PS. Lymphatic function in the yellow nail syndrome. Br J Dermatol 1996;134(2):307–12.

127. Guest PJ, Hansell DM. High resolution computed tomography (HRCT) in emphysema associated with alpha-1-antitrypsin deficiency. Clin Radiol 1992;45(4):260–6.

128. King MA, Stone JA, Diaz PT, et al. Alpha 1-antitrypsin deficiency: evaluation of bronchiectasis with CT. Radiology 1996;199(1):137–41.

129. Dirksen A, Dijkman JH, Madsen F, et al. A randomized clinical trial of alpha(1)-antitrypsin augmentation therapy. Am J Respir Crit Care Med 1999;160(5 Pt 1):1468–72.

130. Greene CM, McElvaney NG. Protein misfolding and obstructive lung disease. Proc Am Thorac Soc 2010;7(6):346–55.

131. Greene CM, Hassan T, Molloy K, et al. The role of proteases, endoplasmic reticulum stress and SERPINA1 heterozygosity in lung disease and α-1 antitrypsin deficiency. Expert Rev Respir Med 2011; 5(3):395–411.

132. Cuvelier A, Muir JF, Hellot MF, et al. Distribution of alpha(1)-antitrypsin alleles in patients with bronchiectasis. Chest 2000;117(2):415–9.

133. Rodriguez-Cintron W, Guntupalli K, Fraire AE. Bronchiectasis and homozygous (P1ZZ) alpha 1-antitrypsin deficiency in a young man. Thorax 1995;50(4):424–5.

134. Longstreth GF, Weitzman SA, Browning RJ, et al. Bronchiectasis and homozygous alpha1-antitrypsin deficiency. Chest 1975;67(2):233–5.

135. Talmud PJ, Martin S, Steiner G, et al. Diabetes Atherosclerosis Intervention Study Investigators. Progression of atherosclerosis is associated with variation in the alpha1-antitrypsin gene. Arterioscler Thromb Vasc Biol 2003;23(4):644–9.

136. Quint JK, Donaldson GC, Kumari M, et al. SERPINA1 11478G→A variant, serum α1-antitrypsin, exacerbation frequency and FEV1 decline in COPD. Thorax 2011;66(5):418–24.

137. Wood AM, Simmonds MJ, Bayley DL, et al. The TNFalpha gene relates to clinical phenotype in alpha-1-antitrypsin deficiency. Respir Res 2008; 9:52.

138. Demeo DL, Campbell EJ, Barker AF, et al. IL10 polymorphisms are associated with airflow obstruction in severe alpha1-antitrypsin deficiency. Am J Respir Cell Mol Biol 2008;38(1): 114–20.

139. Maldonado F, Tazelaar HD, Wang CW, et al. Yellow nail syndrome: analysis of 41 consecutive patients. Chest 2008;134(2):375–81.

140. Battaglia A, di Ricco G, Mariani G, et al. Pleural effusion and recurrent broncho-pneumonia with lymphedema, yellow nails and protein-losing enteropathy. Eur J Respir Dis 1985;66(1):65–9.

141. D'Alessandro A, Muzi G, Monaco A, et al. Yellow nail syndrome: does protein leakage play a role? Eur Respir J 2001;17(1):149–52.

142. Miro AM, Vasudevan V, Shah H. Ciliary motility in two patients with yellow nail syndrome and recurrent sinopulmonary infections. Am Rev Respir Dis 1990;142(4):890–1.

143. Bokszczanin A, Levinson AI. Coexistent yellow nail syndrome and selective antibody deficiency. Ann Allergy Asthma Immunol 2003; 91(5):496–500.

144. Wiggins J, Strickland B, Chung KF. Detection of bronchiectasis by high-resolution computed tomography in the yellow nail syndrome. Clin Radiol 1991;43(6): 377–9.

145. Hoque SR, Mansour S, Mortimer PS. Yellow nail syndrome: not a genetic disorder? Eleven new cases and a review of the literature. Br J Dermatol 2007;156(6):1230–4.

Allergic Bronchopulmonary Aspergillosis

Sonia N. Bains, MD[a], Marc A. Judson, MD[b],*

KEYWORDS

- ABPA • Asthma • Cystic fibrosis • Bronchiectasis

KEY POINTS

- ABPA is a complex hypersensitivity syndrome affecting a small subset of patients with asthma and CF.
- The immunopathogenesis of ABPA remains incompletely understood, and clinical, laboratory, and radiologic findings are varied.
- Because delay in treatment of ABPA can result in permanent lung damage, a high index of suspicion for the disease is warranted in appropriate patients.
- It is hoped that more specific diagnostic assays for ABPA will be developed and novel treatment strategies identified.

Allergic bronchopulmonary aspergillosis (ABPA) is a lung disease resulting from a hypersensitivity response to *Aspergillus fumigatus* (Af) colonization in the airways. ABPA develops almost exclusively in atopic patients with asthma or cystic fibrosis (CF). Hinson and coworkers[1] first described ABPA in 1952 as a syndrome that comprises recurrent chest radiographic infiltrates, peripheral blood, and sputum eosinophilia along with asthma. Clinically, ABPA has a variable course from mild asthma to a destructive lung disease with bronchiectasis and pulmonary fibrosis. This article outlines the immunopathogenesis, clinical features, and treatment options for ABPA.

THE SPECTRUM OF ASPERGILLUS LUNG DISEASE

Aspergillus spores are ubiquitous in the environment. They can be found in high concentrations in fertile soil, decaying vegetation, swimming pool water, leaky basements, crawl spaces, bedding, and dust from homes. Spores may easily become airborne and, when inhaled, deposit in the distal airways. Aspergillus can cause 6 types of lung diseases depending on underlying host characteristics: (1) invasive aspergillosis, which occurs in immunosuppressed patients (especially neutropenia), is often life threatening, and is associated with invasion of the bronchial wall, pneumonia, mycotic abscesses, and systemic spread; (2) chronic necrotizing aspergillosis, a locally invasive pulmonary disease that develops in immunocompromised patients and/or those with an underlying chronic lung disease; (3) aspergilloma, which is a superficial saprophytic colonization of aspergillus mycelia in a bronchiectatic airway or pre-existing cavity; (4) aspergillus-sensitive asthma; (5) extrinsic allergic alveolitis (hypersensitivity pneumonitis)[2]; and (6) ABPA.

The authors have nothing to disclose.
[a] Division of Pulmonary, Critical Care, Allergy & Sleep Medicine, Medical University of South Carolina, 96 Jonathan Lucas Street, CSD 812, Charleston, SC 29425, USA
[b] Division of Pulmonary and Critical Care Medicine, Department of Medicine, Albany Medical College, MC-91, 47 New Scotland Avenue, Albany, NY 12206, USA
* Corresponding author.
E-mail address: judsonm@mail.amc.edu

Clin Chest Med 33 (2012) 265–281
doi:10.1016/j.ccm.2012.02.003
0272-5231/12/$ – see front matter © 2012 Elsevier Inc. All rights reserved.

IMMUNOPATHOGENESIS OF ABPA

ABPA was formerly thought to develop in asthma and CF patients exposed to Af spores who had highly viscid mucus that was conducive to fungal growth. Although the characteristics of mucus may be important in the development of ABPA, this proposed pathogenesis does not account for two important observations. First, ABPA does not necessarily occur in the most severe cases of asthma or CF (with the most viscous mucus). Second, the correlation between the degree of exposure to aspergillus spores and the development of ABPA is weak. For example, ABPA affects urban and rural dwellers with similar frequency.[3] These findings suggest that ABPA is primarily the result of an abnormal host immune response to aspergillus antigens. This abnormal host response likely is influenced by genetic factors because several families have been reported with high rates of ABPA.[4–6]

Host Characteristics

Several host characteristics have been identified to explain the selective development of ABPA in a small subset of individuals who are sensitized to the aspergillus mold. Both allergic asthma and ABPA are characterized by a type 2 helper T cell (T_H2) immune response to aspergillus; however, in patients with ABPA, the T_H2 response is greatly exaggerated.

As the aspergillus mycelia grow in the airways of patients with ABPA, they release allergens that are processed by antigen-presenting cells bearing HLA-DR2 or HLA-DR5 markers.[7,8] The processed allergens are presented to T_H2 lymphocytes, which release cytokines resulting in a type 1 hypersensitivity response. A higher frequency of the HLA-DR2/5 (73%) polymorphism has been reported in patients with ABPA compared with CF and asthmatic patients who are aspergillus sensitive but without ABPA (35%) and with nonatopic controls (35%). Therefore, the exaggerated T_H2 response generated in patients with ABPA may be because individuals who possess HLA-DR2/5 polymorphisms are more effective at presenting allergen to T lymphocytes. Within the HLA-DR2 locus, the DRB1*1501 and DRB1*1503 alleles were found at significantly greater frequencies in patients with ABPA versus the non-ABPA controls.[7,9]

This polymorphism cannot be the sole determinant of ABPA, however, because a significant number of asthmatics and CF patients without ABPA also share the same HLA-DR2/5 genotype. Certain HLA alleles, such as the HLA-DQ2 allele, may be protective against the development of ABPA in CF and asthmatic patients.[9,10]

Mutations in the CF transmembrane conductance regulator (CFTR) gene have been reported in higher frequency in patients with ABPA without CF (normal sweat chloride) compared with non-ABPA controls.[11,12] It is conceivable that these patients may produce mucus with characteristics that promote colonization of Af.

A higher frequency of polymorphisms in the interleukin (IL)-10 promoter region[13] and surfactant protein A[14] has also been reported in patients with ABPA compared with healthy controls. Specific polymorphisms in surfactant protein A result in a diminished host defense against aspergillus, which may allow growth of this fungus in the lungs and thus ABPA. These polymorphisms in surfactant protein A were reported at a higher frequency in severe cases of ABPA. **Box 1** summarizes genes associated with or protective against ABPA.

Immunology

The immunologic response in ABPA begins with the presence of aspergillus spores and hyphae in the airways. Repeated exposure to aspergillus spores may cause allergic diseases, including asthma and allergic sinusitis. In these instances, there is no mycelial colonization or growth of the fungus in the airways, and removal from the environmental source results in clinical improvement. In contrast, ABPA involves mycelial growth of aspergillus in the lungs. This mycelial growth does not invade the bronchial epithelium as is the case with invasive aspergillosis. Although the factors that allow growth of Af in the airways of ABPA patients are unclear, bronchial mucus abnormalities have been implicated. For unknown reasons, the mucus in ABPA becomes extremely viscid and is problematic to extract bronchoscopically.

As the Af mycelia grow in the airways of patients with ABPA, they release allergens that are processed by antigen-presenting cells bearing HLA-DR2 or HLA-DR5 markers, which then present the Af antigen to T lymphocytes.[7,8] In a normal host,

---

Box 1
Genetic factors associated with ABPA

Increased Susceptibility

HLA-DR2 and HLA-DR5[7,8]

IL-10 promoter polymorphisms[13]

Surfactant protein polymorphism[14]

CFTR gene mutation[11,12]

Protective against

HLA-DQ2[9,10]

this results in type 1 helper T cell (T_H1) response that eradicates the organism. Although the T_H1 response is not defective in patients with ABPA, an exaggerated T_H2 response is generated in response to aspergillus antigens causing a chronic eosinophilic and asthmatic-type inflammation.

The spores and hyphae release proteases and antigens, which can (1) activate the innate immune system; (2) damage the bronchial epithelium, causing discrete areas of bronchiectasis[15]; and (3) impair mucociliary clearance. This results in the release of several chemokines into the airways, including thymus-regulated and activation-regulated chemokine (TARC) (CCL17), monocyte chemotactic protein (MCP)-1, eotaxin, RANTES (regulated on activation, normal T-cell expressed, and secreted), IL-8, and macrophage inflammatory protein (MIP)-1α. These cytokines activate an intense T_H2 response, resulting in proliferation of CD4+ T_H2 lymphocytes specific for Af. Factors skewing the inflammatory process toward a T_H2 phenotype include (1) the pattern of chemokine secretion, (2) a history of atopy, and (3) the major histocompatibility complex–restricted phenotype of antigen-presenting cells. These T_H2 lymphocytes produce IL-4, IL-5, IL-9, IL-10, and IL-13, which favor eosinophil growth and survival, mast cell proliferation, and IgG and IgE isotype switching. Aspergillus can serve as a growth factor for eosinophils, which are a major effector of inflammation. There is an exaggerated humoral immune response in ABPA compared with aspergillus-sensitive asthma, with increased total IgE, and increased aspergillus-specific IgE, IgG, and IgA in the serum[16] and bronchoalveolar fluid compartment (**Fig. 1**).[17] Total IgE is increased out of proportion to aspergillus-specific IgE. One explanation for the excessive production of these immunoglobulins is that the B cells from ABPA patients are more sensitive to stimulation with IL-4, which eventually amplifies the CD4+ T_H2 responses.[18] Animal studies have confirmed the longstanding hypothesis that ABPA is characterized by Gell and Coombs type I and type III immunologic reactions.[19,20] These studies have demonstrated that both IgE-Af and IgG-Af are essential for the development of ABPA.[20]

Pathology

Mucoid impaction and eosinophilic pneumonia are common pathologic findings in ABPA. Bronchiectasis may develop in areas of pulmonary infiltrates, especially if corticosteroids are not used to treat the ABPA exacerbation. Upper lobe posterior segments are most commonly affected. It is thought that bronchiectasis and pulmonary fibrosis are sequellae of the mucoid impaction of APBA. The mucus from ABPA contains aspergillus antigens, eosinophilic inflammatory mediators, and inflammatory cells, which may cause airway and parenchymal lung destruction. Despite the similarity of

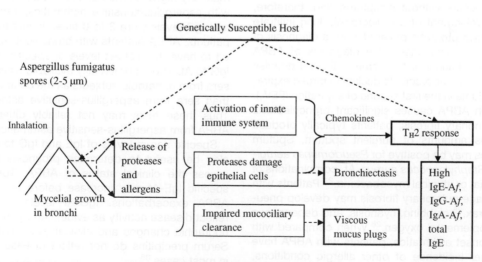

Fig. 1. Immunopathogenesis of ABPA. Certain host characteristics act as susceptibility factors for the development of ABPA. In such patients, inhaled Af spores are able to germinate and grow inside the bronchi (may be due to impaired host defense, thick mucus, or survival factors in Af). This results in the release of several proteases and allergens, which damage epithelial cells and activate the innate immune system. Factors skewing toward a T_H2 response include the pattern of chemokine secretion, atopy, and the HLA-restricted phenotype of antigen-presenting cells. The intense T_H2 response results in increased IgE-Af, IgG-Af, and IgA-Af. Mechanisms underlying bronchiectasis and thick mucus plugs remain incompletely understood.

the clinical and serologic presentation of the disease, the parenchymal responses are varied and include eosinophilic pneumonia, bronchocentric granulomatosis, granulomatous bronchiolitis, exudative bronchiolitis, lipid pneumonia, lymphocytic interstitial pneumonia, desquamative interstitial pneumonia, pulmonary vasculitis, and bronchiolitis obliterans.[21] Individual APBA patients may even develop several of these parenchymal responses concomitantly.[21]

CLINICAL FEATURES
Symptoms

The prevalence of ABPA in asthma ranges from 2% to 32%.[22] Patients with ABPA are usually atopic and have a history of asthma or CF. It is mainly a disease of adults although some cases of patients as young as age of 6 have been described.[23] Symptoms of ABPA include cough, wheezing, shortness of breath, expectoration of tan or brown sputum plugs, low-grade fever, and symptoms of allergic rhinitis. On some occasions, ABPA patients may be completely asymptomatic even when new pulmonary infiltrates develop. Because pneumonia and ABPA may both cause pulmonary infiltrates on a chest radiograph, it may be problematic to distinguish these two entities. Although both conditions may cause fever, the fevers associated with bacterial pneumonia tend to be higher than with ABPA. Bacterial pneumonia may cause rigors and chills, which are unusual with ABPA exacerbations. Pneumonia rarely occurs without symptoms and, therefore, the development of a radiographic lung infiltrate in an asymptomatic patient favors a diagnosis of ABPA. In these cases, the diagnosis of ABPA can be enhanced if the serum IgE level doubles or there is an appreciable decline in forced expiratory volume in the first second of expiration (FEV_1).

When ABPA causes significant bronchiectasis or pulmonary fibrosis, patients typically produce copious amounts of purulent sputum. Sputum cultures may be positive for *Pseudomonas aeruginosa, Staphylococcus aureus*, Af, combinations of bacteria, or atypical mycobacteria.[24] Patients with end-stage pulmonary fibrosis may develop pneumothorax,[25] clubbing, cyanosis, and dependence on supplemental oxygen.[26] When compared with adult-onset asthmatics, patients with ABPA have a higher incidence of other allergic conditions, such as allergic rhinitis, atopic dermatitis, food allergy, and drug allergy.[27]

Laboratory Abnormalities

The diagnosis of ABPA should be suspected in an asthmatic with peripheral eosinophilia, elevated IgE, immediate cutaneous reactivity to Af, recurrent infiltrates, and central bronchiectasis (CB). However, these abnormalities are not specific to ABPA. For example, up to 25% of patients with aspergillus-sensitive asthma (without ABPA) have immediate cutaneous reactivity to Af.[28] Likewise, peripheral eosinophilia may also be observed in asthma without ABPA; however, the degree of eosinophilia can be used to differentiate between the two. Patients with ABPA have higher eosinophil counts generally greater than 1000/µL and commonly greater than 3000/µL, whereas asthmatics without ABPA have mild peripheral eosinophilia with counts lower than 1500/µL[29] and usually below 500/µL.[30]

Serum precipitin reactions to Af are present in the serum of 69% of patients with ABPA, which increases to greater than 90% when the serum is concentrated 3-fold to 4-fold.[31] The presence of serum precipitins, however, is also not specific for ABPA; it has been reported as positive in 3% of healthy individuals, 9% of hospitalized patients, 12% of atopic asthmatics, 27% of patients with farmer's lung,[32] and almost all patients with aspergilloma.

Although total serum IgE may be mildly increased in allergic asthma, it is markedly elevated in ABPA with levels typically exceeding 1000 ng/mL.[33] Elevation of specific serum level of IgE and IgG to Af strongly suggests the diagnosis of ABPA. In a study comparing serum levels of specific IgE and IgG to Af in ABPA patients versus aspergillus-sensitive asthmatics,[34] levels were markedly higher in the ABPA patients. Compared with aspergillus-sensitive asthmatics, serum IgE and IgG levels were 3 to 8 times higher in ABPA patients. APBA patients with bronchiectasis tended to have the highest levels of specific IgE and IgG to Af. The commercially available assays use sera from nonatopic subjects as the control rather than sera from aspergillus-sensitive asthmatics. Thus these tests may not reliably differentiate ABPA from aspergillus-sensitive asthmatics.

Specific serum levels of IgE and IgG to Af may also be useful to determine prognosis and to assess the clinical status of ABPA. Total and specific IgE-Af may increase before and during ABPA exacerbations. IgG-Af levels may also reflect disease activity as evidenced by roentgenographic changes and clinical exacerbations.[35] Serum precipitins do not reflect disease activity in most cases.[35]

Direct examination of sputum plugs from ABPA patients reveals fungal mycelia with healthy cytoplasm (a sign of active growth) and large numbers of eosinophils. This is in contrast to the dead mycelia, which are devoid of cytoplasmic content observed in patients with aspergilloma.[36] A positive sputum culture, however, is not adequately sensitive or specific for the diagnosis of ABPA. Aspergillus-sensitive asthma can be differentiated from ABPA in that there is no saprophytic growth of Af in asthma; hence, fungal sputum cultures are usually negative in aspergillus-sensitive asthma.

Experimental Laboratory Findings

Af has 40 components that can bind IgE. Currently, 22 recombinant Af allergens (Asp f 1 through Asp f 22) have been identified. None of these is available commercially.[37] In one study, the serodiagnosis of ABPA was improved through the use of a battery of Asp f 4, and Asp f 6, whereas Asp f 1 and Asp f 3 were not discriminatory.[38] TARC is secreted by dendritic cells as well as T_H17 cells in the lungs of CF patients. This chemokine recruits T_H2 cells. Latzin and coworkers[39] reported that serum TARC (CCL17) levels can differentiate patients with concomitant CF and ABPA from CF patients who are aspergillus sensitive (but without ABPA). They also reported that monitoring serum TARC levels is superior compared with serial total IgE monitoring for identifying ABPA exacerbations.[39]

Radiographic Imaging

A massive homogeneous shadow without fissure displacement is the most common abnormality seen on a chest radiograph with ABPA; these are most common in the upper and middle lobes. The shadow may be patchy, triangular, oblong, or lobar, and it frequently shifts from one site to another (fleeting).[40] These opacities represent eosinophilic infiltrates, mucous plugging of airways, bronchoceles, atelactasis, and/or lobar collapse.[41] Mucoid impaction in dilated, thickened bronchi may cause the appearance of toothpaste shadows and finger-in-glove opacities (**Fig. 2**).[42] Bronchiectasis is often

observed and has the appearance of a 1 cm to 2 cm diameter ring shadow (dilated bronchus) in an en face orientation and a parallel-line or tramline when viewed in a tangential plane.[37]

The findings of ABPA on high-resolution CT (HRCT) of the chest include centrilobular nodules, CB (inner two-thirds of lung fields) often with mucoid impaction,[43] fibrosis, and cavitation. Although bronchiectasis may occasionally be observed in asthma, bronchiectasis involving 3 or more lobes reliably distinguishes ABPA from asthma. The bronchiectasis observed in ABPA is typically varicose or cystic.[44] When these radiographic findings are present in an asthmatic, the diagnosis of ABPA should be considered.[44] Presence of high-attenuation mucus is characteristic of ABPA (**Fig. 3**) and is another radiographic clue suggesting the diagnosis.[45] High-attenuation mucus and bronchiectasis are predictors of severe disease and frequent exacerbations.[46] Bronchiectasis is also associated with failure to achieve remission.[45]

CLINICAL CLUES SUGGESTING A DIAGNOSIS OF ABPA IN ASTHMA

ABPA should be suspected in asthma that is severe or corticosteroid dependent. Viscous mucus production is common. Pulmonary infiltrates on chest radiograph, peripheral eosinophilia, and serum IgE greater than 1000 ng/mL are also clues suggesting ABPA. Because there are reports of concomitant ABPA and allergic fungal sinusitis,[47] the presence allergic fungal sinusitis may warrant evaluation for ABPA.[48,49] As discussed previously, radiographic findings of CB, the presence of bronchiectasis in 3 or more lobes, and high-attenuation mucus are all highly suggestive of ABPA (**Box 2**).

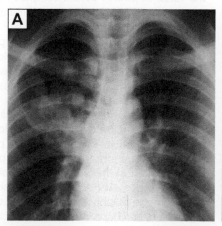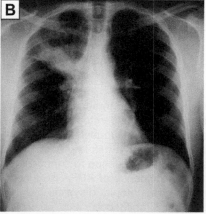

Fig. 2. Chest radiograph of a patient with ABPA showing (A) mucoid impaction in dilated bronchi and (B) finger-in-glove appearance.

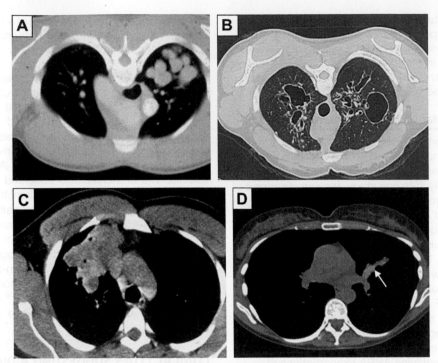

Fig. 3. HRCT images of different patients with ABPA. (*A*) Mucoid impaction of dilated bronchi (same patient shown in **Fig.** 2A), (*B*) central bronchiectasis, (*C*) impacted bronchus, and (*D*) high-attenuation mucus (*arrow*).

CLINICAL CLUES SUGGESTING A DIAGNOSIS OF ABPA IN CF

ABPA should be suspected in a CF patient who develops wheezing or major reductions of FEV_1 without evidence of a CF exacerbation. Additional clues include the development of pulmonary infiltrates, peripheral eosinophilia, and repeatedly positive sputum cultures for Af. The Cystic Fibrosis Foundation Consensus Conference recommended screening with annual or semiannual measurements of total serum IgE levels. If the level is greater than 500 IU/mL, then further testing for ABPA is recommended.

DIAGNOSIS OF ABPA IN PATIENTS WITH ASTHMA

The relationship between asthma and ABPA is complex and incompletely understood. The immunopathogenesis of ABPA suggests that it can result in clinical asthma, and this is probably the typical scenario. Indirect evidence to support this schema is that the incidence of ABPA is highest in adults, unlike other atopic diseases, which are most common in childhood. It is possible, however, that some ABPA patients develop asthma before the onset of ABPA.

The classic clinical findings of ABPA described by Patterson and colleagues[50,51] (mnemonic ART EPICS) include: (1) A: asthma; (2) R: radiographic chest infiltrates, fixed or transient; (3) T: skin test positive (immediate cutaneous reactivity) to Af antigen; (4) E: eosinophilia (>1×10^9/μL in peripheral blood); (5) P: precipitating antibodies against Af antigen; (6) I: IgE in serum elevated greater than 1000 ng/mL; (7) C: CB; and (8) S: serum IgE-Af and/or IgG-Af elevated (more than twice the value of pooled serum samples from patients with aspergillus-sensitive asthmatics without ABPA.

When these clinical findings are present, the diagnosis is certainly established. Most patients with ABPA do not fulfill all criteria, however, especially early in the course of the disease or if they are receiving corticosteroids. In the latter case, several features may be absent, including chest radiographic infiltrates, peripheral blood eosinophilia, elevation in serum IgE, and precipitating antibodies. Therefore, patients who present with only a portion of these diagnostic clinical findings may still have ABPA. The diagnosis of ABPA can be made reliably if the following clinical findings are met: (1) proximal bronchiectasis (in the absence of distal bronchiectasis) and elevated serum IgE-Af and IgG-Af compared with sera

Box 2
Clinical clues that raise suspicion of ABPA

Clinical clues in asthmatics

Signs and symptoms

Worsening asthma control

History of allergic fungal sinusitis

Expectoration of thick mucus plugs

Laboratory findings

Positive skin prick test to Af

Peripheral eosinophilia

Serum IgE >1000 ng/mL

Chest radiograph findings

Fleeting infiltrates

High-resolution CT findings

Central bronchiectasis involving 3 or more lobes

Centrilobular nodules

High-attenuation mucus

Clinical clues in patients with CF

New-onset intermittent wheezing

Sputum cultures repeatedly positive for Af

Unexplained drop in FEV_1

IgE >500 IU/mL

Positive skin prick test to Af

from patients with aspergillus-sensitive asthma (without ABPA) or (2) the presence of CB in an asthmatic along with skin-test reactivity to aspergillus and peripheral eosinophilia. Other combinations of these clinical findings may suggest ABPA but are insufficient for the diagnosis. **Fig. 4** outlines the diagnostic approach suggested by the authors for evaluation of ABPA in patients with asthma.

Although CB (C) is frequently observed in ABPA, it is not a prerequisite for diagnosis.[34,51] The presence of central or proximal bronchiectasis in ABPA is designated ABPA-CB. CB is located in the inner two-thirds of the lung fields on axial sections of CT scans.[43] If sufficient criteria for the diagnosis of ABPA are present except for CB, the patient is classified as having seropositive ABPA (ABPA-S). ABPA-S is thought to be an early stage of the disease. As discussed later, the mucus of ABPA is particularly destructive and is thought to cause bronchiectasis and lung fibrosis. Therefore, ABPA-S tends to be seen in early disease before the lung has been damaged to the point of bronchiectasis or pulmonary fibrosis. This is consistent with the finding that ABPA-S commonly occurs in

patients who have either never or rarely had pulmonary infiltrates detected radiographically.

DIAGNOSIS OF ABPA IN CF

The prevalence of ABPA in CF ranges from 2% to 15%. Establishing the diagnosis of ABPA in patients with CF can be challenging given the similarities between the two conditions. Both diseases can cause airflow obstruction. Both have similar radiographic findings, including hyperinflation, peribronchial inflammatory changes, nodular and branching densities of mucus impaction, atelactasis, predominant upper lobe infiltrates, and bronchiectasis. In addition, CF without ABPA has several features that are seen in ABPA, including atopy (46%), positive skin test to Af (42%), elevated IgE-Af (52%), elevated IgG-Af (58%), precipitins to Af (44%), and elevated total IgE (40%).[52,53] To complicate matters further, patients with concomitant CF and ABPA may spontaneously (in the absence of oral corticosteroid therapy) resolve immunologic markers of Af sensitization, such as a positive skin test to Af (12%), serum precipitins (56%), elevated IgE-Af (51%), elevated IgG-Af (41%), and IgE greater than 1000 IU/mL (86%).[53] As a result of these findings, ABPA may be both underdiagnosed and overdiagnosed in patients with CF.

The Cystic Fibrosis Foundation has established diagnostic criteria for ABPA in CF in an attempt to reconcile these ambiguities[54]: (1) acute or subacute clinical deterioration not attributable to another cause; (2) serum IgE elevated greater than 1000 IU/mL; (3) skin test positive (immediate cutaneous reactivity) to Af antigen or serum IgE-Af positive; (4) precipitating antibodies against Af antigen or serum IgG-Af positive; and (5) abnormalities on chest imaging unresponsive to antibiotics and standard physiotherapy.

Because several of the diagnostic criteria for ABPA are present in asthma and CF, distinguishing between these diseases is problematic. **Table 1** outlines an approach to distinguish these 2 diseases using clinical criteria. It should be noted that although the diagnostic cutoff of the total IgE level is 1000 IU/mL, ABPA should be suspected in patients with a total IgE of greater than 500 IU/ml if they meet some of the other diagnostic criteria.

DIFFERENTIAL DIAGNOSIS

The differential diagnosis of ABPA includes diseases in which 2 of these 3 clinical findings are present: asthma, eosinophilia, and radiographic infiltrates. These diseases are listed in **Table 2**. Although aspergillus-sensitive asthma usually

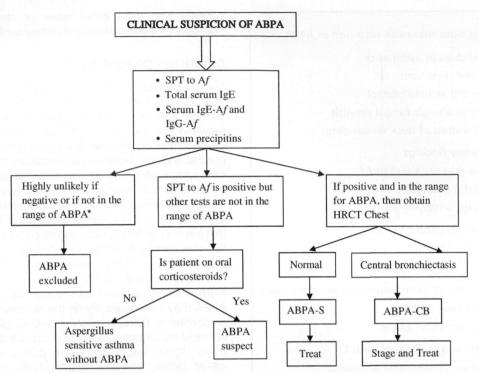

Fig. 4. Diagnostic algorithm for ABPA. SPT, skin prick test. *Serologic parameters may not be abnormal in certain stages of ABPA, including remission, corticosteroid-dependent ABPA, and end-stage ABPA.

does not cause pulmonary infiltrates, it may be problematic to differentiate from serologic ABPA where no radiographic infiltrates are present (ABPA-S). As discussed previously, distinguishing

CF from ABPA may be problematic because many of the clinical, radiologic, and serologic features overlap.

Fungi other than Af may cause an allergic bronchopulmonary mycosis that is clinically identical to ABPA but with antibody and skin testing reflecting allergy to the implicated mold (see **Table 2**). Such fungi include *Curvularia, Fusarium, Drechslera, Stemphylium, Pseudallescheria, Helminthosporium, Torulopsis,* and *Aspergillus* from species other than Af.[16] Bronchocentric granulomatosis is a reaction pattern associated with any condition that causes mucoid impaction. It may be found with ABPA but is not specific for that condition. Hence, histologic evidence of bronchocentric granulomatosis should raise suspicion of ABPA.

Table 1
Distinguishing asthma and CF from ABPA

Diagnostic Criteria for ABPA	Common in Asthma	Common in CF
Asthma	Yes	No
Radiologic chest infiltrates, fixed or transient	No[a]	No[b]
Skin test positive	Yes[c]	Yes[c]
Eosinophilia (>1 × 10⁹/L)	No	No
Precipitating antibodies against Af antigen	No	No
Total IgE elevated or >1000 ng/mL	No	No
Central bronchiectasis	No	Yes
Serum anti-Af IgE and/or IgG elevated	No[d]	No[d]

[a] Except in the case of bacterial pneumonia.
[b] Except in case of chronic suppurative infection.
[c] If skin test is negative, ABPA is excluded.
[d] If sera from aspergillus-sensitive asthmatics without ABPA is used as the negative control.

STAGING OF ABPA

ABPA can be staged based on asthma severity and radiographic and laboratory findings (**Table 3**).[50] These stages do not represent phases of the disease, however; hence, patients do not necessarily progress from one stage to the next. The ABPA staging system is primarily used as a guide for treatment. These stages do not encompass all cases of ABPA because the stages require the presence of CB (ABPA-CB).[43]

Table 2
Differential diagnosis of ABPA

Differential Diagnosis	Clinical Presentation	Laboratory Findings	Radiographic Findings
Chronic eosinophilic pneumonia	Responds readily to prednisone but often recurs if treatment is stopped	Peripheral eosinophilia	Peripheral infiltrates (peripheral negative of pulmonary edema)
Acute eosinophilic pneumonia	Acute respiratory failure	No peripheral eosinophilia; BAL fluid has >25% eosinophils	Diffuse pulmonary infiltrates
Churg-Strauss syndrome	1. Asthma 2. Palpable purpura on hands and legs 3. New onset of sensory or motor neuropathy in an asthmatic (may develop wrist or foot drop) 4. May develop in the setting of administration of LTD4 antagonists	Peripheral eosinophilia, biopsy of infiltrates demonstrate extravascular granulomas and small vessel vasculitis	Pulmonary infiltrates
Asthma with middle lobe syndrome or lobar collapse	1. Status asthmaticus 2. Infiltrates resolve with PO or IV steroids		Middle or upper lobe infiltrates/collapse (due to mucous plugging)
Parasitic infestations (Ascaris, Strongyloides, etc.)	History of travel, diarrhea Resolution with empiric trial of albendazole	Elevated IgE, peripheral eosinophilia, positive serology, positive for stool ova and parasites	Pulmonary infiltrates
Allergic bronchopulmonary mycosis	Identical to ABPA	Immediate cutaneous reactivity to appropriate mold, elevated IgE, peripheral eosinophilia Absence of immediate cutaneous reactivity to Af	Pulmonary infiltrates, central bronchiectasis
Asthma and atopic dermatitis	Asthma without ABPA, may or may not have aspergillus-sensitive asthma	Elevated IgE (due to atopic dermatitis), peripheral eosinophilia, immediate cutaneous reactivity to Af may or may not be present	No abnormalities

Abbreviations: BAL, bronchoalveolar lavage; IV, intravenous; LTD4, leukotriene D4 receptor; PO, oral.

Table 3
Stages of ABPA-CB

Stage	Total Serum IgE	Serum Precipitins	Peripheral Eosinophilia	Radiographic Infiltrates	IgE-Af and IgG-Af
I: Acute *New, active ABPA*	Markedly elevated	Present	Present	Upper or middle lobe	Present
II: Remission *Clinical and serologic remission*	Elevated or normal	Present/absent	Absent	No infiltrate with patient off prednisone >6 months	Present/absent
III: Recurrent exacerbation *Recurrent active ABPA*	Marked increase (>100% increase from baseline)	Present/absent	Present	Upper or middle lobe	Present
IV: Corticosteroid-dependent asthma *Secondary to ABPA*	Elevated or normal	Present/absent	Present/absent	New infiltrates may occur, especially if prednisone dose is <30 mg qOD	Present/absent
V: End-stage fibrocavitary *Secondary to untreated ABPA*	Elevated or normal	Present/absent	Absent	Fibrotic, bullous, or cavitary lesions	Usually present

Abbreviation: qOD, every other day.

Stage I—Acute

Acute ABPA is characterized by the presence of all classic ABPA criteria (ART EPICS) (see **Table 1**). The associated infiltrates seen in APBA usually represent mucoid impaction of dilated airways. An important aspect of the diagnosis is the prompt response to oral corticosteroids. The infiltrates usually clear within 1 to 2 months after a moderate dose of corticosteroids.

Stage 2—Remission

An ABPA remission occurs when an ABPA patient is able to suspend oral corticosteroids for at least 6 months without recurrence or development of radiographic pulmonary infiltrates.[50,55] Some patients may experience a permanent remission.

Stage 3—Recurrent Exacerbation

Recurrent exacerbations of ABPA are defined (1) by the development of new pulmonary infiltrates from ABPA (causes other than ABPA have been excluded) and (2) a 100% increase or more in total serum IgE level.[50,55] Sputum plugs may be expectorated although some patients have no mucus production. Many patients are diagnosed with ABPA in this stage, because prior episodes may have been misdiagnosed as an alternative pulmonary condition.

Stage 4—Corticosteroid Dependent

Corticosteroid-dependent ABPA is defined as a state where discontinuation of oral corticosteroids results in an increase in the serum IgE level and/or development of new infiltrates and/or a worsening asthma.[15,50,55]

Stage 5—End-Stage Fibrocavitary

End-stage fibrocavitary ABPA occurs when results in irreversible fibrosis develops. This is usually associated with airway obstruction and/or a restrictive physiology with a partial or poor response to oral corticosteroids and other bronchodilators.[50,56] These patients may require supplemental oxygen. New radiographic infiltrates are infrequent and may be due to bacterial infections rather than ABPA exacerbations. Chest films may demonstrate cavities, mycetomas within a cavity or bronchiectatic airway, bronchiectasis, volume loss, bullous changes, and chronic interstitial infiltrates.[56] Lung biopsies show areas of eosinophilic pneumonia, mucoid impaction, or interstitial fibrosis with granulomatous inflammation. If the FEV_1 remains below 0.8 L after corticosteroid treatment, the prognosis is poor.[56] This form of ABPA may result from failure to diagnose and treat ABPA at an early stage.

TREATMENT OF ABPA

Timely and aggressive treatment of ABPA has been shown to prevent progression to severe fibrotic lung disease.[51] The goal of treatment with oral corticosteroids is not only to treat asthmatic exacerbations associated with ABPA but also to inhibit the inflammatory response to Af colonization in the lung and thus prevent bronchiectasis and pulmonary fibrosis (**Fig. 5**). Attempts should be made to minimize corticosteroid dependence.

Systemic Corticosteroids

Oral corticosteroids are typically administered for acute ABPA and for APBA exacerbations (stages I and III). Although there are no randomized controlled trials to assess the efficacy of systemic corticosteroids, several large case series and expert opinion support the use of corticosteroids in the management of ABPA. Two regimens have been suggested. Greenberger[37] recommends a corticosteroid dose of prednisone equivalent 0.5 mg/kg/d for 1 to 2 weeks, then on alternate days for 6 to 8 weeks, then a taper by 5 mg to 10 mg every 2 weeks as tolerated until discontinued. Agarwal and coworkers[57] recommend a prednisolone equivalent of 0.75 mg/kg/d for 6 weeks, then 0.5 mg/kg/d for 6 weeks, then a taper by 5 mg every 6 weeks to continue for a total duration of 6 to 12 months. Unfortunately, there are no direct comparisons between the 2 regimens, thus the optimal dose or duration of systemic corticosteroids for the treatment of ABPA is not standardized.

The lowest effective corticosteroid dose should be used to minimize corticosteroid side effects. Compared with the regimen suggested by Greenberger and colleagues,[37] the regimen proposed by Agarwal's group[57] was associated with a lower rate of progression to corticosteroid-dependent asthma (17/126 = 14% vs 38/84 = 45%). Agarwal's regimen requires higher corticosteroid dosing, which may result in greater corticosteroid side effects. These 2 regimens have not been compared in terms of a risk-benefit analysis or in terms of their impact on quality of life.

Corticosteroid-dependent asthma (stage IV ABPA) usually requires a dose of 10 mg to 40 mg of prednisone equivalent either daily or on alternate days. Exacerbations are unlikely to occur until dose is reduced below 15 mg of prednisone equivalent daily.

Monthly pulse intravenous methylprednisolone may have a long-lasting effect in autoimmune diseases with fewer side effects than long-term

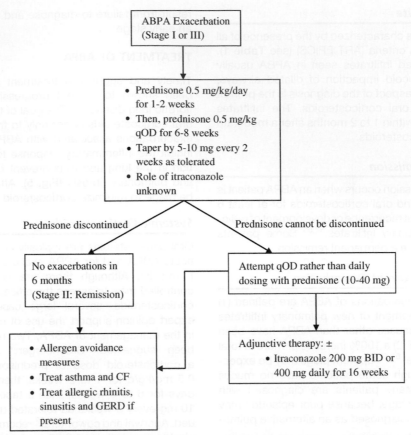

Fig. 5. Management of ABPA. Most patients are diagnosed with ABPA during an exacerbation. Initial management consists of high-dose oral steroids for 2 weeks followed by a taper over several months. The rate at which steroids are tapered has to be individualized and is determined by the rate of relapse. Additional standard asthma therapy should also be used for ABPA, including inhaled corticosteroids, long-acting β-agonists, and allergen avoidance. Other comorbid conditions should be treated if present. If oral steroids cannot be discontinued, then every-other-day dosing should be attempted to reduce side effects. Other adjunctive therapies may also be tried that may be steroid sparing. BID, twice a day; GERD, gastroesophageal reflux disease; qOD, every other day.

administration of oral corticosteroids. Two case series in patients with CF and ABPA have shown that treatment with intravenous methylprednisolone 10 to 20 mg/kg daily for 3 days at 1-month to 2-month intervals for up to 4 years is efficacious and associated with few side effects. Some patients had to discontinue therapy, however, due to corticosteroid side effects.[58,59] Although it has not been evaluated in ABPA, intramuscular administration of corticosteroid may control the symptoms of ABPA on a lower total corticosteroid dose and lessen corticosteroid side effects, as demonstrated with asthma.

Additional standard asthmatic therapy should also be used for ABPA, including a combination of inhaled corticosteroids, long-acting β-agonists, and asthma self-management education.

Antifungal Agents

Persistence of viable Af in the lung seems an important factor in the development and persistence of ABPA. This suggests that antifungal agents may have a role in ABPA to reduce the burden of fungal colonization in the lung, thus attenuating the intense inflammatory response and preventing subsequent lung damage. The currently available antifungal agents with known efficacy against Af are amphotericin B and the azoles (ketoconazole, itraconazole, voriconazole, and posaconazole). The use of amphotericin B is limited by its toxicity and cost. Studies investigating the efficacy of ketoconazole have produced conflicting results in small case series.[60,61] Long-term use of ketoconazole is also associated with significant side effects. There have been 2 randomized placebo-controlled trials that assessed the efficacy of itraconazole in the management of ABPA. Stevens and associates[62] reported that the addition of itraconzole (200 mg twice a day) for 16 weeks versus placebo (n = 55) to the usual management of stage IV ABPA (corticosteroid dependent) resulted in a 50% reduction in oral prednisone dose and led to a 25% reduction in total IgE level. The difference between itraconzole and placebo, however, did not reach statistical significance, and there was no difference between the 2 groups in terms of rates of remission. The investigators also reported that itraconazole was more beneficial in those without bronchiectasis compared with those with bronchiectasis.[62] Wark and colleagues[63] reported that the addition of itraconazole (400 mg daily) compared with placebo (n = 29) resulted in fewer exacerbations in the treatment arm (0.4 vs 1.3, $P = .03$) and reduced markers of immune activation. Neither study demonstrated an improvement in lung function. A limitation of both studies was that the long-term outcomes were not determined. In addition, neither study addresses whether itraconazole was useful for the management of ABPA exacerbations. Itraconazole may aggravate adrenal suppression induced with regular corticosteroid use.[64] In addition, itraconazole is costly, has several significant toxicities, and is occasionally ineffective against Af. For all these reasons, itraconizole is not recommended as a primary therapy for APBA but rather as adjunctive therapy in corticosteroid-dependent patients.[37]

Voriconazole has also been considered in lieu of itraconazole as adjunctive therapy for ABPA because of its slightly superior activity versus Af. Encouraging results were reported in 2 small open trials of voriconazole in patients with CF and ABPA.[65,66] Drug-drug interactions are more common with voriconazole, however, compared with itraconazole, and therapeutic levels are difficult to achieve without toxicity.[67] Voriconazole is also more expensive than itraconazole. Resistance to both of these azoles has been described in ABPA.

Omalizumab

Omalizumab, a humanized monoclonal antibody to IgE, is approved for use in atopic asthmatics with moderate to severe disease and who are over 12 years old. Several case reports and case series have suggested a potential role of omalizumab in CF patients with ABPA.[68–70] The mechanism of action is unclear because the doses of omalizumab reported were inadequate to elute the high serum levels of IgE present in ABPA. A randomized controlled trial of omalizumab has been initiated in CF patients with ABPA.

Allergen Avoidance

Exposure to environments with high aspergillus spore counts is associated with poor control of APBA as assessed by infiltrates and corticosteroid doses requirements.[71] Therefore, mold reduction strategies should be considered, especially in severe or corticosteroid-dependent cases. Mold exposure should be assessed at both an ABPA patient's home and workplace. Major sources of mold include any area of the home or workplace with repeated leaks or flooding. These structural problems should be repaired. Patients should be cautious concerning activities with a high potential for significant mold exposure, such as shoveling moldy bark and mulch.

MONITORING PATIENTS WITH ABPA

Monitoring of ABPA patients begins when the diagnosis is made, which is usually during an exacerbation (stage I or III). Oral corticosteroid therapy should be initiated (as detailed previously). The rate at which corticosteroids are tapered is determined by a patient's clinical, immunologic, and radiologic response. Patients should be re-evaluated at 6-week to 8-week intervals during the first year. Total serum IgE levels, chest radiography (CXR), and spirometry should be performed at each visit. When patients are in remission, they should have regularly scheduled follow-up visits every 3 months (per National Asthma Education and Prevention Program guidelines for routine asthma management). Patients should also be assessed with tests associated with ABPA activity, including serum IgE level, spirometry, and CXR at 6-month intervals.[72] During each monitoring visit, patients should be evaluated for (1) the response to therapy, (2) a possible ABPA exacerbation, (3) the level of asthma control, (4) allergen avoidance, and (5) adverse effects of medications and drug-drug interactions. This evaluation requires a focused history, physical examination, and laboratory and radiologic studies (**Fig. 6**). An exacerbation of ABPA should be considered during these monitoring visits if a patient complains of productive cough with large amounts of purulent sputum, worsening dyspnea, or wheezing. In addition, occult ABPA exacerbations without the development of pulmonary symptoms may occur as evidenced by either a new infiltrate on CXR, a doubling of serum IgE, or an unexplained decline in FEV_1 of at least 15%.

Although there are no established criteria for remission of ABPA, most authorities consider that remission has occurred if the clinical and radiologic features of ABPA have resolved along

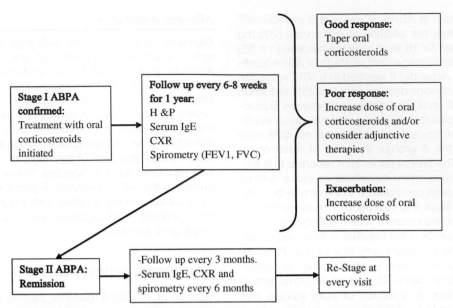

Fig. 6. Monitoring patients with ABPA. Most patients are diagnosed during an exacerbation and oral corticosteroid therapy is initiated. Follow-up should occur every 6 to 8 weeks during the first year. Follow-up may occur quarterly in patients who are in remission. Serial serum IgE measurements are mainly helpful for predicting exacerbations (if the level doubles) rather than predicting response to therapy. HRCT only needs to be repeated if a complication is suspected. FVC, forced vital capacity; H&P, history and physical examination; PO, oral.

with at least a 35% reduction in total serum IgE levels compared with levels during an exacerbation. Agarwal and coworkers[72] recently reported that a 35% reduction in IgE may only be observed in patients with baseline IgE levels exceeding 2500 IU/mL. In patients with lower baseline IgE levels, the decline may be attenuated so that clinical remission occurs with percent reductions as low as 20%.[72] Therefore, serial IgE levels have to be interpreted in the context of clinical and radiologic findings. The total serum IgE levels remain elevated during remissions, and therapy should not directed at reducing the serum IgE level to normal.[56] It has been claimed that the extent of bronchiectasis and the presence of hyperdense mucus on HRCT of the chest are reliable predictors of relapse and inability to achieve complete remission.[45] Therefore, ABPA patients with these radiographic findings should be monitored with heightened vigilance.

SUMMARY

In conclusion, ABPA is a complex hypersensitivity syndrome affecting a small subset of patients with asthma and CF. Despite the similarity in the immune response mounted against Af, ABPA patients have varied pulmonary parenchymal responses. The immunopathogenesis of ABPA remains incompletely understood. The clinical,

laboratory, and radiologic findings of ABPA are varied and not specific, which can delay its diagnosis. Because a delay in diagnosis of ABPA can result in permanent lung destruction, a high index of suspicion for the disease is warranted in appropriate patients. It is hoped that more specific diagnostic assays for ABPA will be developed as well as more insights into the immunopathogenesis of the disease that may identify novel treatment strategies.

REFERENCES

1. Hinson KF, Moon AJ, Plummer NS. Broncho-pulmonary aspergillosis; a review and a report of eight new cases. Thorax 1952;7(4):317–33.
2. Wahner HW, Hepper NG, Andersen HA, et al. Pulmonary aspergillosis. Ann Intern Med 1963;58: 472–85.
3. Vernon DR, Allan F. Environmental factors in allergic bronchopulmonary aspergillosis. Clin Allergy 1980; 10(2):217–27.
4. Shah A, Khan ZU, Chaturvedi S, et al. Concomitant allergic Aspergillus sinusitis and allergic bronchopulmonary aspergillosis associated with familial occurrence of allergic bronchopulmonary aspergillosis. Ann Allergy 1990;64(6):507–12.
5. Starke ID. Asthma and allergic aspergillosis in monozygotic twins. Br J Dis Chest 1985;79(3): 295–300.

6. Mannes GP, van der Heide S, van Aalderen WM, et al. Itraconazole and allergic bronchopulmonary aspergillosis in twin brothers with cystic fibrosis. Lancet 1993;341(8843):492.

7. Chauhan B, Santiago L, Kirschmann DA, et al. The association of HLA-DR alleles and T cell activation with allergic bronchopulmonary aspergillosis. J Immunol 1997;159(8):4072–6.

8. Chauhan B, Knutsen A, Hutcheson PS, et al. T cell subsets, epitope mapping, and HLA-restriction in patients with allergic bronchopulmonary aspergillosis. J Clin Invest 1996;97(10):2324–31.

9. Chauhan B, Santiago L, Hutcheson PS, et al. Evidence for the involvement of two different MHC class II regions in susceptibility or protection in allergic bronchopulmonary aspergillosis. J Allergy Clin Immunol 2000;106(4):723–9.

10. Chauhan B, Hutcheson PS, Slavin RG, et al. MHC restriction in allergic bronchopulmonary aspergillosis. Front Biosci 2003;8:s140–8.

11. Miller PW, Hamosh A, Macek M Jr, et al. Cystic fibrosis transmembrane conductance regulator (CFTR) gene mutations in allergic bronchopulmonary aspergillosis. Am J Hum Genet 1996;59(1):45–51.

12. Eaton TE, Weiner Miller P, Garrett JE, et al. Cystic fibrosis transmembrane conductance regulator gene mutations: do they play a role in the aetiology of allergic bronchopulmonary aspergillosis? Clin Exp Allergy 2002;32(5):756–61.

13. Brouard J, Knauer N, Boelle PY, et al. Influence of interleukin-10 on Aspergillus fumigatus infection in patients with cystic fibrosis. J Infect Dis 2005; 191(11):1988–91.

14. Saxena S, Madan T, Shah A, et al. Association of polymorphisms in the collagen region of SP-A2 with increased levels of total IgE antibodies and eosinophilia in patients with allergic bronchopulmonary aspergillosis. J Allergy Clin Immunol 2003;111(5):1001–7.

15. Patterson R, Greenberger PA, Lee TM, et al. Prolonged evaluation of patients with corticosteroid-dependent asthma stage of allergic bronchopulmonary aspergillosis. J Allergy Clin Immunol 1987;80(5):663–8.

16. Greenberger PA. Allergic bronchopulmonary aspergillosis. J Allergy Clin Immunol 1984;74(5):645–53.

17. Greenberger PA, Smith LJ, Hsu CC, et al. Analysis of bronchoalveolar lavage in allergic bronchopulmonary aspergillosis: divergent responses of antigen-specific antibodies and total IgE. J Allergy Clin Immunol 1988;82(2):164–70.

18. Khan S, McClellan JS, Knutsen AP. Increased sensitivity to IL-4 in patients with allergic bronchopulmonary aspergillosis. Int Arch Allergy Immunol 2000; 123(4):319–26.

19. McCarthy DS, Pepys J. Allergic broncho-pulmonary aspergillosis. Clinical immunology. 2. Skin, nasal and bronchial tests. Clin Allergy 1971;1(4):415–32.

20. Slavin RG, Fischer VW, Levine EA, et al. A primate model of allergic bronchopulmonary aspergillosis. Int Arch Allergy Appl Immunol 1978;56(4):325–33.

21. Bosken CH, Myers JL, Greenberger PA, et al. Pathologic features of allergic bronchopulmonary aspergillosis. Am J Surg Pathol 1988;12(3):216–22.

22. Agarwal R, Aggarwal AN, Gupta D, et al. Aspergillus hypersensitivity and allergic bronchopulmonary aspergillosis in patients with bronchial asthma: systematic review and meta-analysis. Int J Tuberc Lung Dis 2009;13(8):936–44.

23. Mastella G, Rainisio M, Harms HK, et al. Allergic bronchopulmonary aspergillosis in cystic fibrosis. A European epidemiological study. Epidemiologic Registry of Cystic Fibrosis. Eur Respir J 2000; 16(3):464–71.

24. Greenberger PA. Clinical aspects of allergic bronchopulmonary aspergillosis. Front Biosci 2003;8: s119–27.

25. Ricketti AJ, Greenberger PA, Glassroth J. Spontaneous pneumothorax in allergic bronchopulmonary aspergillosis. Arch Intern Med 1984;144(1):151–2.

26. Greenberger PA, Patterson R, Ghory A, et al. Late sequelae of allergic bronchopulmonary aspergillosis. J Allergy Clin Immunol 1980;66(4):327–35.

27. Ricketti AJ, Greenberger PA, Patterson R. Immediate-type reactions in patients with allergic bronchopulmonary aspergillosis. J Allergy Clin Immunol 1983;71(6):541–5.

28. Henderson AH, English MP, Vecht RJ. Pulmonary aspergillosis. A survey of its occurrence in patients with chronic lung disease and a discussion of the significance of diagnostic tests. Thorax 1968;23(5): 513–8.

29. Bousquet J, Chanez P, Lacoste JY, et al. Eosinophilic inflammation in asthma. N Engl J Med 1990; 323(15):1033–9.

30. Schatz M, Wasserman S, Patterson R. The eosinophil and the lung. Arch Intern Med 1982;142(8): 1515–9.

31. Wang JL, Patterson R, Rosenberg M, et al. Serum IgE and IgG antibody activity against Aspergillus fumigatus as a diagnostic aid in allergic bronchopulmonary aspergillosis. Am Rev Respir Dis 1978; 117(5):917–27.

32. Hoehne JH, Reed CE, Dickie HA. Allergic bronchopulmonary aspergillosis is not rare. With a note on preparation of antigen for immunologic tests. Chest 1973;63(2):177–81.

33. Patterson R, Fink JN, Pruzansky JJ, et al. Serum immunoglobulin levels in pulmonary allergic aspergillosis and certain other lung diseases, with special reference to immunoglobulin E. Am J Med 1973; 54(1):16–22.

34. Greenberger PA, Miller TP, Roberts M, et al. Allergic bronchopulmonary aspergillosis in patients with and

without evidence of bronchiectasis. Ann Allergy 1993;70(4):333–8.

35. Rosenberg M, Patterson R, Roberts M, et al. The assessment of immunologic and clinical changes occurring during corticosteroid therapy for allergic bronchopulmonary aspergillosis. Am J Med 1978; 64(4):599–606.

36. Slavin RG, Hutcheson PS, Chauhan B, et al. An overview of allergic bronchopulmonary aspergillosis with some new insights. Allergy Asthma Proc 2004;25(6): 395–9.

37. Greenberger PA. Allergic bronchopulmonary aspergillosis. J Allergy Clin Immunol 2002;110(5):685–92.

38. Fricker-Hidalgo H, Coltey B, Llerena C, et al. Recombinant allergens combined with biological markers in the diagnosis of allergic bronchopulmonary aspergillosis in cystic fibrosis patients. Clin Vaccine Immunol 2010;17(9):1330–6.

39. Latzin P, Hartl D, Regamey N, et al. Comparison of serum markers for allergic bronchopulmonary aspergillosis in cystic fibrosis. Eur Respir J 2008; 31(1):36–42.

40. McCarthy DS, Simon G, Hargreave FE. The radiological appearances in allergic broncho-pulmonary aspergillosis. Clin Radiol 1970;21(4):366–75.

41. Agarwal R, Srinivas R, Agarwal AN, et al. Pulmonary masses in allergic bronchopulmonary aspergillosis: mechanistic explanations. Respir Care 2008;53(12): 1744–8.

42. Agarwal R. Allergic bronchopulmonary aspergillosis. Chest 2009;135(3):805–26.

43. Neeld DA, Goodman LR, Gurney JW, et al. Computerized tomography in the evaluation of allergic bronchopulmonary aspergillosis. Am Rev Respir Dis 1990;142(5):1200–5.

44. Ward S, Heyneman L, Lee MJ, et al. Accuracy of CT in the diagnosis of allergic bronchopulmonary aspergillosis in asthmatic patients. AJR Am J Roentgenol 1999;173(4):937–42.

45. Agarwal R, Gupta D, Aggarwal AN, et al. Clinical significance of hyperattenuating mucoid impaction in allergic bronchopulmonary aspergillosis: an analysis of 155 patients. Chest 2007;132(4):1183–90.

46. Agarwal R, Khan A, Gupta D, et al. An alternate method of classifying allergic bronchopulmonary aspergillosis based on high-attenuation mucus. PLoS One 2010;5(12):e15346.

47. Dykewicz MS, Hamilos DL. Rhinitis and sinusitis. J Allergy Clin Immunol 2010;125(2 Suppl 2):S103–15.

48. Sher TH, Schwartz HJ. Allergic Aspergillus sinusitis with concurrent allergic bronchopulmonary Aspergillus: report of a case. J Allergy Clin Immunol 1988;81(5 Pt 1):844–6.

49. Erwin GE, Fitzgerald JE. Case report: allergic bronchopulmonary aspergillosis and allergic fungal sinusitis successfully treated with voriconazole. J Asthma 2007;44(10):891–5.

50. Patterson R, Greenberger PA, Radin RC, et al. Allergic bronchopulmonary aspergillosis: staging as an aid to management. Ann Intern Med 1982; 96(3):286–91.

51. Patterson R, Greenberger PA, Halwig JM, et al. Allergic bronchopulmonary aspergillosis. Natural history and classification of early disease by serologic and roentgenographic studies. Arch Intern Med 1986;146(5):916–8.

52. Milla CE. Allergic bronchopulmonary aspergillosis and cystic fibrosis. Pediatr Pulmonol 1999;27(2): 71–3.

53. Hutcheson PS, Rejent AJ, Slavin RG. Variability in parameters of allergic bronchopulmonary aspergillosis in patients with cystic fibrosis. J Allergy Clin Immunol 1991;88(3 Pt 1):390–4.

54. Stevens DA, Moss RB, Kurup VP, et al. Allergic bronchopulmonary aspergillosis in cystic fibrosis—state of the art: Cystic Fibrosis Foundation Consensus Conference. Clin Infect Dis 2003;37(Suppl 3):S225–64.

55. Patterson R, Greenberger PA, Ricketti AJ, et al. A radioimmunoassay index for allergic bronchopulmonary aspergillosis. Ann Intern Med 1983;99(1): 18–22.

56. Lee TM, Greenberger PA, Patterson R, et al. Stage V (fibrotic) allergic bronchopulmonary aspergillosis. A review of 17 cases followed from diagnosis. Arch Intern Med 1987;147(2):319–23.

57. Agarwal R, Gupta D, Aggarwal AN, et al. Allergic bronchopulmonary aspergillosis: lessons from 126 patients attending a chest clinic in north India. Chest 2006;130(2):442–8.

58. Thomson JM, Wesley A, Byrnes CA, et al. Pulse intravenous methylprednisolone for resistant allergic bronchopulmonary aspergillosis in cystic fibrosis. Pediatr Pulmonol 2006;41(2):164–70.

59. Cohen-Cymberknoh M, Blau H, Shoseyov D, et al. Intravenous monthly pulse methylprednisolone treatment for ABPA in patients with cystic fibrosis. J Cyst Fibros 2009;8(4):253–7.

60. Shale DJ, Faux JA, Lane DJ. Trial of ketoconazole in non-invasive pulmonary aspergillosis. Thorax 1987; 42(1):26–31.

61. Fournier EC. Trial of ketoconazole in allergic bronchopulmonary aspergillosis. Thorax 1987;42(10):831.

62. Stevens DA, Schwartz HJ, Lee JY, et al. A randomized trial of itraconazole in allergic bronchopulmonary aspergillosis. N Engl J Med 2000;342(11): 756–62.

63. Wark PA, Hensley MJ, Saltos N, et al. Anti-inflammatory effect of itraconazole in stable allergic bronchopulmonary aspergillosis: a randomized controlled trial. J Allergy Clin Immunol 2003;111(5):952–7.

64. Skov M, Main KM, Sillesen IB, et al. Iatrogenic adrenal insufficiency as a side-effect of combined treatment of itraconazole and budesonide. Eur Respir J 2002;20(1):127–33.

65. Hilliard T, Edwards S, Buchdahl R, et al. Voriconazole therapy in children with cystic fibrosis. J Cyst Fibros 2005;4(4):215–20.

66. Glackin L, Leen G, Elnazir B, et al. Voriconazole in the treatment of allergic bronchopulmonary aspergillosis in cystic fibrosis. Ir Med J 2009; 102(1):29.

67. Berge M, Guillemain R, Boussaud V, et al. Voriconazole pharmacokinetic variability in cystic fibrosis lung transplant patients. Transpl Infect Dis 2009; 11(3):211–9.

68. van der Ent CK, Hoekstra H, Rijkers GT. Successful treatment of allergic bronchopulmonary aspergillosis with recombinant anti-IgE antibody. Thorax 2007; 62(3):276–7.

69. Zirbes JM, Milla CE. Steroid-sparing effect of omalizumab for allergic bronchopulmonary aspergillosis and cystic fibrosis. Pediatr Pulmonol 2008;43(6): 607–10.

70. Kanu A, Patel K. Treatment of allergic bronchopulmonary aspergillosis (ABPA) in CF with anti-IgE antibody (omalizumab). Pediatr Pulmonol 2008;43(12): 1249–51.

71. Radin RC, Greenberger PA, Patterson R, et al. Mould counts and exacerbations of allergic bronchopulmonary aspergillosis. Clin Allergy 1983;13(3):271–5.

72. Agarwal R, Gupta D, Aggarwal AN, et al. Clinical significance of decline in serum IgE levels in allergic bronchopulmonary aspergillosis. Respir Med 2010; 104(2):204–10.

Bronchiectasis and Nontuberculous Mycobacterial Disease

David E. Griffith, MD[a],*, Timothy R. Aksamit, MD[b]

KEYWORDS

- Nontuberculous mycobacteria • Bronchiectasis • *Mycobacterium avium* complex
- *Mycobacterium abscessus*

KEY POINTS

- Bronchiectasis and nontuberculous mycobacterial (NTM) lung disease are inextricably linked pathophysiologically.
- *Mycobacterium avium* complex (MAC) is the most frequently encountered NTM respiratory pathogen in bronchiectasis patients.
- Therapy for NTM respiratory pathogens in bronchiectasis patients should be guided by published guidelines.
- Diagnosis of NTM lung disease in bronchiectasis patients does not always necessitate therapy directed against the NTM pathogen.
- Optimal management of patients with bronchiectasis and NTM lung disease requires carefully considered treatment of both conditions.

To paraphrase that underappreciated philosopher Forrest Gump, nontuberculous mycobacterial (NTM) lung infections and bronchiectasis "goes together like peas and carrots."[1] Although this assertion may seem self-evident now, it has in fact only recently become widely accepted. As a corollary, it is also axiomatic that many patients with NTM lung disease have at least one additional lung disease, either bronchiectasis or chronic obstructive pulmonary disease (or both), necessitating treatment of more than one disease process in most patients with NTM lung disease. The interplay between NTM lung infections and bronchiectasis is growing progressively more complex and encompasses fundamental pathophysiologic and management considerations, including assessment of

which is the primary disease process, which disease is a predisposition to the other, when and how should NTM disease be treated in the presence of bronchiectasis, and what are the optimal management strategies for bronchiectasis. In the relatively brief time that has elapsed since the recognition that these 2 diseases are intimately related, a deepening appreciation is evolving for the complex interaction between them. There is, however, little lingering doubt that NTM infections and bronchiectasis are inextricably linked (**Fig. 1**).

Two impediments had to be overcome before the association of NTM disease and bronchiectasis would be widely embraced. The first, and most important, was the description of NTM lung disease in patients who did not present with the expected

The authors have no financial conflicts of interest to disclose.

D.E.G. is supported in part by the W.A. and E.B. Moncrief Distinguished Professorship.

[a] Pulmonary and Critical Care Division, Department of Medicine, University of Texas Health Science Center, Tyler, 11937 U.S. Highway 271, Tyler, TX 75708, USA

[b] Department of Internal Medicine, Mayo Clinic College of Medicine, 200 First Street SE, Rochester, MN 55905, USA

* Corresponding author.

E-mail address: david.griffith@uthct.edu

Clin Chest Med 33 (2012) 283–295

doi:10.1016/j.ccm.2012.02.002

0272-5231/12/$ – see front matter © 2012 Elsevier Inc. All rights reserved.

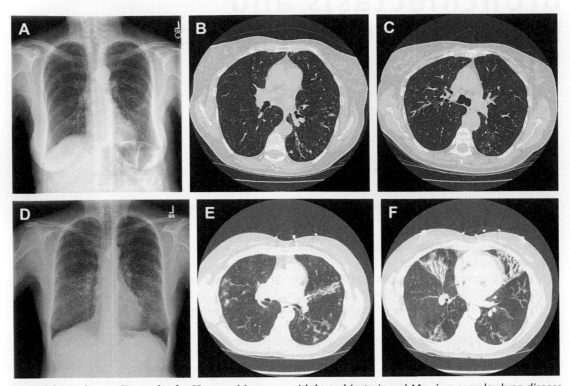

Fig. 1. (*A*) P/A chest radiograph of a 62-year-old woman with bronchiectasis and *M avium* complex lung disease, showing bilateral primarily midlung nodular and reticulonodular densities. (*B, C*) HRCT images of the same patient demonstrating bronchiectasis, nodular densities, and tree-in-bud densities. (*D*) Posteroanterior (P/A) chest radiograph of a 74-year-old woman with bronchiectasis and *Mycobacterium avium* complex lung disease, showing bilateral primarily midlung nodular and reticulonodular densities. (*E, F*) High-resolution chest CT (HRCT) images of the same patient demonstrating bronchiectasis with destruction of the right middle lobe and lingula, nodular densities, and tree-in-bud densities characteristic of mycobacterial lung infection.

radiographic findings typical of reactivation tuberculosis (TB) and traditionally accepted to be also typical of NTM lung disease.[2] Credit for this observation is generally attributed to Prince and colleagues,[3] who published a seminal article describing *Mycobacterium avium* complex (MAC) lung infection in older women without underlying lung disease other than bronchiectasis. In retrospect, there was some anticipation for this observation evident in previous work. In 1979, as part of the first comprehensive description of NTM diseases, Emanuel Wolinsky[2] wrote, "The average case of *M kansasii* or *M avium-intracellulare* disease would be a 48-year-old white man with longstanding lung disease, such as chronic obstructive pulmonary disease or silicosis... The chest roentgenogram shows fibrosis and a thin walled cavity in the right upper lobe and sputum is positive for AFB on smear." Wolinsky added, "It must be emphasized, however, that cases do occur in women, in younger men, and in middle aged men without apparent lung disease or deficiency of cellular immunity" and that bronchiectasis was

among the "most common predisposing conditions..." for NTM pulmonary disease.[2]

Also in 1979, Rosenzweig[4] published the findings from a series of 100 consecutive patients with MAC lung disease in Wisconsin. Although there is limited detail about the radiographic abnormalities in this cohort, 24 patient radiographs were described as either "minimal" or "moderate noncavitary." Of additional interest, all but 1 of the women in this series older than 50 years were Caucasian, whereas in other age groups, for both men and women, there was a more diverse racial distribution. In a statement all too familiar today, Rosenzweig noted, "While the tuberculosis caseload has declined steadily in the past 10–15 years in our clinic, cases of atypical mycobacterial infection, especially with *M intracellulare-avium*, have grown from a trickle to numbers which currently rival those of tuberculosis." In 1982, Ahn and colleagues[5] described a group of 66 patients with sputum cultures that were repeatedly positive for MAC or *Mycobacterium kansasii*, who also had noncavitary radiographic changes described as "…changes resembling infiltration of some type, mostly fibrotic." These patients were noted to attain more rapid conversion of sputum to acid-fast bacilli (AFB) culture negativity with therapy when compared with patients with cavitary radiographic abnormalities, although the apparent rapid microbiological response to therapy was not associated with significant radiographic improvement. Longitudinal follow-up of these patients, a step necessary to show convincingly that they had MAC infection and disease rather than "colonization," was unfortunately not reported. That important step was, however, accomplished by Prince and colleagues,[3] who described patients with noncavitary MAC lung disease including a subpopulation who had progressive lung disease resulting in death. It subsequently became clear that this form of MAC lung disease, henceforth referred to as the nodular/bronchiectatic form of NTM lung disease, could be seen not only with MAC, but with essentially any NTM respiratory pathogen, albeit most commonly with MAC.[6–9]

The second and perhaps less well appreciated barrier that was overcome was a technological one. Until approximately 25 years ago, the diagnostic proof for bronchiectasis required the performance of bronchography (bronchograms), a rather medieval radiographic procedure that requires instillation of radiographic dye into the tracheobronchial tree, an experience that few patients would voluntarily repeat. The technological advance was the advent of computed tomography (CT) of the chest and, specifically, high-resolution chest CT (HRCT) scanning.[10,11] It is interesting that widespread acceptance of CT scanning of the chest as a reliable diagnostic test for bronchiectasis was not immediate, and as late as the mid-1990s some reviewers were hesitant to accept CT abnormalities alone as diagnostic for bronchiectasis.[12] At present, HRCT scanning is the standard for diagnosing bronchiectasis, as well as following the course of the disease and related comorbidities such as NTM infections.

With the advent of better diagnostic tools, bronchiectasis has emerged as a much more readily recognized and more frequently diagnosed disease entity, perhaps not coincidentally in tandem with increased recognition of NTM lung disease. As previously noted, this association was not immediately demonstrated or widely appreciated. In some initial studies assessing the microbiological findings from patients with bronchiectasis, the isolation prevalence of NTM ranged from 0% to 40%.[12–16] Some of this discrepancy might be explained by geographic differences, particularly between the United States and Europe, but it is also possible that the application of uniform and rigorous microbiological methodology would yield more consistent NTM isolation from patients in disparate geographic locations.

PATHOPHYSIOLOGY: CHICKEN AND EGG

Is NTM pulmonary disease a consequence or the cause (or both) of bronchiectasis? There are lines of evidence that support both contentions. First, it is clear that patients with severe generalized bronchiectasis, for whatever reason, are predisposed to acquiring NTM infection and in some instances progressive NTM disease. The best-described bronchiectasis-associated disease that is recognized as a predisposition for NTM infection is cystic fibrosis (CF). Olivier and colleagues[17,18] reported the results of a multicenter study evaluating the prevalence of NTM respiratory isolates in CF patients. These studies found that 13% of the CF patients had NTM respiratory isolates, including 72% MAC and 16% Mycobacterium abscessus. A reliable algorithm that can predict which CF patients with NTM respiratory isolates will have progressive NTM disease and which patients, especially those with MAC respiratory isolates, require therapy directed against the NTM pathogen, has not emerged to date. The pathogen of most concern is M abscessus, because of case reports describing rapid clinical deterioration and even death in some CF patients infected by M abscessus.[19] This concern is unfortunately confounded by the difficulty in effectively treating M abscessus, resulting in a complicated risk/benefit decision in the absence of a mechanism for accurately predicting those patients who will have disease progression and those likely to have satisfactory treatment response. In addition to CF patients, NTM respiratory isolates have been reported in 10% of patients with cilial dyskinesia syndromes and bronchiectasis.[20]

It has long been postulated that prior TB is a risk factor for NTM respiratory disease, and it has been assumed that postinflammatory bronchiectasis was likely responsible for this association.[2,21] A question that is still debated is whether mycobacterial pathogens other than M tuberculosis can cause postinflammatory bronchiectasis. For a pathogen such as M kansasii, which is the NTM that causes lung disease clinically and radiographically most similar to reactivation TB, it is perhaps easier to accept this association than with a less virulent NTM pathogen such as MAC. In a series of reports from Japan, Fujita and colleagues[22,23] described the pathologic findings after partial lung resections from a small number of patients diagnosed with MAC lung disease. All patients had presurgical cavitary MAC lung disease radiographically. Pathologic findings from these patients included bronchiectasis, bronchiolitis, nodules, and extensive granuloma formation throughout the airways. These findings suggested that at least for cavitary MAC lung disease, bronchiectasis was a common and expected pathologic consequence of MAC infection.

It is perhaps relatively easy to accept that cavitary NTM disease caused by any NTM pathogen might result in postinflammatory bronchiectasis. It is clear, however, that the nodular/bronchiectatic form of the disease is more difficult to accept in this role. In a brief but tantalizing report, Tanaka and colleagues[24] reported a small group of patients with nodular/bronchiectatic MAC disease who appeared to have the initial appearance of nodules followed temporally by bronchiectasis formation in the bronchi subtending these nodules. Unfortunately, aside from this incomplete and inconclusive report, there is little current evidence to support the evolution of bronchiectasis in patients with nodular/bronchiectatic lung disease resulting from an initial peripheral MAC infection, granulomatous inflammation, and nodule formation.

The debate has recently been intensified by the demonstration of a disproportionately large prevalence of NTM lung disease patients with primarily nodular/bronchiectatic NTM lung disease who are heterozygous for CF or α_1-antitrypsin (AAT) mutations.[25–28] Kim and colleagues[25] recently reported a characteristic body habitus in 63 patients with nodular/bronchiectatic NTM lung disease evaluated at the National Institutes of Health. In this population of mostly postmenopausal Caucasian women, the body mass index was significantly lower and the height significantly greater than in matched controls. There were no recognized immune defects, cell-mediated dysfunction, or cytokine-pathway abnormalities identified in these patients, and no significant or unusual correlations regarding environmental water exposure. This population did have higher rates of scoliosis, pectus excavatum, and mitral valve prolapse, compared with a matched control population. In this select population, cystic fibrosis transmembrane conductance regulator (CFTR) gene mutations were found significantly more commonly than in the general population but with no consistent correlation between sweat chloride concentrations and CFTR variants. It has also recently been noted in a study from Japan[29] that patients presenting with pulmonary NTM disease have mutations in the CFTR gene significantly more frequently than in the general population.

Prior dogma has suggested that patients with single CFTR mutations do not have sufficient bronchial mucosal ion and water-transport disturbance to cause clinically detectable CF with abnormal chloride test results for sweat. Recent data, however, suggest that even heterozygous CFTR mutations may be associated with abnormalities of bronchial epithelial ion transport. Patients with bronchiectasis without CF mutations, patients heterozygous for CFTR mutations, and patients with homozygous CFTR mutations were found to have a continuum of nasal mucosal potential differences compatible with a spectrum of abnormalities related to mucosal ion transport.[30] This apparent bronchial mucosal ion and water-transport abnormality seems plausible as a possible mechanism for bronchiectasis development and a potential explanation for why an apparently high percentage of women with nodular/bronchiectatic disease have CFTR mutations without frank CF. An alternative explanation might be that these patients are not truly heterozygous for CFTR mutations but have an additional unidentified CFTR mutation or polymorphism that would indicate actual CF, and more readily explain a pathway to bronchiectasis development. To date, no clear mechanistic connections have been discovered between the characteristic body habitus described earlier, single CFTR mutations, and the pathogenesis of bronchiectasis. These patients are undeniably intriguing, and may provide clues to the pathogenesis of NTM lung disease in at least a subset of patients.

These data also beg 2 important questions. First, should all patients with bronchiectasis and NTM disease be screened for genetic or hereditary predispositions for bronchiectasis, such as CF, AAT deficiency, or immune globulin deficiency? It is arguable that immune globulin deficiency and AAT deficiency are treatable and, even if rarely identified, would lead to a specific therapeutic intervention. The CF evaluation, however, is expensive, and even with a 20% to 30% yield in selected populations may not be a cost-effective strategy other than as a guide for genetic counseling for a patient's family.[25] Outside of research settings this remains an unsettled question, although there is some agreement among experts that younger patients with bilateral and/or diffuse bronchiectasis are the population most likely to yield positive results with these analyses. The second question is perhaps somewhat less controversial: should all patients with bronchiectasis be screened for NTM pathogens? This question takes on perhaps even more urgency with the current recommendation for the use of a macrolide as an immune-modulating agent in patients with CF, and the recent suggestion that macrolide might also benefit some patients with frequent exacerbations of chronic obstructive pulmonary disease (COPD).[31,32] The use of macrolide monotherapy for patients also at risk for NTM lung disease raises the specter that macrolide-resistant NTM isolates, especially MAC isolates, might emerge in a patient with occult or unrecognized NTM (MAC) lung disease. It seems reasonable that any patient with bronchiectasis considered for macrolide monotherapy should have sputum collected for AFB analysis initially and then intermittently afterward, as recommended for CF patients.[20] In addition, it also seems reasonable that sputum should be evaluated for NTM in any patient with bronchiectasis with unexplained clinical deterioration or new and unexplained radiographic abnormalities.

PATHOPHYSIOLOGY: NTM ACQUISITION

The source of NTM respiratory pathogens is still assumed to be the environment, with increasing concern that biofilms that form in municipal water sources may be a significant source for NTM. Feazel and colleagues[33] recently analyzed rRNA gene sequences from 45 showerhead biofilm sites around the United States. Sequences indicating *M avium* were identified in 20% of showerhead swabs. Using a quantitative polymerase chain reaction with *M avium*–specific primers, *M avium* DNA was detected in 20 additional biofilm swab samples in which *M avium* was not encountered in their RNA gene libraries.

Using microbiological techniques, Nishiuchi and colleagues[34] reported the recovery of MAC from residential bathrooms of patients in Japan with pulmonary MAC disease. MAC was isolated from 10 of 371 patient residence cultures versus 1 of 33 control households. Two patients with MAC lung disease were found to have identical sputum and bathroom MAC genotypes. Falkinham[35] recently reported that NTM were isolated from the household water systems of 59% of patients with NTM lung disease. In 7 households, the patient isolate and 1 plumbing isolate showed similar genotype patterns. Two additional reports have demonstrated identical genotypes of MAC isolated from plumbing and MAC isolates obtained from humans with MAC lung disease, including one with conventional MAC lung infection and one with hypersensitivity-like lung disease.[36,37]

Even in the context of this provocative data, it is still unknown how much of a risk NTM in plumbing presents and whether municipal plumbing in general, and showerheads specifically, represent a significant or common source of NTM for patients with NTM lung disease. The ubiquity of the organisms in the environment, along with what appears to be inevitable and universal environmental exposure and the seemingly endless variety of NTM (especially MAC) genotypes, makes the task of matching environmental and patient NTM isolate genotypes challenging to say the least. In the context of this daunting task, patients inevitably ask if they should continue to take showers, knowing that NTM are part of the flora of modern municipal water systems. In the opinion of the authors there is likely some risk of NTM infection and disease transmission via this route, but NTM organisms are ubiquitous and exposure is unavoidable even if patients abstain from showering or bathing, also an unsavory public health prospect.

DIAGNOSIS: NTM LUNG DISEASE IN BRONCHIECTASIS PATIENTS

The diagnosis of NTM lung disease is dependent on 3 components: patient symptoms, radiographic findings, and microbiological results. In the setting of bronchiectasis, symptom evaluation is complicated because of the shared symptoms of bronchiectasis and NTM lung disease, including cough, sputum production, fatigue, and weight loss. A change or progression of symptoms may presage the diagnosis of NTM lung disease. Similarly, the radiographic abnormalities of bronchiectasis may mask or confuse radiographic changes associated with NTM disease and infection. Again, new or progressive radiographic abnormalities, not thought to be due to an acute bacterial process such as pneumonitis or bronchiectatic exacerbation, would provide a clue to possible NTM infection and disease. Certainly some radiographic patterns such as tree-in-bud abnormalities, nodules, and cavitation would raise suspicion for NTM lung disease, even in the absence of symptomatic change (see **Fig. 1**).[38–41]

Ultimately the microbiological evaluation will be the final arbiter of NTM disease diagnosis in patients with bronchiectasis. The NTM are all found in 1 or multiple niches in the environment so that isolation of any NTM species can be the consequence of environmental contamination, especially contamination by nonsterile (tap) water sources. Hence, diagnostic criteria for respiratory NTM isolates are necessary to aid in the determination of which NTM isolates are clinically significant (**Box 1**).[21] It is readily conceded that one set of diagnostic criteria could not be and is not appropriate or applicable to more than 100

Box 1
Suggested microbiological diagnostic criteria for NTM lung disease

1. Pulmonary symptoms associated with either cavitary or nodular/bronchiectatic radiographic (chest radiograph or HRCT scan) abnormalities.

2. Exclusion of other diagnoses such as tuberculosis

3. Positive AFB culture results from at least 2 separate expectorated sputum samples

4. Positive culture result from at least one bronchial wash or lavage

5. Transbronchial or other lung biopsy with compatible histopathologic features (granulomatous inflammation or AFB smear positive) and positive AFB culture for NTM, OR biopsy showing compatible histopathologic features and one or more sputum or bronchial washings that are culture positive for NTM

Data from Griffith DE, Aksamit T, Brown-Elliott BA, et al. ATS Mycobacterial Diseases Subcommittee; American Thoracic Society; Infectious Disease Society of America. An official ATS/IDSA statement: diagnosis, treatment, and prevention of nontuberculous mycobacterial diseases. Am J Respir Crit Care Med 2007;175(4):367–6 [review. erratum in: Am J Respir Crit Care Med 2007;175(7):744–5].

species of NTM. A clinician evaluating these patients cannot uncritically apply these diagnostic criteria, and must have knowledge about the virulence of the NTM species isolated and the host from which the organism was isolated.

The diagnosis of NTM lung disease based on a single positive NTM culture from a bronchoscopic specimen merits particular attention (see Box 1). This criterion was adopted specifically for application to patients with nodular/bronchiectatic NTM disease who are frequently unable to produce sputum for AFB analysis and for whom serial bronchoscopies would be either impractical or risky. The important caveat for this recommendation is that common NTM pathogens such as MAC, M kansasii, Mycobacterium simiae, Mycobacterium fortuitum, and M abscessus can be found in municipal (tap) water so that contamination of a bronchoscopic specimen with tap water can result in a false-positive bronchoscopic culture (pseudoinfection), triggering unnecessary and potentially toxic therapy. Again, uncritical application of the diagnostic guidelines may cause more harm than benefit.

There are NTM species such as M kansasii and Mycobacterium szulgai that are almost always associated with significant disease when isolated from respiratory specimens.[21] In some cases, lung disease might be diagnosed on the basis of one positive culture for these organisms (especially M kansasii). Conversely, there are NTM such M simiae and M fortuitum that are usually not respiratory pathogens, even if the NTM diagnostic criteria are met.[6,42] Lastly there are NTM species such as Mycobacterium gordonae and Mycobacterium terrae complex, which almost always represent contamination of respiratory specimens.[21]

Other diagnostic techniques to augment the current diagnostic criteria remain under investigation but are not currently recommended for general use. Skin testing with NTM antigens has been of interest for many years, especially in the context of NTM disease prevalence, but the role of skin testing for diagnosing NTM disease in individual patients is not established.[21] Another novel approach is a serologic test based on an enzyme immunoassay (EIA) kit detecting serum immunoglobulin A (IgA) antibody to glycopeptidolipid core antigen specific for MAC.[43] This technique offers promise in identifying patients with MAC lung disease and differentiating patients with MAC lung disease from TB patients. There is, however, considerable overlap in serum IgA-antibody levels between the patient groups. It remains to be determined as to where this test will fit in the overall evaluation of patients with suspected MAC lung disease. Certainly in this population of sometimes frail, elderly individuals with bronchiectasis and NTM lung disease who have difficulty producing sputum for AFB analysis, some type of noninvasive, nonmicrobiological-based diagnostic test would be of great value.

Time and patience are perhaps the only two luxuries in the diagnostic evaluation of these patients, owing to the indolence of nodular/bronchiectatic NTM disease. Careful evaluation of the microbiological and radiographic data over time in conjunction with the patient's symptoms is invaluable and can boost the diagnostic confidence of the physician and patient who is, after all, facing many months of potentially toxic therapy. It cannot be overstressed, however, that making the diagnosis of NTM lung disease in a bronchiectasis patient does not, per se, necessitate the institution of therapy. Alternatively, the coexistence of bronchiectasis and NTM infection does not in any way preclude treatment of the NTM, as some patients may experience an accelerated respiratory decline without such therapy. The decision to initiate treatment for patients with

NTM lung disease is ultimately a decision based on risk/benefit analysis, taking into account patient symptoms, radiographic findings (progression), and microbiological results versus the adverse effects of multiple potentially toxic and relatively weak drugs. In addition, the authors do not recommend empiric treatment of suspected NTM lung disease in the absence of isolation and identification of an NTM pathogen.

THERAPY FOR NTM LUNG DISEASE

It has been approximately 25 years since the newer macrolides, clarithromycin and the closely related azalide azithromycin, were recognized as the key element in successful treatment regimens for multiple NTM species, especially MAC. The limitations of macrolide-containing regimens for NTM pathogens are now abundantly clear, and it is equally clear that new, more potent medications are needed to improve therapy for NTM disease.

An especially frustrating problem in the management of patients with NTM lung disease is the observation that in vitro susceptibility testing may not be a reliable predictor for in vivo response to antibiotics, as it is in the therapy for TB. The most clinically vexing example is MAC, where there is, so far, only evidence to support a correlation between in vitro macrolide susceptibility and in vivo clinical response.[21,44–47] Both the Clinical and Laboratory Standard Institute and the American Thoracic Society (ATS) recommend that new MAC isolates should be tested in vitro only for susceptibility to macrolides.[21] Understandably, clinicians still cling to in vitro susceptibility reports for MAC isolates that list multiple agents as either "susceptible" or "resistant" based on in vitro minimum inhibitory concentrations (MICs), even though those MICs have not been shown to correlate with in vivo response to the antibiotics tested. Perhaps not surprisingly, there are multiple other NTM species and pathogens that share this frustrating property with MAC, including, among many others, M simiae, Mycobacterium xenopi, Mycobacterium malmoense, and M abscessus.[21] It should be noted as well that there are several species for which in vitro susceptibility testing can be a reliable guide for successful therapy, including M kansasii, Mycobacterium marinum, Mycobacterium szulgai, and M fortuitum.[21]

The explanation for this somewhat inconvenient aspect of NTM behavior is not yet clear, but recent work with rapidly growing mycobacteria (RGM) may offer a window into the complex relationship between in vitro responses and the in vivo effect of antibiotics for NTM. Macrolide antimicrobial agents act by binding to the 50S ribosomal subunit and inhibiting peptide synthesis. Erythromycin methylase (erm) genes, a diverse collection of methylases that impair binding of macrolides to ribosomes, reduce the inhibitory activity of these agents. The primary mechanism of acquired clinically significant macrolide resistance for some mycobacteria, especially RGM, is the presence of an inducible erm gene (erm 41).[48,49] All isolates of M abscessus and M fortuitum, but not Mycobacterium chelonae, contain an inducible erm gene. The most interesting and frustrating aspect of this inducible gene is that if an M fortuitum or M abscessus isolate is exposed to macrolide, the erm gene activity is induced, with subsequent in vivo macrolide resistance that may not be reflected by the initial in vitro MIC of the organism for the macrolide! In other words, the organism may appear to be susceptible in vitro to the macrolide but will not respond to the macrolide in vivo.

To expose this inducible macrolide resistance, termed cryptic resistance, requires incubation of an NTM isolate with macrolide before determining an MIC for the macrolide. This discovery offers one explanation for the discrepancy between in vitro susceptibility results and in vivo responses for M abscessus and M fortuitum. There is no erm gene in MAC, and the primary mechanism for the emergence of macrolide-resistant MAC strains is still the selection of 23S rRNA gene mutations with macrolide monotherapy. It is important to ask, however, if there could be other inducible genes that confer in vivo resistance to antibiotics for MAC. It is an intriguing, if unproved, possibility.

Mycobacterium avium Complex Lung Disease

The decision to treat patients with MAC lung disease, especially the nodular/bronchiectatic form of MAC lung disease, should be based on potential risks and benefits of therapy for individual patients. Treatment of MAC lung disease is long, expensive, frequently associated with drug-related toxicities, and requires considerable commitment on the part of the patient and physician. Clinical improvement and sputum conversion to AFB-culture negativity for 12 months while on therapy are the main treatment goals, but for many patients may not be attainable. Recent guidelines suggest that MAC treatment regimens should include a rifamycin (rifampicin or rifabutin), ethambutol, and a macrolide (azithromycin or clarithromycin).[21] An example of successful MAC therapy with a macrolide-based regimen is illustrated in **Fig. 2**. Multidrug regimens can be given daily or intermittently, depending on the disease type and severity. Cavitary disease and disease caused by documented relapse after previous

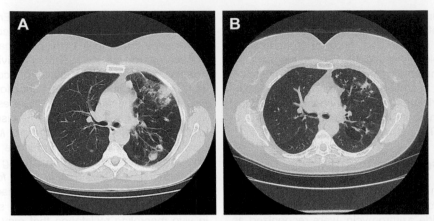

Fig. 2. (A) HRCT image of a 60-year-old woman with bronchiectasis diagnosed with *M avium* complex (MAC) lung disease before initiation of therapy, demonstrating primarily large nodular densities. (B) Comparable HRCT image after successful treatment of MAC lung disease with a macrolide-based regimen for a duration including 12 months of sputum AFB-culture negativity while on therapy.

successful therapy should be treated with daily drug dosing, as intermittent therapy is frequently not effective in these patients.[50] For moderate or severe disease, or for patients not responding to standard oral drug regimens, parenteral agents such as streptomycin or amikacin can be included in the treatment regimen. The optimal duration for parenteral therapy is not established, but in the authors' experience, patients may require these drugs for 6 months or longer to determine their efficacy. The inclusion of parenteral agents in MAC treatment regimens increases culture conversion rates, but does not appear to improve long-term outcome.[51]

A critical element in the management of patients with MAC lung disease is prevention of the emergence of macrolide-resistant MAC. While the role of in vitro susceptibility for other agents remains controversial, it is clear that the development of macrolide resistance in a MAC isolate (MIC >16 μg/mL) is strongly associated with treatment failure and increased mortality.[52] The most important risk factors for developing macrolide-resistant MAC are macrolide monotherapy and the combination of a macrolide and fluoroquinolone without an effective third companion drug. It is a therapeutic imperative that clinicians protect patients from the emergence of macrolide-resistant MAC isolates.

Several aspects of therapy for MAC lung disease remain controversial, including the roles of clofazimine, fluoroquinolones, and inhaled amikacin. There are limited data that suggest a possible role for clofazimine and nebulized amikacin in the treatment of MAC lung disease, but no large or convincing trials that would support routine or first-line use of these agents.[53,54] There

are essentially no data demonstrating the efficacy of fluoroquinolones for the treatment of MAC lung disease.

Other inconvenient aspects of the treatment of MAC lung disease include the observation that after an initial treatment failure, even if a MAC isolate remains macrolide susceptible, subsequent treatment efforts will be less effective.[44,46] In addition, patients who are successfully treated with sputum conversion to AFB-culture negativity are likely to have new MAC genotypes (strains) if the sputum again becomes culture-positive for MAC as opposed to recurrence of the original MAC genotype (disease relapse).[55] It has been proposed that this phenomenon can be explained by reinfection of the patient by a new MAC genotype, although polyclonal infections cannot be completely discounted. These "reinfection" MAC isolates are uniformly macrolide susceptible. Some patients with bronchiectasis and NTM infections do not respond, for unclear reasons, to what seem to be appropriate multidrug regimens (**Fig. 3**). These patients are perhaps the most challenging and frustrating for clinicians who manage NTM lung disease.

Mycobacterium abscessus Lung Disease

Jeon and colleagues[56] recently reported the results of therapy in a series of 69 patients, 84% female, with *M abscessus* lung disease. The patients were treated with a regimen consisting of an initial 1 month of parenteral therapy with amikacin and cefoxitin while hospitalized, in combination with oral medications including clarithromycin, ciprofloxacin, and doxycycline for a median of 24 months. Forty-seven of 69 patients (68%)

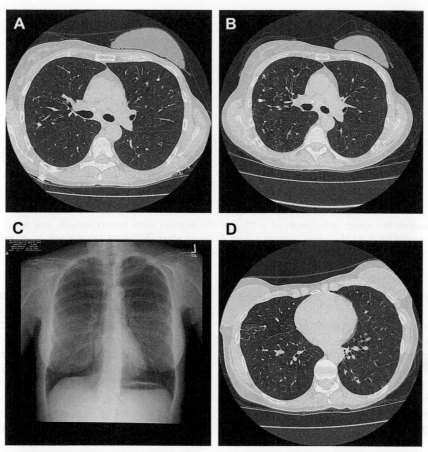

Fig. 3. (*A*) HRCT image of a 62-year-old woman with bronchiectasis and one cystic fibrosis transmembrane regulator (CFTR) gene mutation diagnosed with MAC lung disease before initiation of therapy. (*B*) Comparable HRCT image after 24 months of treatment for MAC lung disease including 12 months' therapy with a parenteral agent and right middle lobe lobectomy, and with persistently positive sputum AFB cultures for MAC. (*C*) P/A chest radiograph of a 64-year-old woman with minimal mid-lung field densities before initiating multidrug MAC therapy with a macrolide-based regimen. (*D*) HRCT image showing minimal right middle lobe tree-in-bud abnormalities from the same patient after 12 months of multidrug macrolide-containing therapy, with sputum still AFB-culture–positive for MAC.

converted sputum to negative, with a median time to sputum conversion of 1 month. Nine of 47 patients (19%) relapsed after a median of 12 months. Sputum conversion with macrolide-resistant strains occurred in 27% of patients versus 71% with macrolide-susceptible strains, while relapse occurred in 100% of patients with macrolide-resistant strains. These sputum-conversion rates and the rapidity of sputum conversion are surprising, given the very poor in vitro susceptibility pattern of *M abscessus* previously reported with fluoroquinolones and doxycycline, and the relatively short period of parenteral therapy administered to patients in this study.[20,56]

Jarand and colleagues[57] published a retrospective analysis of treatment outcomes for 107 patients with *M abscessus* lung disease. Sixty-

four percent of the patients were followed for an average of 34 months. Antibiotic treatment was individualized based on drug-susceptibility results and patient tolerance. Sixteen different antibiotics were used in 42 different combinations for an average of 4.6 drugs per patient over the course of therapy with a median of 6 months on intravenous antibiotics. At least 1 drug was stopped because of side effects or toxicity in most patients, most commonly amikacin or cefoxitin. Twenty-four patients had surgery in addition to medical therapy. Forty-nine patients converted sputum cultures to negative but 16 relapsed. There were significantly more surgical patients who became culture negative compared with medically treated patients. Seventeen (15.9%) deaths occurred in the study population, remarkably similar to results

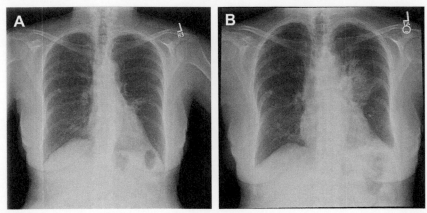

Fig. 4. (*A*) Baseline P/A chest radiograph of a 70-year-old woman with bronchiectasis and MAC lung disease. (*B*) P/A chest radiograph of the same patient taken 4 weeks after the chest radiograph in *A*, and after acute onset of increased cough, sputum production, pleuritic chest pain, and fever.

of a previous study of *M abscessus* lung disease from 1993.

The bottom line for therapy for *M abscessus* is murky at best. To date, there is no predictably or reliably effective regimen with or without parenteral agents or guided by in vitro susceptibility results. In the authors' opinion, if the regimen suggested by Jeon and colleagues[56] is chosen then patients must be followed very closely for evidence of disease progression and treatment failure.

Treatment of Bronchiectasis in Patients with NTM Lung Disease

Because chronic lung disease is inevitably and unavoidably present in patients with NTM lung

disease, management of the underlying or concomitant chronic lung disease is an inevitable and unavoidable complicating aspect of the overall care of patients with NTM lung disease, and can sometimes be the most important and effective therapy for the patient. The comprehensive management of bronchiectasis is beyond the scope of this manuscript so that comments in this section are focused on the bronchietasis management specifically for patients with NTM pulmonary disease.

First, and perhaps most importantly, bronchiectasis is literally a separate disease and presents its own treatment challenges that often arise unexpectedly during the course of therapy for NTM lung disease. Symptoms of bronchiectasis including

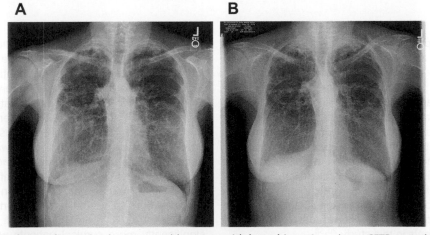

Fig. 5. (*A*) P/A chest radiograph of a 62-year-old woman with bronchiectasis and one CFTR mutation and *Mycobacterium abscessus* lung disease, demonstrating bilateral nodular and reticulonodular densities in mid- and upper-lung fields. (*B*) P/A chest radiograph after 2 months of twice-daily nebulized hypertonic (7%) saline, showing improvement in the bilateral radiographic densities.

cough, sputum production, fatigue, weight loss, and bronchospasm are not just nuisances but also significantly overlap with symptoms caused by NTM lung infection, complicating the interpretation of NTM treatment response.

Bronchiectasis is also associated with its own sometimes severe complications and exacerbating factors, such as infectious exacerbation of bronchiectasis (frequently due to drug-resistant bacteria such as *Pseudomonas*), pneumonia, hemoptysis (±mycetoma) and bronchospastic exacerbations of bronchiectasis, all of which require either adjustments to therapy or introduction of new therapeutic strategies in a patient already on 2 to 3 antibiotics. Infectious (bacterial) processes, either exacerbation of underlying bronchiectasis or frank pneumonitis, are perhaps the most common and troublesome bronchiectasis sequelae, partly because of the symptomatic and radiographic overlap with NTM lung disease (**Fig. 4**). Usually the time course of these infections provides a major clue to their origins, with relatively acute symptom or radiographic changes being caused by bronchiectasis rather than NTM infection, but careful clinical judgment is still necessary to ensure that a worsening of the NTM infection is not overlooked or that symptoms are inappropriately attributed to NTM disease. Based on clinical observations, the acute onset of purulent sputum with increased respiratory symptoms in those with NTM lung disease and bronchiectasis most often heralds an exacerbation of bronchiectasis rather than a flare of NTM lung disease. The use of oral fluoroquinolones in the management of bronchiectatic exacerbations caused by *Pseudomonas* is a frequent occurrence and has been conditionally recommended by the British Thoracic Society.[58] Because fluoroquinolones have limited activity against MAC and an unclear association between in vitro susceptibility and in vivo response, there does not appear to be a risk, as seen with *Mycobacterium tuberculosis*, that fluoroquinolone therapy for bronchiectasis exacerbations will result in delayed diagnosis of MAC disease or induce fluoroquinolone MAC resistance, although these possibilities have not been rigorously tested.

Airway-clearance therapies such as inhaled hypertonic saline or mannitol, as well as sputum clearance devices, chest percussion with postural drainage, and use of a percussion vest can also have a significant, if somewhat unpredictable, beneficial effect (**Fig. 5**). Prolonged administration of inhaled antipseudomonal antibiotics can also offer symptomatic improvement to some patients. The pros and cons of macrolide monotherapy in this patient population was discussed earlier.

However, the authors wish to emphasize the importance of addressing treatment opportunities and strategies for bronchiectasis as well as NTM disease.

SUMMARY

The challenges for the clinician managing patients with NTM lung disease with bronchiectasis were summarized eloquently in a recent editorial.

Thus, the decision is made by the clinician, who may, in view of sometimes rather uncomfortable effects the drugs can have, be wise enough to keep under observation even some of those patients who fulfill consensus criteria for mycobacterial disease. Optimal conservative treatment of underlying disease should not be underestimated, either in this or other contexts, despite the fact that drug treatment has improved over the decades, and patients with bronchiectasis and chronic bronchitis...should profit from such an approach.[59]

The insightful commentator added, "Is this a mere opinion? The ATS statement is full of opinions, and rightly so!"[59] Major challenges for the future include better, more effective treatment modalities for both NTM and bronchiectasis, better understood disease pathophysiology, and better strategies for disease prevention.

REFERENCES

1. Forrest Gump. Paramount Pictures; 1994.
2. Wolinsky E. Nontuberculous mycobacteria and associated diseases. Am Rev Respir Dis 1979; 119(1):107–59.
3. Prince DS, Peterson DD, Steiner RM, et al. Infection with *Mycobacterium avium* complex in patients without predisposing conditions. N Engl J Med 1989;321(13):863–8.
4. Rosenzweig DY. Pulmonary mycobacterial infections due to *Mycobacterium intreacellulare-avium* complex (clinical features and course in 100 consecutive cases). Chest 1979;75:115–9.
5. Ahn CH, McLarty JW, Ahn SS, et al. Diagnostic criteria for pulmonary disease caused by *Mycobacterium kansasii* and *Mycobacterium intracellulare*. Am Rev Respir Dis 1982;125(4):388–91.
6. Valero G, Peters J, Jorgensen JH, et al. Clinical isolates of *Mycobacterium simiae* in San Antonio, Texas. An 11-yr review. Am J Respir Crit Care Med 1995;152(5 Pt 1):1555–7.
7. Griffith DE, Girard WM, Wallace RJ Jr. Clinical features of pulmonary disease caused by rapidly

growing mycobacteria. An analysis of 154 patients. Am Rev Respir Dis 1993;147(5):1271–8.

8. Griffith DE, Brown-Elliott BA, Wallace RJ Jr. Thrice-weekly clarithromycin-containing regimen for treatment of *Mycobacterium kansasii* lung disease: results of a preliminary study. Clin Infect Dis 2003;37(9): 1178–82.

9. Polverosi R, Guarise A, Balestro E, et al. High-resolution CT of nontuberculous mycobacteria pulmonary infection in immunocompetent, non-HIV-positive patients. Radiol Med 2010;115(2):191–204.

10. Grenier P, Maurice F, Musset D, et al. Bronchiectasis: assessment by thin-section CT. Radiology 1986;161(1):95–9.

11. Joharjy IA, Bashi SA, Adbullah AK. Value of medium-thickness CT in the diagnosis of bronchiectasis. AJR Am J Roentgenol 1987;149(6):1133–7.

12. Nicotra MB, Rivera M, Dale AM, et al. Clinical, pathophysiologic, and microbiologic characterization of bronchiectasis in an aging cohort. Chest 1995; 108(4):955–61.

13. Pasteur MC, Helliwell SM, Houghton SJ, et al. An investigation into causative factors in patients with bronchiectasis. Am J Respir Crit Care Med 2000; 162(4 Pt 1):1277–84.

14. Scala R, Aronne D, Palumbo U, et al. Prevalence, age distribution and aetiology of bronchiectasis: a retrospective study on 144 symptomatic patients. Monaldi Arch Chest Dis 2000;55(2):101–5.

15. Wickremasinghe M, Ozerovitch LJ, Davies G, et al. Non-tuberculous mycobacteria in patients with bronchiectasis. Thorax 2005;60(12):1045–51.

16. Fowler SJ, French J, Screaton NJ, et al. Nontuberculous mycobacteria in bronchiectasis: prevalence and patient characteristics [erratum in: Eur Respir J 2007;29(3):614–5]. Eur Respir J 2006;28(6):1204–10.

17. Olivier KN, Weber DJ, Lee JH, et al, Nontuberculous Mycobacteria in Cystic Fibrosis Study Group. Nontuberculous mycobacteria. II: nested-cohort study of impact on cystic fibrosis lung disease. Am J Respir Crit Care Med 2003;167(6):835–40.

18. Olivier KN, Weber DJ, Wallace RJ Jr, et al, Nontuberculous Mycobacteria in Cystic Fibrosis Study Group. Nontuberculous mycobacteria. I: multicenter prevalence study in cystic fibrosis. Am J Respir Crit Care Med 2003;167(6):828–34.

19. Griffith DE. Emergence of nontuberculous mycobacteria as pathogens in cystic fibrosis. Am J Respir Crit Care Med 2003;167(6):810–2.

20. Noone PG, Leigh MW, Sannuti A, et al. Primary ciliary dyskinesia: diagnostic and phenotypic features. Am J Respir Crit Care Med 2004;169(4):459–67.

21. Griffith DE, Aksamit T, Brown-Elliott BA, et al, ATS Mycobacterial Diseases Subcommittee, American Thoracic Society; Infectious Disease Society of America. An official ATS/IDSA statement: diagnosis, treatment, and prevention of nontuberculous mycobacterial diseases. Am J Respir Crit Care Med 2007;175(4):367–416 [review. erratum in: Am J Respir Crit Care Med 2007;175(7):744–5].

22. Fujita J, Ohtsuki Y, Shigeto E, et al. Pathological analysis of the cavitary wall in *Mycobacterium avium* intracellulare complex pulmonary infection. Intern Med 2002;41(8):617–21.

23. Fujita J, Ohtsuki Y, Shigeto E, et al. Pathological findings of bronchiectases caused by *Mycobacterium avium* intracellulare complex. Respir Med 2003; 97(8):933–8.

24. Tanaka E, Lee WJ, Juba Y, et al. Computed tomography findings of pulmonary infections caused by *Mycobacterium avium* complex in patient without predisposing conditions. Am Rev Respir Dis 1994; 149:A108.

25. Kim RD, Greenberg DE, Ehrmantraut ME, et al. Pulmonary nontuberculous mycobacterial disease: prospective study of a distinct preexisting syndrome. Am J Respir Crit Care Med 2008;178(10): 1066–74.

26. Ziedalski TM, Kao PN, Henig NR, et al. Prospective analysis of cystic fibrosis transmembrane regulator mutations in adults with bronchiectasis or pulmonary nontuberculous mycobacterial infection. Chest 2006;130(4):995–1002.

27. Chan ED, Kaminska AM, Gill W, et al. Alpha-1-antitrypsin (AAT) anomalies are associated with lung disease due to rapidly growing mycobacteria2 and AAT inhibits *Mycobacterium abscessus* infection of macrophages. Scand J Infect Dis 2007;39(8):690–6.

28. Kim JS, Tanaka N, Newell JD, et al. Nontuberculous mycobacterial infection: CT scan findings, genotype, and treatment responsiveness. Chest 2005;128(6): 3863–9.

29. Mai HN, Hijikata M, Inoue Y, et al. Pulmonary *Mycobacterium avium* complex infection associated with the IVS8-T5 allele of the CFTR gene. Int J Tuberc Lung Dis 2007;11(7):808–13.

30. Bienvenu T, Sermet-Gaudelus I, Burgel PR, et al. Cystic fibrosis transmembrane conductance regulator channel dysfunction in non-cystic fibrosis bronchiectasis. Am J Respir Crit Care Med 2010;181(10): 1078–84.

31. Saiman L, Marshall BC, Mayer-Hamblett N, et al, Macrolide Study Group. Azithromycin in patients with cystic fibrosis chronically infected with *Pseudomonas aeruginosa*: a randomized controlled trial. JAMA 2003;290(13):1749–56.

32. Albert RK, Connett J, Bailey WC, et al, COPD Clinical Research Network. Azithromycin for prevention of exacerbation of COPD. N Engl J Med 2011;365: 689–98.

33. Feazel LM, Baumgartner LK, Peterson KL, et al. Opportunistic pathogens enriched in showerhead biofilms. Proc Natl Acad Sci U S A 2009;106: 16393–9.

34. Nishiuchi Y, Maekura R, Kitada S, et al. The recovery of Mycobacterium avium-intracellulare complex (MAC) from the residential bathrooms of patients with pulmonary MAC. Clin Infect Dis 2007;45(3):347–51.

35. Falkinham JO 3rd. Nontuberculous mycobacteria from household plumbing of patients with nontuberculous mycobacteria disease. Emerg Infect Dis 2011;17(3):419–24.

36. Falkinham JO 3rd, Iseman MD, de Haas P, et al. Mycobacterium avium in a shower linked to pulmonary disease. J Water Health 2008;6:209–13.

37. Marras TK, Wallace RJ Jr, Koth LL, et al. Hypersensitivity pneumonitis reaction to Mycobacterium avium in household water. Chest 2005;127(2):664–71.

38. Tanaka E, Kimoto T, Tsuyuguchi K, et al. Effect of clarithromycin regimen for Mycobacterium avium complex pulmonary disease. Am J Respir Crit Care Med 1999;160:866–72.

39. Hartman TE, Swensen SJ, Williams DE. Mycobacterium avium-intracellulare complex: evaluation with CT. Radiology 1993;187(1):23–6.

40. Swensen SJ, Hartman TE, Williams DE. Computed tomographic diagnosis of Mycobacterium avium-intracellulare complex in patients with bronchiectasis. Chest 1994;105(1):49–52.

41. Patz EF Jr, Swensen SJ, Erasmus J. Pulmonary manifestations of nontuberculous Mycobacterium. Radiol Clin North Am 1995;33(4):719–29.

42. Park S, Suh GY, Chung MP, et al. Clinical significance of Mycobacterium fortuitum isolated from respiratory specimens. Respir Med 2008;102:437–42.

43. Kitada S, Kobayashi K, Ichiyama S, MAC Serodiagnosis Study Group. Serodiagnosis of Mycobacterium avium-complex pulmonary disease using an enzyme immunoassay kit. Am J Respir Crit Care Med 2008;177:793–7.

44. Wallace RJ Jr, Brown BA, Griffith DE, et al. Clarithromycin regimens for pulmonary Mycobacterium avium complex: the first 50 patients. Am J Respir Crit Care Med 1996;153:1766–72.

45. Kobashi Y, Abe M, Mouri K, et al. Clinical usefulness of combination chemotherapy for pulmonary Mycobacterium avium complex disease. J Infect 2010. [Epub ahead of print].

46. Kobashi Y, Yoshida K, Miyashita N, et al. Relationship between clinical efficacy of treatment of pulmonary Mycobacterium avium complex disease and drug-sensitivity testing of Mycobacterium avium complex isolates. J Infect Chemother 2006 Aug; 12(4):195–202.

47. Research Committee of the British Thoracic Society. First randomised trial of treatments for pulmonary disease caused by M avium intracellulare, M malmoense, and M xenopi in HIV negative patients: rifampicin, ethambutol and isoniazid versus rifampicin and ethambutol. Thorax 2001;56(3):167–72.

48. Nash KA, Brown-Elliott BA, Wallace RJ Jr. A novel gene, erm(41), confers inducible macrolide resistance to clinical isolates of Mycobacterium abscessus but is absent from Mycobacterium chelonae. Antimicrob Agents Chemother 2009;53(4):1367–76.

49. Nash KA, Andini N, Zhang Y, et al. Intrinsic macrolide resistance in rapidly growing mycobacteria. Antimicrob Agents Chemother 2006;50(10):3476–8.

50. Lam PK, Griffith DE, Aksamit TR, et al. Factors related to response to intermittent treatment of Mycobacterium avium complex lung disease. Am J Respir Crit Care Med 2006;173(11):1283–9.

51. Kobashi Y, Matsushima T, Oka M. A double-blind randomized study of aminoglycoside infusion with combined therapy for pulmonary Mycobacterium avium complex disease. Respir Med 2007;101: 130–8.

52. Griffith DE, Brown-Elliott BA, Langsjoen B, et al. Clinical and molecular analysis of macrolide resistance in Mycobacterium avium complex lung disease. Am J Respir Crit Care Med 2006;174(8):928–34.

53. Field SK, Cowie RL. Treatment of Mycobacterium avium-intracellulare complex lung disease with a macrolide, ethambutol, and clofazimine. Chest 2003;124:1482–6.

54. Davis KK, Kao PN, Jacobs SS, et al. Aerosolized amikacin for treatment of pulmonary Mycobacterium avium infections: an observational case series. BMC Pulm Med 2007;7:2.

55. Wallace RJ Jr, Zhang Y, Brown-Elliott BA, et al. Repeat positive cultures in Mycobacterium intracellulare lung disease after macrolide therapy represent new infections in patients with nodular bronchiectasis. J Infect Dis 2002;186(2):266–73.

56. Jeon K, Kwon O, Lee N, et al. Antibiotic treatment of Mycobacterium abscessus lung disease: a retrospective analysis of 65 patients. Am J Respir Crit Care Med 2009;180:896–903.

57. Jarand J, Levin A, Zhang L, et al. Clinical and microbiologic outcomes in patients receiving treatment for Mycobacterium abscessus pulmonary disease. Clin Infect Dis 2011;52(5):565–71.

58. Hill AT, Pasteur M, Cornford C, et al. Primary care summary of the British Thoracic Society Guideline on the management of non-cystic fibrosis bronchiectasis. Prim Care Respir J 2011;20(2):135–40.

59. Schönfeld N. The mycobacterial mystery. Eur Respir J 2006;28(6):1076–8.

Diffuse Panbronchiolitis

Shoji Kudoh, MD, PhD[a,b,*], Naoto Keicho, MD, PhD[c]

KEYWORDS

- Diffuse panbronchiolitis • Chronic airway infection • Macrolide antibiotics • Asian disease

KEY POINTS

- This chronic airway disease mainly involves Japanese, Korean, Chinese, and other Asian people.
- Main symptoms are a large amount of sputum and progressive exertional dyspnea in patients with nonallergic chronic paranasal sinusitis.
- Centrilobular nodular shadows, frequently with peripheral bronchiectasis, in high-resolution computed tomography (CT) images are characteristic.
- Long-term treatment with 14-membered or 15-membered ring macrolides is effective.

In the mid1960s, a new disease entity, diffuse panbronchiolitis (DPB), distinct from chronic bronchitis or bronchiectasis, was established from clinicopathologic investigation by Homma and Yamanaka.[1] The first comprehensive report of DPB was published in the English language literature in 1983.[2] Prognosis of DPB was dismal in the advanced stages after superinfection with *Pseudomonas aeruginosa*.[3] The prognosis of this life-threatening airway disease has improved greatly since the initial success of long-term treatment with low-dose erythromycin was reported by Kudoh and colleagues[4] in 1984. The disease is now regarded as curable. Although the cause of the disease is still unknown, recent advances in cellular and molecular biology have helped in the understanding of the mechanisms underlying the efficacy of macrolides.

EPIDEMIOLOGY

According to a population-based survey in 1980, the incidence of physician-diagnosed DPB was 11.1 per 100,000 in Japan.[5] However, the incidence of disease seems recently to have decreased. The peak of the age distribution is among patients in their 40s to 50s. No sex predominance is noted.

Two-thirds of the patients did not smoke tobacco. There was no history of inhalation of toxic fumes.[3]

DPB has been also described in other east Asian populations such as the Koreans and Chinese.[6,7] A limited number of cases have been reported from outside Asia,[8,9] and about half the patients were Asian immigrants in reports from Western countries. Currently, it is reasonable to conclude that DPB is a chronic airway disease predominantly affecting east Asians.

CAUSE

Development of DPB in east Asians, including Asian emigrants, indicates that disease susceptibility is possibly determined by a genetic predisposition unique to Asians. Human leukocyte antigen (HLA)-B54, known as an ethnic antigen unique to east Asians, was strongly associated with the disease in Japan.[10,11] In contrast, Korean patients with DPB showed a positive association with HLA-A11.[12] Keicho and colleagues,[13] analyzed genetic markers and predicted that the most likely region for the major disease susceptibility gene was between the 2 HLA loci on chromosome 6. They recently cloned 2 novel mucinlike genes designated panbronchiolitis-related mucinlike 1 and 2

a Japan Anti-Tuberculosis Association, Fukujuji Hospital, 3-1-24 Matsuyama, Kiyose, Tokyo 204-8522, Japan
b Nippon Medical School, 1-1-5 Sendagi, Bunkyo-ku, Tokyo 113-8602, Japan
c Department of Respiratory Diseases, Research Institute, National Center for Global Health and Medicine, 1-21-1 Toyama, Shinjuku-ku, Tokyo 162-8655, Japan
* Japan Anti-Tuberculosis Association, Fukujuji Hospital, 3-1-24 Matsuyama, Kiyose, Tokyo 204-8522, Japan.
E-mail address: kudous@fukujuji.org

Clin Chest Med 33 (2012) 297–305
doi:10.1016/j.ccm.2012.02.005
0272-5231/12/$ – see front matter © 2012 Elsevier Inc. All rights reserved.

(PBMUCL1 and PBMUCL2) in the candidate region.[14]

PATHOLOGY

Cut surfaces of autopsied lung tissue in DPB are characterized by fine yellowish nodules in the parenchymal area (**Fig. 1**).[15] These nodules consist of thickened walls of the respiratory bronchioles with infiltrations of lymphocytes, plasma cells, and histiocytes. These inflammatory changes extend to the peribronchiolar tissues, whereas alveolar walls are not affected with accumulation of foamy histiocytes in the walls of the respiratory bronchioles adjacent to the alveolar ducts. DPB in the advanced stages is difficult to distinguish from diffuse bronchiectasis because of secondary ectasia of proximal bronchioles.

PATHOGENESIS
Lymphocyte Accumulation Around the Small Airway

It is important to characterize lymphocyte and macrophage accumulation around respiratory bronchioles to elucidate the pathogenesis of DPB. Sato and colleagues[16] showed that bronchus-associated lymphoid tissue hyperplasia is frequently observed in the lung biopsy samples from patients with DPB. Surface immunoglobulin

(Ig) M–positive B lymphocytes are distributed in the follicular area and T lymphocytes, mainly CD4+ cells, are located in the parafollicular area. In subsequent studies, it was reported that cytotoxic T cells expressing CD8+/CDIIb- were activated, and activated cell numbers correlated with the levels of the chemokine, MIP-1α, in the bronchial fluid.[17–19]

Neutrophil Accumulation into the Large Airway

Neutrophil accumulation in the proximal airway is another important feature of the disease.[20] Neutrophil numbers and their elastase activity were significantly elevated in the bronchial fluid from patients with DPB.[21] Kadota and colleagues[22] also showed that chemotactic activity was significantly increased in the bronchial fluid from patients with DPB. Subsequent investigations clarified that these chemotaxins were interleukin (IL)-8, leukotriene B4 (LTB4), and other chemotactic substances. Leukocyte adherent surface molecule Mac1 of neutrophils in the peripheral blood and bronchial fluid of patients with DPB expressed significantly higher levels. In addition, serum levels of soluble forms of other adhesion molecules, members of the selectin and the immunoglobulin supergene family, were found to be significantly increased in patients with

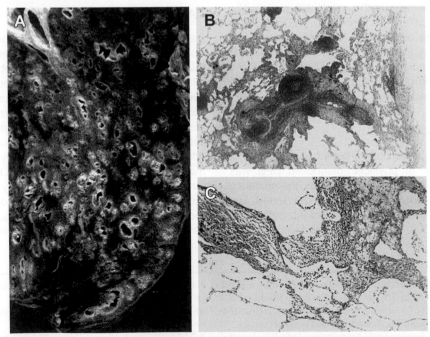

Fig. 1. Pathologic findings of DPB. Fine yellowish nodules with bronchiectasis are scattered on the cut surface of autopsied lung (*A*). Respiratory bronchioles with infiltrations of lymphocytes, plasma cells (*B*), and accumulation of foamy histiocytes (*C*).

DPB.[23,24] These results suggest that, in DPB, excessive neutrophil chemotactic factors at the site of inflammation and upregulation of adhesion molecules in the circulation are followed by recruitment of neutrophils into the proximal airway.

DIAGNOSIS
Clinical Manifestations

More than 80% of patients with DPB have a history or coexistence of chronic paranasal sinusitis. In their second to fifth decade, patients usually present with chronic cough and copious purulent sputum production. Exertional dyspnea develops subsequently. Physical examination of the lungs reveals coarse crackles. In about a half of patients with no intervention, sputum volume is greater than 50 mL/d.[3] In a review of 81 histologically proven cases of diffuse panbronchiolitis in 1980, 44% had *Haemophilus influenzae* in their sputum at presentation and 22% had *P aeruginosa*.[22] *Streptococcus pneumoniae* and *Moraxella catarrhalis* have been detected in sputum. The detection rate of *P aeruginosa* increases, on average, to 60% after 4 years of the disease.

Radiological Manifestations

A plain chest radiograph reveals bilateral, diffuse, small nodular shadows in the lower lung field with hyperinflation of the lung. Ring-shaped or tramline shadows suggesting bronchiectasis are frequently noted in advanced cases. High-resolution CT (HRCT) is useful for the detection of characteristic pulmonary lesions associated with DPB (**Fig. 2**).[25,26] Centrilobular nodular opacities, which suggest inflammatory lesions of the peripheral airway, are observed with bronchiectasis.

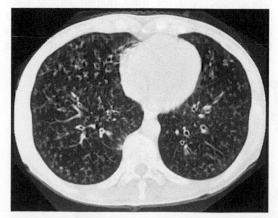

Fig. 2. Typical CT findings of DPB. Centrilobular nodular shadows (tree in bud) are diffusely distributed with bronchiectasis.

Pulmonary Functions

Pulmonary function measurements show significant airflow limitation that is resistant to bronchodilators.[3,27] Forced expiratory volume in 1 second (FEV$_1$)/forced vital capacity (FVC) are less than 70% from the early stages. Vital capacity (VC) decreases and residual volume (RV) increases in advanced stages. However, diffusing capacity (DLco) is not decreased, as distinct from chronic obstructive pulmonary disease (COPD). Arterial blood gas analysis has revealed hypoxemia from the early stage of the disease. Hypercapnia progresses in the advanced stage. In addition, pulmonary hypertension develops and is associated with the development of cor pulmonale.

Laboratory Findings

Laboratory findings suggest immunologic abnormalities reflecting chronic bacterial infection.[3] The titer of cold hemagglutinin is continuously increased in most Japanese patients with no evidence of mycoplasma infection.[28] Serum IgA levels are increased and a positive rheumatoid factor is often observed. Other laboratory abnormalities suggesting nonspecific inflammation include mild neutrophilia, increased erythrocyte sedimentation rate, and positive findings for C-reactive protein.

Diagnostic Criteria

Diagnostic criteria for DPB proposed[29] by a working group of the Ministry of Health and Welfare of Japan are as follows:

1. Persistent cough, sputum, and exertional dyspnea
2. History of, or current, chronic sinusitis
3. Bilateral, diffuse, small nodular shadows on a plain chest radiograph or centrilobular micronodules on chest CT images
4. Coarse crackles
5. FEV$_1$/FVC less than 70% and Pao$_2$ less than 80 mm Hg
6. Titer of cold hemagglutinin equal to or greater than 64.

Definite cases should fulfill the first 3 criteria (1–3) and at least 2 other remaining criteria (4–5).

TREATMENT
History

In the 1970s, none of the medications for DPB was effective in preventing a fatal outcome. Antibiotics such as β-lactams were administered against *H influenzae* and other bacteria, but failed to change the natural course of the disease. The overall 5-year survival rate of histologically proven cases of DPB was 51% and 8% in advanced DPB with *P aeruginosa* superinfection.[3]

In 1984, Kudoh and colleagues[4] first reported efficacy of low-dose, long-term erythromycin therapy for DPB, which was discovered from an open trial as a reexamination of the records of a patient with DPB treated by a general physician. After 6 months to 3 years of treatment with erythromycin 600 mg/d, 18 patients with DPB showed improvement in symptoms and clinical parameters of lung function. FEV_1 was increased from 1.61 to 2.17 L ($P<.01$) and Pao_2 was increased on average from 65.2 to 75.1 mm Hg ($P<.01$). Small nodular shadows on chest radiographs disappeared in more than 60% of the cases after therapy (**Fig. 3**).

Erythromycin Therapy

The favorable effect of erythromycin in the treatment of DPB was soon confirmed by others. The beneficial effects of erythromycin was also confirmed in a prospective double-blind, placebo-controlled study conducted by Yamamoto,[30] with the support of the Ministry of Health and Welfare of Japan in 1990. In the 1970s, the overall 5-year survival rate of patients with DPB was 63%. Between 1980 and 1984, fluoroquinolones were administered for the treatment of *P aeruginosa* superinfection and the survival rate was increased to 72%. After 1985, when erythromycin therapy was widespread, the 5-year survival rate was significantly increased to 91% (**Fig. 4**).[31]

Other Macrolides

Recently, 14-membered ring macrolides other than erythromycin have also been used in the treatment of patients with DPB. Clinicians administered clarithromycin and roxithromycin for the treatment of DPB in the 1990s, and obtained similar clinical benefits.[32,33] Azithromycin, a 15-membered ring macrolide, was in limited use in Japan until it was made freely available in 2001.

It seems to have similar beneficial effects to other macrolides on DPB.[34] Sixteen-membered ring macrolides (eg, josamycin) have been ineffective against DPB.[35] A recent clinical guideline for macrolide therapy for DPB is designated in **Box 1**.[36]

POTENTIAL MECHANISM OF ACTION

In the treatment of DPB, it seems that bactericidal activity is not a major determinant of the clinical efficacy of 14-membered ring macrolides.[4] First, irrespective of bacterial clearance, clinical parameters are significantly improved by the treatment. Second, even in cases with superinfection with *P aeruginosa*, which is resistant to macrolides, treatment with macrolides is effective. Third, at the recommended dosage, peak levels of macrolides in the sputum and serum are less than the minimum inhibitory concentrations for major pathogenic bacteria colonizing the airway. Moreover, long-term usage of potent antimicrobial agents including fluoroquinolones was less effective than low-dose erythromycin in the treatment of patients with DPB.[37] Investigations for the potential mechanisms underlying the effectiveness of macrolide therapy in DPB have commenced. An association for studying novel actions of macrolides was established in Japan and has had annual meetings since 1994, and many clinicians and researchers are studying the mechanism of action of macrolides. Several reviews[38–41] are now available on the antiinflammatory effects of macrolides.

Inhibition of Hypersecretion

Copious sputum production is one of the major characteristics in DPB. The sputum volume is reduced with erythromycin therapy. Goswami and associates[42] first reported that erythromycin dose dependently suppressed the secretion of respiratory glycoconjugates from human airway cells in vitro. Tamaoki and colleagues[43] measured a short-circuit current representing in vitro ion transport across airway epithelial cells and showed

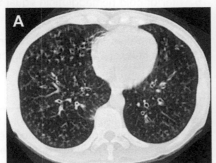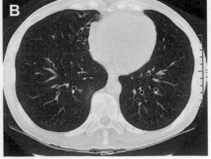

Fig. 3. CT findings of before (*A*) and after (*B*) 3 years of erythromycin therapy.

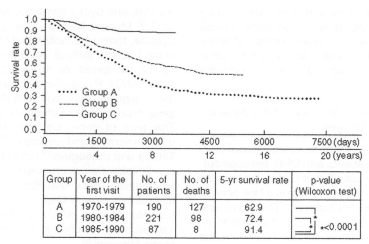

Group	Year of the first visit	No. of patients	No. of deaths	5-yr survival rate	p-value (Wilcoxon test)
A	1970-1979	190	127	62.9	
B	1980-1984	221	98	72.4	*<0.0001
C	1985-1990	87	8	91.4	

Fig. 4. Survival curves of DPB by the years of first examination; 5-year survival significantly improved after the first report on erythromycin therapy in 1984.

that erythromycin from the submucosal side suppressed the current in a dose-dependent manner. They showed that the chloride channel was blocked by erythromycin, leading to suppression of water secretion into the airway lumen.

Inhibition of Neutrophil Accumulation

As mentioned previously, a large number of neutrophils, frequently reaching 70% to 80% of the total lavage cells, are found in the bronchial fluid in patients with DPB.[20] After treatment with erythromycin, neutrophil numbers and elastase activity in the lower respiratory tract of patients with DPB are decreased.[21] Kadota and colleagues[22] showed that neutrophil chemotactic activity in the bronchoalveolar lavage fluid is reduced in patients with DPB treated with erythromycin. Oishi and colleagues[44] and Sakito and colleagues[45] showed that levels of IL-8, a major neutrophil chemoattractant, are decreased in the airways of patients with DPB after erythromycin therapy. Takizawa and colleagues[46] reported that erythromycin suppressed the expression of IL-8

Box 1
Guidelines for therapy for DPB

- One would think that therapy should be started soon if clinical response is better in the early stage
- Choice of drug:
  - First choice: erythromycin 400–600 mg/d, orally
  - Second choice: clarithromycin 200–400 mg/d or roxithromycin 150–300 mg/d, orally, in the event of poor efficacy or adverse events associated with erythromycin
  - Azithromycin is also acceptable, but 16-membered ring macrolides seem to be ineffective
- Assessment of response and duration of treatment:
  - Clinical response is usually obvious within 2 or 3 months of commencing therapy; however, treatment should be continued for at least 6 months and the overall response evaluated
  - Therapy should be completed after 2 years when clinical manifestations, radiological findings, and pulmonary function measurements are improved or stable without significant impairment of daily activity
  - Therapy should be restarted if symptoms reappear after cessation of erythromycin treatment.
  - In advanced cases with extensive bronchiectasis or respiratory failure, therapy should be continued for more than 2 years if there is a response to treatment

Based on the clinical guidelines on macrolide therapy for diffuse panbronchiolitis (Diffuse Lung Disease Committee of the Ministry of the Health and Welfare in Japan, 2000[36]; revised by the authors).

and other inflammatory cytokines from airway epithelial cells in vitro. They subsequently showed that this suppression of inflammatory cytokines was the result of inhibition of the transcription factors nuclear factor (NF)-κB or activator protein-1.[47]

Inhibition of Lymphocyte Accumulation and Effects on Macrophages

It is difficult to obtain tissue samples of respiratory bronchioles from patients with DPB, because surgical lung biopsy is usually not necessary to make a diagnosis for the therapy. There is a lack of information on lymphocytes and macrophages around respiratory bronchioles. As mentioned earlier, an increase in the number of activated CD8+ cells is observed in the bronchial fluid of patients with DPB, and these cell numbers decrease after the therapy.[18] Keicho and colleagues[48,49] showed that erythromycin partially suppresses lymphocyte proliferation when these cells are activated by lectins and antigens. They[50] also showed that differentiation of monocyte-derived macrophages was promoted by erythromycin, although the mechanism was unknown. Currently, the mechanism by which macrolide therapy can resolve nodular lesions consisting of lymphocytes and foamy macrophages in patients with DPB remains unknown.

Modulation of Bacterial Virulence

Many investigators have shown that the macrolides at less than the minimum inhibition concentrations (MICs) exert inhibitory effects on a variety of potential virulence factors such as elastase and pyocyanin produced by P aeruginosa.[51,52] Mucoid type of P aeruginosa produces alginate, forming a biofilm that makes eradication of the bacteria difficult. Alginate can be disrupted by 14-membered or 15-membered macrolides at sub-MICs. P aeruginosa uses extracellular chemical signals that cue cell-density-dependent gene expression to coordinate biofilm formation. This type of gene regulation has been termed quorum sensing and response.[53] In a recent study, Tateda and colleagues[54] reported that azithromycin inhibits the quorum-sensing circuitry of P aeruginosa. These anti-Pseudomonas effects of macrolides at sub-MICs may be beneficial for patients infected with P aeruginosa in the advanced stage of chronic lung diseases including cystic fibrosis.[55]

Fig. 5 shows the change of bacterial species in sputum of patients with DPB before and after treatment. With the conventional therapy, mainly using β-lactam antibiotics, the frequency of isolation of H influenzae declined and the frequency of isolation of P aeruginosa increased after the treatment. Conversely, the isolation of both H influenzae and P aeruginosa declined after erythromycin therapy, whereas the frequency of isolation of only nonpathogenic bacteria increased. This changing to normal flora is considered to be a result of improvement in chronic airway inflammation by erythromycin, as mentioned previously.

RECENT ADVANCEMENTS IN CLINICAL APPLICATIONS OF MACROLIDE THERAPY

Recently, 14-membered and 15-membered ring macrolides have been used for many other

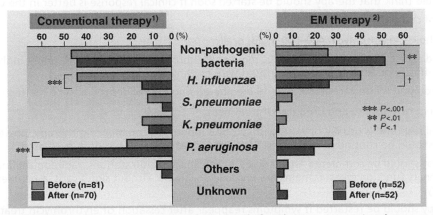

Fig. 5. Changes of isolated pathogens from sputum before and after therapy. Comparison between erythromycin and conventional therapy; frequency of pathogenic bacteria including P aeruginosa isolated from sputum decreased, and nonpathogenic bacteria increased (normalization of bacterial flora) after erythromycin therapy. (*Data from* Nakata K, Inatomi K. The 1981 Annual Report of Interstitial Lung Disease Research Committee, Japanese Ministry of Health and Welfare; 1982. p. 25; and Kudoh S, Yamaguchi T, Kurashima A, et al. The 1988 Annual Report Diffuse Parenchymal Lung Disease Research Committee, Japanese Ministry of Health and Welfare; 1989. p. 175.)

diseases. Recent reviews discussed long-term macrolide therapy for chronic inflammatory airway diseases including cystic fibrosis, bronchiectasis, bronchial asthma, COPD and posttransplant obstructive bronchiolitis other than DPB.[38,39]

Suzuki and colleagues[56] first reported that erythromycin inhibits exacerbation of COPD by inhibiting rhinovirus infection to the airway. Seemangal and colleagues[57] recently reported that long-term erythromycin therapy was associated with a significant reduction in exacerbations of COPD from a 12-month cohort study. In addition, Albert and colleagues[58] reported that azithromycin decreased the frequency of exacerbations and improved quality of life among patients with COPD. Recently, preventive effects for seasonal and swine (H1N1) influenza infection have been discussed.[59,60]

SUMMARY

More than 40 years have passed since DPB was first described in Japan. Studies on the cause of the disease have progressed in the context of a genetic predisposition unique to Asians. The advent of macrolide therapy has changed the prognosis of DPB, and has clarified various antiinflammatory actions of 14-membered and 15-membered ring macrolides and the pathogenesis of airway inflammation in DPB. The beneficial effects are now being applied in other chronic inflammatory diseases.

ACKNOWLEDGMENTS

This work supported by the Japanese Association of Nobel Action of Macrolides.

REFERENCES

1. Yamanaka A, Saiki S, Tamura S, et al. [Problems in chronic obstructive bronchial diseases, with special reference to diffuse panbronchiolitis]. Naika 1969; 23(3):442–51 [in Japanese].
2. Homma H, Yamanaka A, Tanimoto S, et al. Diffuse panbronchiolitis. A disease of the transitional zone of the lung. Chest 1983;83(1):63–9.
3. Homma H. Diffuse panbronchiolitis. Jpn J Med 1986;25(3):329–34.
4. Kudoh S, Uetake T, Hagiwara K, et al. [Clinical effects of low-dose long-term erythromycin chemotherapy on diffuse panbronchiolitis]. Nihon Kyobu Shikkan Gakkai Zasshi 1987;25(6):632–4215 [in Japanese].
5. Odaka M, Saito N, Hosoda Y, et al. [An epidemiological study of DPB in a large company. Annual report on the study of interstitial lung disease in 1980].

Tokyo: Ministry of Health and Welfare of Japan; 1981. p. 25–8 [in Japanese].
6. Kim YW, Han SK, Shim YS, et al. The first report of diffuse panbronchiolitis in Korea: five case reports. Intern Med 1992;31(5):695–701.
7. Tsang KW, Ooi CG, Ip MS, et al. Clinical profiles of Chinese patients with diffuse panbronchiolitis. Thorax 1998;53(4):274–80.
8. Fitzgerald JE, King TE Jr, Lynch DA, et al. Diffuse panbronchiolitis in the United States. Am J Respir Crit Care Med 1996;154(2 Pt 1):497–503.
9. Brugiere O, Milleron B, Antoine M, et al. Diffuse panbronchiolitis in an Asian immigrant. Thorax 1996; 51(10):1065–7.
10. Sugiyama Y, Kudoh S, Maeda H, et al. Analysis of HLA antigens in patients with diffuse panbronchiolitis. Am Rev Respir Dis 1990;141(6):1459–62.
11. Keicho N, Tokunaga K, Nakata K, et al. Contribution of HLA genes to genetic predisposition in diffuse panbronchiolitis. Am J Respir Crit Care Med 1998; 158(3):846–50.
12. Park MH, Kim YW, Yoon HI, et al. Association of HLA class I antigens with diffuse panbronchiolitis in Korean patients. Am J Respir Crit Care Med 1999; 159(2):526–9.
13. Keicho N, Ohashi J, Tamiya G, et al. Fine localization of a major disease-susceptibility locus for diffuse panbronchiolitis. Am J Hum Genet 2000;66(2):501–7.
14. Hijikata M, Matsushita I, Tanaka G, et al. Molecular cloning of two novel mucin-like genes in the disease-susceptibility locus for diffuse panbronchiolitis. Hum Genet 2011;129(2):117–28.
15. Maeda M, Saiki S, Yamanaka A. Serial section analysis of the lesions in diffuse panbronchiolitis. Acta Pathol Jpn 1987;37(5):693–704.
16. Sato A, Chida K, Iwata M, et al. Study of bronchus-associated lymphoid tissue in patients with diffuse panbronchiolitis. Am Rev Respir Dis 1992;146(2):473–8.
17. Todate A, Chida K, Suda T, et al. Increased numbers of dendritic cells in the bronchiolar tissues of diffuse panbronchiolitis. Am J Respir Crit Care Med 2000; 162(1):148–53.
18. Mukae H, Kadota J, Kohno S, et al. Increase in activated CD8+ cells in bronchoalveolar lavage fluid in patients with diffuse panbronchiolitis. Am J Respir Crit Care Med 1995;152(2):613–8.
19. Kawakami K, Kadota J, Iida K, et al. Phenotypic characterization of T cells in bronchoalveolar lavage fluid (BALF) and peripheral blood of patients with diffuse panbronchiolitis; the importance of cytotoxic T cells. Clin Exp Immunol 1997;107(2):410–6.
20. Ichikawa Y, Koga H, Tanaka M, et al. Neutrophilia in bronchoalveolar lavage fluid of diffuse panbronchiolitis. Chest 1990;98(4):917–23.
21. Ichikawa Y, Ninomiya H, Koga H, et al. Erythromycin reduces neutrophils and neutrophil-derived elastolytic-like activity in the lower respiratory tract of

bronchiolitis patients. Am Rev Respir Dis 1992;
146(1):196–203.

22. Kadota J, Sakito O, Kohno S, et al. A mechanism of
erythromycin treatment in patients with diffuse panbronchiolitis. Am Rev Respir Dis 1993;147(1):153–9.

23. Kusano S, Kadota J, Kohno S, et al. Effect of roxithromycin on peripheral neutrophil adhesion molecules in patients with chronic lower respiratory
tract disease. Respiration 1995;62(4):217–22.

24. Mukae H, Kadota J, Ashitani J, et al. Elevated levels of
soluble adhesion molecules in serum of patients with
diffuse panbronchiolitis. Chest 1997;112(6):1615–21.

25. Akira M, Kitatani F, Lee YS, et al. Diffuse panbronchiolitis: evaluation with high-resolution CT. Radiology 1988;168(2):433–8.

26. Nishimura K, Kitaichi M, Izumi T, et al. Diffuse panbronchiolitis: correlation of high-resolution CT and
pathologic findings. Radiology 1992;184(3):779–85.

27. Koyama H, Nishimura K, Mio T, et al. Bronchial
responsiveness and acute bronchodilator response
in chronic obstructive pulmonary disease and
diffuse panbronchiolitis. Thorax 1994;49(6):540–4.

28. Takizawa H, Tadokoro K, Miyoshi Y, et al. [Serolog-
ical characterization of cold agglutinin in patients
with diffuse panbronchiolitis]. Nihon Kyobu Shikkan
Gakkai Zasshi 1986;24(3):257–63 [in Japanese].

29. Nakata K. Revision of clinical guidelines for DPB.
Annual report on the study of diffuse lung disease
in 1998. Tokyo: Ministry of Health and Welfare of
Japan; 1999. p. 109–111 [in Japanese].

30. Yamamoto M. A double-blind placebo-controlled
study on the therapeutic effect of erythromycin on
DPB. Annual report on the study of diffuse lung
disease in 1990. Tokyo: Ministry of Health and
Welfare of Japan; 1991. p. 18–20 [in Japanese].

31. Kudoh S, Azuma A, Yamamoto M, et al. Improvement of survival in patients with diffuse panbronchiolitis treated with low-dose erythromycin. Am J Respir
Crit Care Med 1998;157(6 Pt 1):1829–32.

32. Tamaoki J, Takeyama K, Tagaya E, et al. Effect of clarithromycin on sputum production and its rheological
properties in chronic respiratory tract infections. Antimicrobial Agents Chemother 1995;39(8):1688–90.

33. Nakamura H, Fujishima S, Inoue T, et al. Clinical and
immunoregulatory effects of roxithromycin therapy
for chronic respiratory tract infection. Eur Respir J
1999;13(6):1371–9.

34. Kobayashi H, Takeda H, Sakayori S, et al. [Study on azithromycin in treatment of diffuse panbronchiolitis]. Kansenshogaku Zasshi 1995;69(6):711–22 [in Japanese].

35. Oritsu M. [Effectiveness of macrolide antibiotics
other than erythromycin]. Ther Res 1990;11:545–6
[in Japanese].

36. Nakata K, Taguchi Y, Kudoh S. Therapeutic guidelines for DPB. Annual Report on the study of diffuse
lung disease in 1999. Tokyo: Ministry of Health and
Welfare of Japan; 2000. p. 111 [in Japanese].

37. Yamamoto M, Kondo A, Tamura M, et al. [Long-term
therapeutic effects of erythromycin and newquinolone
antibacterial agents on diffuse panbronchiolitis]. Nihon Kyobu Shikkan Gakkai Zasshi 1990;28(10):
1305–13 [in Japanese].

38. Crosbie PA, Woodhead MA. Long-term macrolide
therapy in chronic inflammatory airway diseases
[review]. Eur Respir J 2009;33:171–81.

39. Friedlander AL, Albert RK. Chronic macrolide
therapy in inflammatory airways diseases [review].
Chest 2010;138:1202–12.

40. Altenburg J, de Graaff CS, van der Werf TS, et al.
Immunomodulatory effects of macrolide antibiotics-
part1: biological mechanisms [review]. Respiration
2011;81(1):67–74.

41. Altenburg J, de Graaff CS, van der Werf TS, et al.
Immunomodulatory effects of macrolide antibiotics-
part 2: advantages and disadvantages of long-term,
low-dose macrolide therapy [review]. Respiration
2011;81(1):75–87.

42. Goswami SK, Kivity S, Marom Z. Erythromycin
inhibits respiratory glycoconjugate secretion from
human airways in vitro. Am Rev Respir Dis 1990;
141(1):72–8.

43. Tamaoki J, Isono K, Sakai N, et al. Erythromycin
inhibits Cl secretion across canine tracheal epithelial
cells. Eur Respir J 1992;5(2):234–8.

44. Oishi K, Sonoda F, Kobayashi S, et al. Role of
interleukin-8 (IL-8) and an inhibitory effect of erythromycin on IL-8 release in the airways of patients with
chronic airway diseases. Infect Immun 1994;62(10):
4145–52.

45. Sakito O, Kadota J, Kohno S, et al. Interleukin 1
beta, tumor necrosis factor alpha, and interleukin 8
in bronchoalveolar lavage fluid of patients with
diffuse panbronchiolitis: a potential mechanism of
macrolide therapy. Respiration 1996;63(1):42–8.

46. Takizawa H, Desaki M, Ohtoshi T, et al. Erythromycin
modulates IL-8 expression in normal and inflamed
human bronchial epithelial cells. Am J Respir Crit
Care Med 1997;156(1):266–71.

47. Desaki M, Takizawa H, Ohtoshi T, et al. Erythromycin
suppresses nuclear factor-kappaB and activator
protein-1 activation in human bronchial epithelial cells.
Biochem Biophys Res Commun 2000;267(1):124–8.

48. Keicho N, Kudoh S, Yotsumoto H, et al. Antilympho-
cytic activity of erythromycin distinct from that of
FK506 or cyclosporin A. J Antibiot (Tokyo) 1993;
46(9):1406–13.

49. Morikawa K, Oseko F, Morikawa S, et al. Immunomodulatory effects of three macrolides, midecamy-
cin acetate, josamycin, and clarithromycin, on
human T-lymphocyte function in vitro. Antimicrobial
Agents Chemother 1994;38(11):2643–7.

50. Keicho N, Kudoh S, Yotsumoto H, et al. Erythromycin
promotes monocyte to macrophage differentiation.
J Antibiot (Tokyo) 1994;47(1):80–9.

51. Kita E, Sawaki M, Oku D, et al. Suppression of virulence factors of *Pseudomonas aeruginosa* by erythromycin. J Antimicrob Chemother 1991;27(3):273–84.

52. Sakata K, Yajima H, Tanaka K, et al. Erythromycin inhibits the production of elastase by *Pseudomonas aeruginosa* without affecting its proliferation in vitro. Am Rev Respir Dis 1993;148(4 Pt 1): 1061–5.

53. Davies DG, Parsek MR, Pearson JP, et al. The involvement of cell-to-cell signals in the development of a bacterial biofilm. Science 1998;280(5361): 295–8.

54. Tateda K, Comte R, Pechere JC, et al. Azithromycin inhibits quorum sensing in *Pseudomonas aeruginosa*. Antimicrobial Agents Chemother 2001;45(6):1930–3.

55. Jaffe A, Francis J, Rosenthal M, et al. Long-term azithromycin may improve lung function in children with cystic fibrosis. Lancet 1998;351(9100):420.

56. Suzuki T, Yanai M, Yamaya M, et al. Erythromycin and common cold in COPD. Chest 2001;120(3): 730–3.

57. Seemungal TA, Wilkinson TM, Hurst JR, et al. Long-term erythromycin therapy is associated with decreased chronic obstructive pulmonary disease exacerbations. Am J Respir Crit Care Med 2008;178:1139–47.

58. Albert RK, Connett J, Bailey WC. Azithromycin for prevention of exacerbations of COPD. N Engl J Med 2011;365:689–98.

59. Yamaya M, Shinya K, Hatachi Y, et al. Clarithromycin inhibits type a seasonal influenza virus infection in human airway epithelial cells. J Pharmacol Exp Ther 2010;333(1):81–90.

60. Bermejo-Martin JF, Kelvin DJ, Eiros JM, et al. Macrolides for the treatment of severe respiratory illness caused by novel H1N1 swine influenza viral strains. J Infect Dev Ctries 2009;3(3):159–61.

Recent Advances in Cystic Fibrosis

Jason Lobo, MD[1], Juan M. Rojas-Balcazar, MD[1],
Peadar G. Noone, MD, FCCP, FRCPI*

KEYWORDS

- Cystic fibrosis • CFTR • Gene modifiers • *Pseudomonas aeruginosa* • Bronchiectasis
- Mucociliary clearance

KEY POINTS

- Cystic fibrosis (CF) is an inherited chronic disease that remains a common cause of morbidity and mortality in affected patients.
- Since its first description in 1938, study of the genetics, pathophysiology, and clinical manifestation of the disease has led to the creation of new therapies and significantly improved quality of life and survival.
- Improvements in the delivery of care to patients with CF have developed by using a team-based approach, and continuous quality improvement projects.
- The outcome for patients with CF has never been brighter and will undoubtedly continue to improve.

Cystic fibrosis (CF) is an inherited chronic disease that affects approximately 30,000 children and adults in the United States and approximately 80,000 individuals worldwide.[1] CF is characterized by mutations in the gene encoding the CF transmembrane conductance regulator (CFTR), with resultant abnormalities in airway epithelial ion transport, dysregulation of airway surface liquid (ASL), and abnormalities in airway host defense. The presence of gram-negative bacteria, such as mucoid *Pseudomonas aeruginosa*, leads to an inflammatory response, airway damage, bronchiectasis, and progressive obstructive airway disease. Although a multisystem disease, most of the morbidity and mortality in patients with CF is a result of severe lung disease and respiratory failure. Disease of the upper respiratory tract (rhinosinusitis) is a significant cause of morbidity, but not usually mortality. Other systems involved in CF include the hepatobiliary system, the gastrointestinal tract, the pancreas, the endocrine system, and less commonly skin and joint disease.

Research into the pathophysiology of CF has been intense for several decades, especially in recent years, although much remains to be understood. The first comprehensive description of the disease occurred in 1938 by Dorothy Andersen, followed by the discovery of abnormalities in sweat electrolytes in CF in the 1950s by Gibson and Cooke. The same decade saw the creation of the Cystic Fibrosis Foundation (CFF), now a major force in driving innovation in research into, and treatments of, the disease. The early 1980s saw the discovery of airway ion channel abnormalities, later followed by cloning of the gene in 1989. This led to an understanding of CFTR structure and function, genotype–phenotype relations, and CFTR interactions with other proteins. The years since the 1990s have seen novel therapeutic strategies including gene transfer studies, the development of clinical research networks, and the establishment of quality improvement (QI) and standardized protocols for treating populations of patients with CF. Studies of animal models have set the stage for

Disclosures: The authors have nothing to disclose.
Division of Pulmonary and Critical Care Medicine, Department of Medicine, University of North Carolina, CB 7020, Chapel Hill, NC 27599–7020, USA
[1] Contributed equally to the manuscript.
* Corresponding author.
E-mail address: pnoone@med.unc.edu

Clin Chest Med 33 (2012) 307–328
doi:10.1016/j.ccm.2012.02.006
0272-5231/12/$ – see front matter © 2012 Elsevier Inc. All rights reserved.

further work on understanding the complexities of CF. In parallel with this explosion of work and knowledge, the survival of patients with CF has improved significantly over the last 40 years. Aggressive therapies to prevent loss of pulmonary function and to maintain adequate nutrition, together with early identification and treatment of CF-related complications, and application of a multidisciplinary team approach in specialized CF centers (using best practice and consensus protocols) have improved the median survival age to approximately 37.5 years.[2,3]

In terms of the recent interest in CF, a glance at the published work over the years provides a glimpse into the evolution of the process. A brief survey of CF-related publications in prominent respiratory journals (*Chest*, *American Journal of Respiratory and Critical Care Medicine*, *Thorax*, and *European Respiratory Journal*) during one random month, at 10-yearly intervals, shows no CF-related publication in July 1991, one publication in July 2001, and 10 publications in July 2011. The *Journal of Cystic Fibrosis* emerged as a subspecialty journal in 2002; in July 2011, this journal contained seven original articles, three short communications, and one comprehensive review of a CF topic.

This article addresses recent advances in CF, in the context of what has been learned previously, but focuses on new insights into the disease. The article starts by looking at advances in the molecular basis of disease expression in conjunction with non-genetic factors, moving through disease pathogenesis, infectious issues, and finally examining recently developed and future therapies and the institution of QI in the delivery of care.

DISEASE EXPRESSION: GENETIC AND NONGENETIC FACTORS

CF is an autosomal-recessive disease characterized by mutations of the CFTR gene located on the long arm of chromosome 7. The most common mutation is the ΔF508 mutation, with an allele frequency of approximately 70% in white patients with CF worldwide.[4] A small number of other gene mutations ($\sim$ 15–20) accounts for another 15% to 20% of mutations, depending on the ethnic backgrounds of the population in question. The disease exhibits locus heterogeneity, also known as allelic variation (ie, although it is a single-gene recessive disorder, involving one gene [CFTR], more than 1800 different mutations have been described in CF). CFTR mutations have been divided into classes I to V depending on the level of CFTR function: classes I to III are "severe" (no CFTR function) and classes IV and V are "mild" (some residual

CFTR function).[5] Other factors, such as the length of the polythymidine tract in intron 8 (IVS8), also influence CFTR expression.[6]

After the discovery of the gene, efforts commenced to identify relationships between genotype and phenotype. Establishing such relations proved elusive in the sinopulmonary tract, although early on it was recognized that severe CFTR mutations are strongly associated with pancreatic insufficiency, whereas mild mutations are associated with pancreatic sufficiency. Similarly, observations in males with infertility caused by absence of the vas deferens, a phenotypic feature of CF, suggested that the level of functioning CFTR is related to disease expression, but in an organ-specific manner; thus, even minor reductions in CFTR function in utero resulted in congenital absence of the vas deferens, but commonly with no, or mild, pulmonary disease. Thus, allelic variations in CFTR accounts for only a minor part of phenotypic variations, especially in the lung.[4] At a clinical level this results in some patients with null mutations (eg, ΔF508) having mild lung disease well into adulthood, whereas other patients with mutations associated with retained CFTR function and pancreatic sufficiency may have severe lung disease early in life. This early observation of the lack of an obvious link to between genotype and lung phenotype has led researchers in recent years to search for causes of phenotypic variation independent of CFTR genotype. These causes include genetic factors (non-CFTR) and a range of environmental factors.

Genetic Factors

Although it is often assumed that the CF population is homogeneous, and mostly of northern European descent, recent studies have shown that a surprising proportion of patients are of mixed African-Mexican-Indian-white ancestries.[7] Thus, ethnic diversity in the population of patients with CF in North America implies the need for caution when studying any aspect of CF genetics, especially genetic association studies. An obvious place to start, to try to measure the effect of genetics on disease expression as independently as possible of nongenetic factors, is with family members (siblings) and twin siblings. The assumption is that it should be possible to tease out the genetic versus environment effects on phenotypic expression, in persons sharing similar or identical DNA. Twin studies, involving dizygous and monozygous twins, showed a high degree of heritability in forced expiratory volume in 1 second (FEV_1) measures, in those with and without identical CFTR mutations (ΔF508 homozygotes).[4] In all, the heritability factor (h^2) was greater than 0.5

(range, 0.54–1), implying that genetic traits outside of the CFTR gene influence to a significant degree the FEV_1, which has an impact on survival.[8] To further narrow the search for these genetic contributions, a significant effort was required. This led to the formation of the North American Gene Modifier Consortium, with collaboration from centers in the United States and Canada. The formation of this consortium was designed to ensure inclusion of sufficient lung function data to be able to accurately classify disease severity, and to ensure that the appropriate study designs were selected.[9] The initial challenge was to deal with the difficulties in analysis of multiple FEV_1 measures, with attendant effects of age and death as confounders. The FEV_1 is currently the measure of choice in determining lung disease severity, and using sophisticated techniques, the Consortium has done tremendous work in refining use of the FEV_1 as a measure by which patients can be segregated into "mild" versus "severe" disease (ie, into the extremes of the phenotype). Segregation of large numbers of patients with similar genotypes, but with different severity of lung disease, allows a search for non-CFTR genetic influences on disease expression

(gene modifiers). Any positive findings in these studies are required to be replicated in separate populations of patients. Several studies, involving sufficient numbers of patients and sophisticated genetic and molecular techniques, have by now shown gene variants that have an influence on the heritability of CF lung disease, such as MBL2, TGFβ1, IFRD1, IL-8, and EDNRA (**Table 1**). A more recent study by the consortium using a genome-wide association and linkage approach identified two new loci (APIP and EHF) that contribute to the variation of the lung function in patients with CF. APIP interacts with the apoptotic protease-activating factor 1 (APAF1) and can inhibit apoptosis, possibly leading to a delay in the resolution of neutrophilic inflammation.[9] EHF is known to be an important regulator of differentiation under conditions of stress and inflammation. Variants in TLR5, an important gene in the inflammatory response of the airway epithelium against *P aeruginosa* infection, are associated with less inflammation of the airway epithelial cells and with improvement of the nutritional status of patients with CF, but with no association with lung function.[10] Finally, SLC9A3 is a gene that

Table 1
Modifier genes in cystic fibrosis (see text for details[4])

Modifier Gene	Gene Description	Modifier Gene Effect
MBL2	Mannosa binding lectin	FEV_1 and risk of bacterial infection
EDNRA	Endothelin receptor type A	Increased smooth muscle proliferation and FEV_1
TGFβ1	Transforming growth factor β1	FEV_1
IL-8	Interleukin-8	Possible association FEV_1 and neutrophil function
IFRD1	Interferon-related developmental regulator 1	Possible regulation of neutrophil effector function and bacterial infection
APIP	Apaf-1–interacting protein	Possible association with inhibition of apoptosis and worsening of lung disease
EHF	Epithelial-specific ETS transcription factor	Regulator of cellular differentiation under conditions of stress and inflammation
TLR5	*P aeruginosa* flagellin receptor, involved in the airway inflammatory response	Possible reduction of the inflammatory response and improvement of nutritional status
SLC9A3	Gene encoding for a sodium and bicarbonate exchanger protein	Possible association with age of bacterial infection acquisition and decline in FEV_1
SERPINA 1	Serpin peptidase inhibitor, (α_1-antiproteinase, -antitrypsin)	Possible association with severe liver disease
MSRA	Methionine sulfoxide reductase A	Probable association with meconium illeus obstruction
TGF7L2	Transcription factor 7–like 2	Increased risk for CF-related diabetes

encodes for a Na^+/H^+ exchanger and can influence the salt and water balance in the ALS.[11] Durie and colleagues found a significant association between variants in the SLC9A3 gene and age at acquisition of *P aeruginosa* infection and lung disease.[12] Thus, children with CF with the T allele (45%) of variant rs4957061 in the gene have significantly earlier age of onset of *P aeruginosa* infection and reduced lung function. Examples of gene variants that seem to have no association with the lung phenotype, but with a possible association with liver disease, include SERPINA 1. Variants in the MSRA gene on chromosome 8 exhibit a likely association with meconium ileus obstruction. TGF7L2 seems to exert a modifier effect on CF-related diabetes, independent of steroid use.[13] Although these studies are incredibly resource intensive, they have already yielded exciting data, which ultimately should help in the identification of therapeutic targets.

Nongenetic Factors

CF was predominantly a disease of childhood in prior decades, whereas recent decades have seen the median survival climb from approximately 27 years in 1986 to approximately 37 years as of 2009 (http://www.cff.org/). The improvement over several decades since the 1950s has been attributed to multiple factors, such as the development of pancreatic enzyme replacement therapies, better and more aggressive use of antibiotic therapies, nutritional support, and the development of healthcare teams and CF centers dedicated to the care of large populations of patients with the disease, from birth to late adulthood. Most adult CF clinics now have patients well into older age, with some patients achieving geriatric status. This change in the patient spectrum has resulted in a paradigm shift over the past few decades, with adults (>18 years) now comprising 47% of patients, requiring the training of adult pulmonologists with an expertise in CF, and the development of adult CF healthcare teams. The CFF tracks the demographics of these patients by a national registry, as do other countries. A total of 33% of US adults with CF in 2009 were college graduates, 35% were in full-time employment, and 39% were either married or living with a life partner.

Although the data generated by the CFF database are largely descriptive, there has been much work in recent years attempting to more specifically identify the various factors that influence disease expression and survival. An important factor in disease severity long term is infectious complications. Thus, acquisition of different infectious organisms influences the severity and progression of disease.

For example, acquisition of *P aeruginosa* early in life leads to accelerated declines in lung function and increased mortality.[14] Early acquisition of the bacteria is in turn related to several other factors, such as use of antibiotics, especially antistaphylococcal drugs, infectious contacts, hospitalizations with viral infections, and use of nebulizers.[15,16] This shows the complexity of the relationships, but also highlights points at which intervention might make a long-term difference. Methicillin-resistant *Staphylococcus aureus* (MRSA) has also shown to be related to poor health outcomes, and *Burkholderia cepacia* complex (BCC) organisms have long been known to be associated with poor outcomes, especially with *Burkholderia cenocepacia*.[17] There are emerging data that *Stenotrophomonas maltophilia* is related to worse outcomes, specifically FEV_1 and risk of pulmonary exacerbation.[18] Fungal organisms in the airway may also be deleterious, specifically *Aspergillus fumigatus*, with various studies showing relations to lower lung function (with *P aeruginosa*), hospitalizations, older age, and use of inhaled antibiotics.[19] Finally, nontuberculous mycobacteria (NTM), especially *Mycobacterium abscessus*, have been linked to lung function declines, which are not unexpected given the difficulty this organism can pose clinically.[20] Thus, it is clear that multiple studies have shown links between the presence (and acquisition) of a variety of organisms in the lung and the likelihood of having worse disease.[21] These data not only confirm clinical suspicions, but also open the door for studies that evaluate therapies for either eradication or control of such infections, with the ultimate goal of improving mid- and long-term outcomes.

Many non-infectious factors are also at play, which may influence the course of CF (see the section on "outcomes" later).[22] Age at diagnosis is an interesting issue to study, because newborn screening has recently been instituted throughout the United States and in other countries. Emerging evidence supports the hypothesis that early (newborn) diagnosis is associated with better nutritional and pulmonary outcomes, although reports also suggest that adults diagnosed later in life have milder disease overall (this may reflect at least in part the presence of non-classic disease patients in such populations).[23,24] As with other chronic diseases, socially and economically deprived patients tend to have worse lung disease and survival, for multiple reasons (eg, poor health insurance, less access to care, poorer compliance, and psychological reasons).[21,22] Other factors, such as air pollution, ozone, and tobacco smoke exposure, influence the severity of disease in children. Gender is also related to severity of disease; females generally do worse, at least when diagnosed early in life, possibly related to hormonal influences, and other inherent differences in the genders (body image and attitudes to life).[25] Although most patients are white, minority patients, such as Hispanic and African Americans, report worse emotional and social functioning, which in turn might have a bearing on medical outcomes. Finally, as Wolfenden and Schechter[21] so elegantly state, the nongenetic "mileu" imposes a significant effect, with the interactions of the environment *in toto* (the social and cultural setting and the healthcare delivery system surrounding the patient [eg, attending vs not attending a CFF-accredited center]) all resulting in an unpredictable outcome for any given individual.

PATHOPHYSIOLOGY

Since the discovery of the CFTR gene in 1989, major efforts have been made to explain the relationship between alterations in the epithelial ion transport and the development of airway inflammation and infection in the lung. Much work has been done in the past two decades that has substantially increased the understanding of the pathophysiology of CF lung disease. Nevertheless, many aspects of the pathogenesis of the disease still remain unclear, or remain somewhat controversial.[1]

Although the structure and function of the CFTR protein were unknown before cloning of the gene, characterization of the protein rapidly followed. CFTR belongs to the adenosine triphosphate (ATP)-binding cassette transporter protein family, which regulates transmembrane transport of small molecules. CFTR is expressed in the apical plasma membrane of the airway epithelial cells and in the serous cells of submucosal glands of the lungs. CFTR is known to work as a regulated chloride (Cl^-) and bicarbonate channel, and affects the activity of other plasma membrane channels (eg, the epithelial sodium channel [ENaC]). Although the structure, function, biosynthetic processing, intracellular trafficking, and five classes of gene mutations of the CFTR protein have been extensively described, understanding how the absence of functional CFTR protein translates into the spectrum of the CF disease phenotype has been more challenging.[26] To address the challenge, studies in in vitro human cell cultures and in animal models and humans with CF have been performed and are reviewed in this section. This section also briefly addresses non-pulmonary disease pathophysiology.

ASL and Ion Transport Defects

Since the ion transport defects in CF were described in the early 1980s, it had long been believed that disease resulted from abnormalities in salt and water transport across airway epithelia, with disruption in mucociliary clearance. Proof of concept was more difficult. In the late 1990s, two opposing theories arose to explain the development of lung disease. The first suggested that a high salt content on airway surfaces led to inactivation of airway defensins (broad-spectrum antimicrobial peptides), leading to susceptibility to chronic infection.[27] An alternate hypothesis suggested that ion transport defects led to depletion of ASL resulting in a significant reduction in mucociliary transport, leading to a major breach in airway host defense at a mechanical level.[28] Mechanical clearance of mucus is a major defense mechanism of the airways against inhaled microorganisms. Normal mucociliary clearance is mediated by a two-layer liquid system known as ASL. The upper phase is the mucus layer, which is composed of high-molecular-weight secreted mucins, and the lower layer is known as the periciliary liquid layer (PCL). The interaction between these two-layers facilitates effective ciliary function and airway clearance. Adequate hydration of this airway surface fluid depends on the balance between sodium (Na^+) absorption by ENaC, and Cl^- secretion mediated by CFTR, augmented by non-CFTR chloride channels (alternative chloride channels). In this way, ion transport exerts osmotic forces that regulate the water content of ASL, more specifically the height (or depth) of the layer, which seems to be critical for function of the entire system. In CF airways, abnormal CFTR function leads to excessive Na^+ reabsorption, with failure of secretion of Cl^-, leading to a reduction in salt mass on the airway. Osmotic forces are thus in favor of less water moving into the airway lumen, hence the term "dehydration hypothesis" for this model concept. The depletion of the PCL water content makes this layer collapse and lose its lubricant activity that separates the mucus layer from epithelial cells, producing adhesion of mucus to airway surfaces, impairing airway clearance of thick mucus secretions, and facilitating colonization with respiratory pathogens, generating chronic infection and inflammation of the airways.[29] Although studies of ASL in vivo are technically challenging, much work has been performed in the past several years to lend credence to the dehydration hypothesis, including studies of the composition of ASL (non-CF and CF are both isotonic), the height of the ASL layer (reduced in CF vs normal), and studies in vitro and in vivo where addition of an osmotic load to the airway restores normal ASL height by "hydrating" the airway, which can temporarily at least improve mucociliary clearance.[30,31] To complicate matters, alternative (non-CFTR) chloride transport channels in CF have also been described. The two pathways of chloride secretion in the respiratory airways are the CFTR and the calcium-activated chloride conductance channel (CaCC; see later).

Human Cell-Culture Models

Measures of ASL physiology are very difficult in humans in vivo given the complexity of airway structures and the very shallow depth of ASL ($\sim$25 μm) and PCL ($\sim$7 μm).[7] However, the development of human-cultured bronchial epithelial cells has provided much information about the bioelectric and fluid transport properties of airway epithelial cells, and the interactions with the ASL volume. Different methods to measure the composition and properties of airway gland secretion in human bronchial–tracheal cells have been developed, and submucosal gland secretions, in non-CF airway human cell cultures compared with CF.[31] Most work over the past several years using these model systems has shown that CFTR is predominantly expressed in ciliated cells of airway epithelia and in submucosal glands. Evidence now supports CFTR contributing to ASL volume, but that regulation of ASL volume (by the mechanisms alluded to previously regarding rates of Na^+ and Cl^- secretion controlling ASL water content) rests mostly with surface epithelia, given its massive surface area. To further complicate matters, regulation of ASL volume is also influenced by other mediators' actions on ENaC and other chloride channels, such as proteases and protease inhibitors. How alternative secretory channel pathways can modulate the ASL secretion in CF is still under investigation. The CaCC is an alternative ATP-activated chloride channel that contributes to the mucociliary clearance (MCC) and is positively affected by shear stress conditions (by ATP-mediated shear stress signaling). Studies in human epithelial cells have demonstrated that chloride secretion mediated by CaCC involves the activation of $P2Y_2$ receptors, which are located in the apical membrane of airway epithelial cells and are activated by ATP, rising intracellular calcium concentrations, and enhancing chloride secretion. Other proteins have been identified in the calcium-dependent chloride transport arena (eg, TMEM16A) and are under further research.[32]

Mucus production with decreased MCC is also a hallmark of CF airway disease. Mucins are high-molecular-weight glycoconjugates and are major macro-components of normal mucus that are secreted by the superficial epithelial cells and the submucosal glands of the respiratory airways, and provide viscoelastic properties to the airway mucus secretions. Human and CF airway epithelial cell culture models have shown similar mucin composition. However, mucin overproduction and hypersecretion in the CF epithelial cultures have been seen in response to chronic infection and inflammation.[33] In addition, defective secretion of bicarbonate has been linked to abnormal mucus hydration. Experiments in cultured-airway cells showed evidence that abnormal bicarbonate secretion leads to decreased mucin expansion and hydration. Bicarbonate was found to decrease calcium cross-linking in mucins, reducing mucin viscosity and dehydrated airway mucus production. Impairment in bicarbonate secretion has been reported in many organs in CF; thus, these results suggest that not only the CFTR-dependent electrolyte abnormalities are implicated in the pathogenesis of CF, but also that diminished epithelial bicarbonate transport and abnormalities of mucus biology may play an important role in mucus formation and development of CF disease.[34]

Finally, the role of endoplasmic reticulum stress and the intracellular calcium mobilization in the CF airway epithelia have been demonstrated in cultured CF bronchial epithelial cells. Intracellular calcium mobilization has been implicated in regulating airway defense functions including calcium-dependent chloride secretion, ciliary activity, mucin secretion, and inflammatory responses. Up-regulation of proinflammatory pathways seems to be a key component in CF airway inflammation and whether increased calcium mobilization is triggered by chronic infection, or is an intrinsic property of the CF epithelial cells, remains under debate. The unfolded protein response is a form of endoplasmic reticulum stress, and is also involved in the calcium-mediated amplification of the airway inflammatory response.[35]

Animal Models

The early development of CF animal models, initially the mouse model, together with the more recent development of pig and ferret models, has added to opportunities for a better understanding of CF pathophysiology.[36,37] Other non-CF models (eg, the transgenic mouse model with airway-specific overexpression of βENaC) have also shed insights at an in vivo level into normal and abnormal airway ion transport and its contributions to health and disease. Studies in mice with mutant CFTR protein showed that the airways of the animal do not exhibit the same ion transport abnormalities as seen in humans with CF. Furthermore, the phenotypic manifestations are different: the CF mouse model does not develop significant lung disease, but tends to show early mortality with gastrointestinal disease. Because of these research limitations, new animal models have been generated that share specific characteristics of human CF, or CF-like disease. In the transgenic βENaC mouse, for example, the β subunit of the epithelial sodium channel was overexpressed, to determine how the various ion transport activities (Na^+ vs Cl^-) relate to disease pathophysiology.[38] This model shows increased epithelial Na^+ absorption, similar to CF, causing ASL volume depletion and reduced mucociliary clearance. These changes resulted in airway mucus obstruction, goblet cell metaplasia, mucus hypersecretion with chronic airway inflammation, reduced clearance of bacterial pathogens, and a high pulmonary mortality in βENaC mice. Although this is not a CFTR-knockout model, βENaC mice address the hypothesis that Na^+ channels play a significant role in the development of CF and CF-like airway disease.

Initial studies in CFTR knockout pigs demonstrated defective Cl^- epithelial transport with the subsequent development of meconium ileus, exocrine pancreatic dysfunction, and focal biliary cirrhosis, all clinical manifestation seen in humans with CF.[39–41] However, the lungs of newborn pigs with mutated CFTR genes were found (at birth) to have no signs of airway inflammation, remodeling, mucus accumulation, or infection. However, a few hours after birth, the lungs of CF pigs were rapidly colonized with multiple bacteria, suggesting a host defense impairment to eradicate airway pathogens in absence of inflammation. This suggests that chronic bacterial infection precedes inflammation and initiates the progression of the CF lung disease. Moreover, the respiratory airways have shown significant reduction in size and circularity of the tracheal lumen, abnormal smooth muscle, and hypoplastic submucosal glands. These changes can be seen in newborns and young children with CF. This airflow obstruction might influence the progression of the CF disease in postnatal life. Recent data suggest that electrolyte transport in porcine CF epithelia showed reduced Cl^- and $HCO3^-$ transport, but no increase in Na^+ or liquid absorption in the nasal and tracheal or bronchial epithelia. These findings challenge the prevailing hypothesis of the specific roles of various ion transport mechanisms in the pathophysiology in CF. Although these observations suggest that the pig model can help to set the stage for the development of target therapies and preventive strategies in CF, further studies are necessary to elucidate the intricate pathways involved.

Similar results have been obtained in the recently created ferret CFTR-knockout model of CF.[42] Sun and colleagues[42] described the phenotype of the CFTR-knockout neonatal ferrets, which shares many organ abnormalities seen in human CF disease, including meconium ileus, pancreatic disease, liver disease, pulmonary disease, absence of the vas deferens, severe impaired nutrition, and malabsorbtion. Tracheal epithelia from newborn CF ferrets showed evidence of defective cAMP-induced Cl^- transport and reduced submucosal gland fluid secretion. Cultures of bronchoalveolar lavage (BAL) fluid in newborn CF ferrets show a predisposition to develop pulmonary infections soon after birth caused by S aureus, Streptococcus pneumonia, and enterobacteria. Outside the lung, liver function tests were noted to be elevated in newborn CF ferrets that were normalized by the administration of ursodeoxycholic acid, a situation similar to humans. Because of the similarities in anatomy and physiology with the CF human disease, the CF ferret model is another useful model that may improve understanding of the pathophysiology of CF disease.

Human Studies

Research studies in human subjects with CF have provided important information about the abnormalities in ion transport, mucus secretion, and MCC in the pathogenesis of CF airway disease. By now classic studies in the respiratory epithelia of patients with CF found increased transepithelial electric potential difference, suggesting an abnormality in Na^+ and Cl^- ion transport.[1] Interestingly, some years later another human disease involving Na^+ channel dysfunction shed insight into the relative contribution of this ion channel to epithelial dysfunction in human disease. Patients with systemic pseudohypoaldosteronism were found to have defective ENaC function, with absence of Na^+ transport in the respiratory airways and increased ASL fluid content, and enhanced mucociliary clearance.[43] These observations in a human disease (not CF) involving ion channels reveal crucial evidence of how the Na^+ channel plays an important role in the regulation of ASL height, and how ASL fluid hydration plays an important role in maintaining adequate airway mucus clearance.

The relationship between airway inflammation and worsening of lung function was recently demonstrated in the pediatric population. Neutrophilic airway inflammation found in BAL of infants with CF was associated with lower pulmonary function tests. At the same time, infection with S aureus and P aeruginosa was correlated with a more rapid decline in lung function. These results suggest that airway inflammation and infection are key pathogenic features in the development and progression of CF lung disease.[44]

Other theories have arisen as to the development of disease. Membrane lipid abnormalities have been proposed to explain the predisposition to inflammation and infection on epithelial surfaces (eg, low linoleic acid and docosahexaenoic acid). More recently, the role of ceramides in the pathophysiology of CF lung disease has been explored. Ceramides are molecules that belong to the sphingolipid family and are an essential component of the plasma membranes, and high levels of ceramide have been found in the airway epithelial cells of knockout mice deficient in CFTR with the subsequent development of inflammation and susceptibility to *P aeruginosa* infection.[45] However, data to date have been conflicting, with high and low levels of ceramide found in mice and humans. Nonetheless, the concept of ceramide in the immunomodulation of CF lung disease remains under investigation as a possible therapeutic target.

Extrapulmonary CF Disease Pathophysiology: Liver, Pancreas, and Gastrointestinal Tract

Liver disease occurs in 27% to 41% of patients with CF, with severe disease occurring in approximately 5% of patients.[46] Hepatobiliary complications of CF liver disease are caused by bile duct obstruction, resulting in periductal inflammation, bile duct proliferation, and periportal fibrosis leading to cirrhosis and portal hypertension. The CFTR protein is localized in the apical membrane of the cholangiocytes and cholecystocytes and regulates the Cl^-, Na^+, and bicarbonate transport and the fluid content of the bile. Absence of functional CFTR produces abnormal secretion of Cl^- and bicarbonate generating thick bile secretions and favoring the bile duct plugging. Recent studies in the CF mouse model showed evidence of increased bilirubin conjugates and unconjugated bilirubin, lower gallbladder bile pH levels, and elevated levels of calcium bilirubinate, favoring the likelihood of supersaturating bile and formation of black pigment gallstones.[47] Studies in the CF pig model demonstrated signs of biliary cirrhosis including cellular inflammation, ductal hyperplasia, and fibrosis.[48] In the ferret model, there were elevations of alanine aminotransferase and bilirubin that normalized with ursodeoxycholic acid, like the response seen in infants with CF, suggesting similar pathophysiologic mechanisms. Recent studies in patients with CF with and without liver involvement suggest that CF liver disease represents a phenotype as a result of altered nutrition, carrying a poorer prognosis and a higher risk of developing CF-related diabetes.[49,50] CF liver disease is an important complication, severe in some patients with CF (likely related to genetic factors), which warrants more research in animal models to generate novel therapies that prevent

and treat effectively hepatobiliary complications in CF.

The pathophysiology of exocrine pancreatic disease in CF is related to abnormal pancreatic secretions, decreased intraluminal bile salt and increased bile salt fecal loss, abnormal composition of bile secretions, and intestinal mucosal abnormalities, which lead to chronic fat malabsorbtion, hypoalbuminemia, fat-soluble vitamin deficiency, and malnutrition.[51] Pancreatic and duodenal bicarbonate levels are decreased in CF because of CFTR dysfunction. Endocrine pancreatic insufficiency is characterized by reduction in the number of islets of Langerhans, reduced β cells, islet architecture disruption, sclerosis, and amyloid deposit. Human studies have shown the association between the severity of CFTR genotype and the risk of pancreatitis. Thus, patients with CF with mild CFTR genotypes were found to have a higher risk of developing pancreatitis compared with patients with CF with moderate to severe CFTR genotypes, suggesting that residual CFTR function increases the risk of pancreatitis.[52,53] From the endocrine pancreas function perspective, in a large retrospective cohort study, CF-related diabetes was associated with a higher mortality rate in patients with CF.[54] Studies in the CF knockout mouse model showed improvement in the lipolytic activity and lipid absorption after pharmacologic gastric acid reduction. In the CF pig model, there is evidence of severe exocrine tissue destruction at birth with the endocrine pancreatic tissue apparently intact. The CF ferret model shows a relatively lower degree of exocrine pancreatic insufficiency with dilation of acini and ductules and eosinophilic zymogen secretions. Of note, the CF pig and ferret models have shown more similarities in the pathophysiology of the CF pancreatic disease in humans than the mouse model, and will likely be useful for further research to understand the mechanisms of CF pancreatic insufficiency.

Meconium ileus, distal intestinal obstruction syndrome, and significant constipation are difficult complications in the gastrointestinal tract in CF.[55] In the intestinal epithelia, CFTR dysfunction leads to decreased Cl^- and fluid volume secretion, and increased Na^+ absorption by ENaC (followed by fluid absorption), producing more viscous intestinal contents and predisposing to obstruction.[50] Meconium ileus occurs in 13% to 17% of patients with CF, with significant morbidity and occasional mortality.[56] New evidence of CF-related enteropathy has been recently described by direct observations of the intestinal mucosa in subjects with CF, showing evidence of intestinal mucosa inflammation, causing chronic intestinal malabsorbtion.[57] The CF mouse, pig, and ferret models have demonstrated gastrointestinal obstructive pathology; however, they both exhibit more meconium ileus than in human infants with CF (100% of pigs and 75% of ferrets have meconium ileus at birth). Other intestinal abnormalities seen in CF disease have been found in CF pigs and ferrets, including intestinal atresia, diverticulosis, and microcolon, as yet not commonly noted in humans with CF.[37]

MICROBIOLOGY

Understanding of the microbiology of the CF lung has evolved over time, because of advances in clinical microbiology laboratory techniques, therapeutic strategies, and possibly changes in infectious patterns.[58] In the 1930s, it was thought that the primary infection associated with CF was S aureus, but by the 1950s P aeruginosa was recognized as an important pathogen, followed by BCC in the 1990s with the latter pathogens recognized as being associated with rapid decline in pulmonary function, bacteremia, and an increased mortality. With dramatic improvements in life expectancy in CF, there has been an increasingly broad spectrum of microbes that have been recognized to infect the CF airways. Some of these organisms are pathogenic, whereas others have less well-defined roles in the pathogenesis in the CF lung.[59] Work to more specifically define the role of the various organisms in CF is critical, given the prognostic and therapeutic implications. Despite a consistent pathogen burden, most patients respond to therapy, suggesting essential changes in the pathogen population that cannot be detected by current quantitative cultures. Quantitative changes may occur in unrecognized or underappreciated organisms during antibiotic therapy, which are now being increasingly recognized. Organisms not considered pathogens on their own may alter the pathogenesis of the microbe community through microbe-to-microbe and polymicrobe-to-host interactions.

Prevalence of Organisms and Detection Techniques

Bacterial culture from sputum and antibiotic susceptibility testing has generally been the mainstay in defining the microbiology of CF airways. The CFF compiles the results of respiratory cultures from patients with CF seen at accredited CF centers and publishes the results annually.[3] Although patients with CF are infected at an early age and often with multiple pathogens, the data demonstrate how the predominant organisms change with age, with S aureus and Haemophilus influenzae occurring most commonly in younger patients, followed later by P aeruginosa. BCC

organisms are problematic in some adults. Other organisms, such as A fumigatus, Achromobacter (Alcaligenes) xylosoxidans, S maltophilia, and NTM, are reported with increasing frequency.[18]

Sampling the lower respiratory tract generally involves acquiring expectorated sputum, although other methods may be used. Oropharyngeal swab sampling is another method, and assumes that the upper respiratory tract flora matches the lower respiratory tract flora. Induced sputum may be used, but is of limited value on younger patients, especially infants. BAL is generally reserved for patients with compelling reasons to obtain a lower respiratory sample. A previous study compared oropharyngeal swabs with BAL samples for the common CF organisms previously mentioned, and found the correlation to be only about 40%.[60] CF sputum protocols have been developed in microbiology laboratories to identify the common CF pathogen by optimizing incubation times and growth conditions, but may have limitations in evaluating the complete diversity of the CF airway's microflora.[61] For example, organisms that are fastidious or difficult to culture may be missed using standard techniques. Newer molecular approaches, such as ribosomal DNA sequencing and terminal restriction fragment length polymorphism, have the potential to greatly improve microbe detection rates and may allow the full classification of the microbial presence in the CF airway.[62,63] Using these techniques, Rogers and colleagues[64] showed that a typical CF airway harbors approximately 13 different species of bacteria. The largest sequence-based analysis of bacteria associated with human airways used pediatric patients with CF.[65] These data showed that molecular approaches provide a more comprehensive view of the microbiology of the lower airways than standard laboratory cultures. The significance of this is still undefined, particularly with respect to the need to treat this diverse population of microbes.[64] A drawback to DNA sequencing is an inability to determine physiologic properties, such as bacterial antibiotic resistance. Nonetheless, this technique promises to open up new avenues in the understanding of the diversity of CF lung flora.

Pseudomonas Aeruginosa

In the adult CF population, P aeruginosa is the most common pathogen cultured chronically in adults, although early eradication treatments may delay the onset of chronic infection.[66] Some more pathogenic strains of P aeruginosa are hyperproducers of pyocyanin, which affects the cilia of the respiratory epithelium and induces neutrophils apoptosis. It is regulated by quorum sensing (QS), a mechanism by which individual bacteria communicate with one another, to alter gene expression in response to changes in population density by secreting molecules referred to as "autoinducers."[67] In *P aeruginosa*, these genes encode for pathogenicity, biofilm formation, and motility. This mechanism allows for precise regulation of genes in response to environmental stimuli and cell density. Bacteria isolated from the chronically infected patient with CF differ from the usual *P aeruginosa* cultured from acute infections in the non-CF population. For example, clonal *P aeruginosa* can form colonies with differing morphotypes. The classic CF isolate is mucoid, caused by the overproduction of alginate; other morphotypes include coliforms, nonpigmented forms, and slow-growing small-colony variants (SCVs). The mucoid phenotype is advantageous because it enhances biofilm formation (see later) and provides immunomodulatory properties that lead to dysregulation of the immune system, which impedes opsonization, phagocytosis, and killing. SVCs are hydrophobic, poorly motile, biofilm formers and are frequently missed in routine culture because of their prolonged culture time. Other phenotypes, such as type III secretors, showing lipopolysaccharide modification (smooth to rough) may enhance pathogenicity and antibiotic resistance. Interestingly, as *P aeruginosa* evolves in the chronically infected patient, the phenotype may become less virulent, enabling the microbe to hide from the immune system, with less tissue damage, allowing it to grow more efficiently and rapidly.[68] Thus, because of the wide range of *P aeruginosa* phenotypes and morphotypes, susceptibility testing may be relatively inaccurate.[69] At a clinical level, there may be poor correlation between antimicrobial susceptibility and successful treatment of an acute exacerbation. For example, Smith and colleagues[70] correlated antibiotic resistance with clinical response and showed that FEV_1 improved in patients despite in vitro antibiotic *P aeruginosa* resistance. Even with resolution of symptoms, antibiotics seldom eradicate chronic *P aeruginosa* infections, and frequently there is little or no demonstrable reduction in the bacterial load. One hypothesis to explain a clinical response despite the presence of resistant bacteria is that antibiotics inhibit bacterial attachment to cells, reducing alginate production (and thus biofilm formation), and may reduce pathogenicity by inhibiting QS.[71] However, the presence of hypermutator strains has led to rapid antibiotic resistance. These strains have defects in their ability to correct mistakes in DNA replication because of a range of selected mutations, such as the mutation in the mismatch repair gene, *mutS*. It has been shown that infection with *P aeruginosa* is associated with worse clinical outcomes in patients with CF.[66] Several small studies suggest that eradication of *P aeruginosa* from the airways of newly or intermittently infected patients with CF results in improved outcomes (see later). Taccetti and colleagues[72] treated 58 newly infected patients with CF with inhaled colomycin and oral ciprofloxacin for 3 weeks. Eradication was achieved in 81% of these patients and was maintained for a median of 18 months with a reduction the annual decline in FEV_1 compared with well-matched controls. Whether *P aeruginosa* is a marker, rather than the cause, of respiratory deterioration may be open to speculation; nevertheless, antipseudomonal therapy does seem to decrease morbidity in chronically infected individuals in the absence of eradication.

Burkholderia Cepacia Species

Phenotypically similar to *Pseudomonas*, isolates of the species BCC have now been classed into their own distinct genomovars. Currently, there are at least 17 different species of *Burkholderia*. They are all natural soil bacteria found in the rhizosphere and they can be plant symbionts or pathogens. *Burkholderia* spp survive well in natural and healthcare environments and may easily spread between patients. Their ability to survive in human epithelial cells and macrophages makes them difficult to eradicate. They are complex microbes with a wide range of pathogenicity factors (lipopolysaccharide, cytotoxin, and biofilm formation), which are regulated by QS mechanisms. *Burkholderia* spp are generally opportunistic pathogens affecting patients who are severely immune-suppressed, or after contamination of fluids or medical devices. The reason for the association with CF is unclear, because patients with non-CF bronchiectasis do not seem to become infected. Infection is more common in older patients with CF, and symptoms may occur when the organism is first acquired, or many years after the initial exposure. Initially recognized in the United Kingdom and Canada in the 1980s, the first strain, *Burkholderia cenocepacia* (ET12 strain; Edinburgh-Toronto), was highly transmissible and pathogenic, leading to many deaths because of severe pneumonia and bacteremia.[73] Currently, the most prevalent strain in patients with CF is *Burkholderia multivorans*. Most new documented infections show unrelated clones, suggesting a decrease in patient-to-patient contamination (possibly as a result of better infection control measures). The gradual decline in lung function with increasing severity of disease may be strain-specific rather than species-specific, or dependent on host (patient) factors or interactions with other pathogens.[73] Infections with *B cepacia* can cause significant decreases in FEV$_1$ in the first 12 months, with increased mortality.[74] B cenocepacia is the genomovar most closely associated with increased morbidity and mortality and the development of the "cepacia syndrome."[17] The impact of B multivorans on CF outcomes remains poorly defined but seems less severe than that of B cenocepacia. A naturally occurring nonmucoid isolate was shown to overexpress several virulence factors relative to the mucoid phenotype, with the most prevalent strain of B cenocepacia being nonmucoid. Interestingly, BCC strains may convert from a mucoid to a nonmucoid morphology during the course of an infection and this may be spurred by the onset of antibiotics. The impact of B cenocepacia on the survival of patients with CF after lung transplantation has resulted in this being considered a relative, or at some centers an absolute, contraindication to the procedure.[75,76] B multivorans has not shown to be associated with similar increases in mortality, although there may be high morbidity.[77]

Staphylococcus Aureus

Staphylococcus aureus is found in approximately 30% of infants with CF by 3 months and persists despite appropriate antibiotic therapy. The SCV phenotype is common in patients with CF and its adaptations include increased antibiotic resistance, resistance to killing by cationic proteins of the innate immune system, and an ability to survive inside host cells.[78] These adaptations enable this phenotype to persist in the CF airways. The SCV colonies are hard to identify and make susceptibility testing in automated systems unreliable. There are higher rates of genome alterations in persisting clones of S aureus in CF sputum compared with healthy individuals, most likely secondary to repeated antibiotic courses and selective pressure of the host response. These S aureus strains have higher rates of mutations presumably to inactivation of a DNA mismatch repair gene, mutS, so mutations are more common and when a favorable mutation occurs these are selected for. One of the more concerning mutations is the increase in MRSA, not because it is more pathogenic, but because treatment options are limited. Despite attempts to control the spread of MRSA, the prevalence in patients with CF is increasing.[79] There are multiple studies relating MRSA infections in CF to overall outcomes, with varying results, although recent studies suggest slightly worse clinical outcomes.[15] A rare strain of S aureus that is vancomycin resistant has been shown in soft tissue infections in non-CF, although none have yet been reported in the CF patient population. S aureus also has the ability to form biofilm, which enhance

their survival and make treatment difficult. The pathogenicity of S aureus is clear in children and is associated with higher mortality and a decreased FEV$_1$; however, in adults it is less clear. In a cross-sectional analysis of the European Epidemiologic Registry of Cystic Fibrosis, analysis of the data did not detect an association between S aureus and concurrent impaired pulmonary status in children or adults.[80] A further study followed the courses of 142 patients with CF and noted that infection with S aureus alone (in the absence of other pathogens) was only associated with mild disease and had improved long-term survival after the age of 18 years.[81] A multivariate logistic regression model of 5820 children and adults in the US CFF Patient Registry identified S aureus infection as a marker for improved survival, suggesting that infection with S aureus may prevent infection with more virulent pathogens, such as P aeruginosa.[74]

Haemophilus Influenzae

Haemophilus influenzae is common in infants (38%) and young children with CF but less common as the population ages. There is little information available on long-term infections with H influenza, and studies have shown that most patients with recurrent H influenzae infections tend to acquire different strains. A study examining the sputum of 30 patients with CF showed that 90% of the patients had two or more distinct strains over a 7-year period.[82] In patients with CF, this organism is usually unencapsulated (nontypeable) and not covered by the H influenzae type b vaccine. Antibiotic resistance has increased with time with up to 37% of H influenzae strains being quinolone resistant, rarely seen outside of the CF population. Similar to S aureus, its increased mutation rates stem from the mutS gene and its persistence enhanced with biofilm formation. Interestingly, azithromycin inhibits biofilm formation in vitro, and reduces established biofilm in H influenzae without affecting bacterial growth. In contrast to most organisms, the pathogenicity of the CF strains of H influenzae is debatable because they are common colonizers of the upper airways of healthy children. A cross-sectional analysis of 7010 patients from the European Epidemiologic Registry of Cystic Fibrosis found that isolation of H influenzae from the respiratory tract was not associated with a decrease in FEV$_1$; however, several other studies suggest that H influenzae may play a role in CF disease progression.[80] One older study observed a rise in the rate of isolation of H influenzae before and during acute exacerbations in patients with CF and noted that clinical improvement after antimicrobial therapy coincided with a reduction in bacterial load.[83]

Miscellaneous Bacteria and Anerobes

With increasing life expectancy, prolonged use of antibiotics, and improvement in laboratory identification, including the application of molecular non–culture-based techniques designed for characterizing bacterial communities, such as 16S rRNA gene profiling by terminal restriction fragment length polymorphism or pyrosequencing, there has been an increasing prevalence and recognition of other microbes (largely gram-negative) in the CF population, most notably S maltophilia, A xylosoxidans, Bordetella, Enterobacteriaceae, Acinetobacter, and Pandoraea apista. The clinical significance of many of these is uncertain, without a clear association with outcomes, such as FEV$_1$.[84] These microbes may be relatively harmless colonizers, but correct identification is key because they can be mistakenly identified for known pathogens. The recent use of species-specific polymerase chain reaction and ribosomal RNA gene sequencing has greatly increased the sensitivity of microbial identification.[85] Sputum and sometimes BAL samples grow bacteria that maybe labeled "normal mouth/upper airway flora." Initially, they were thought contaminated with saliva; however, recent data show that the microbe density is too great to be explained from contamination alone.[63] Using 16s rRNA gene profiling by terminal restriction fragment length polymorphisms directly from the high density CF sputum exposes a diverse population of anaerobic and aerobic species.[86] The significance of this observation is also unknown. It is possible that they are normal flora with no clinical importance, but alternatively they could be pathogenic and overshadowed by other assumed pathogens, such as P aeruginosa. They may also interact with other pathogens making them more virulent. This could account for the clinical improvement seen in patients with CF despite using antibiotics to which their primary pathogen is resistant. Analysis of CF airway samples by strict anoxic culture and culture-independent molecular methods have consistently isolated anaerobic species in numbers comparable with the typical aerobic bacterial pathogens.[62] This suggests that anaerobes are persistent rather than transient. The relative abundance of anaerobes in samples, and differences in composition of anaerobic species between purely oral specimens and sputum samples, suggests that they originate from the lower respiratory tract with no significant oral contamination.[87] In the CF lung, there are extreme oxygen gradients with regions of hypoxia within mucus plugs. There are new studies that support a potential pathogenic role for some anaerobic organisms. Field and colleagues showed that Prevotella, a species commonly found in CF airways, are able to produce β-lactamses and an auto-inducer molecule,[87] and Ulrich and colleagues[88] showed that patients with CF, unlike healthy patients, have antibodies against Prevotella antigens. Even if anaerobic bacteria are not virulent, they could influence the virulence of other microorganisms by QS. Targeting anaerobes with specific antibiotics is challenging because susceptibility testing of gram-positive and negative anaerobes shows the specific CF isolates are extremely resistant to antibiotics commonly used to treat anaerobic infections, including amoxicillin–clavulinate, metronidazole, clindamycin, and pipercillin–clavulinate. Tunney and colleagues[89] showed that antibiotic treatment targeted against aerobes had minimal effect on most anaerobes despite an improvement in the clinical status. This was redemonstrated by Worlitzsch and colleagues,[90] who showed an improvement in lung function after treatment with intravenous antibiotics despite no reduction in obligate anaerobe density. Although there are emerging data for the relative importance of anaerobes in CF and non-CF lung disease, there is some uncertainty as to their exact role in disease course and management, although it is believed that they have the potential to be pathogenic.

Nontuberculous Mycobacteria

As the prevalence of NTM increases in the aging CF population, it has been increasingly recognized as a clinical problem. With increased surveillance and new automated liquid laboratory systems more NTM are being seen in the CF population. In a classic study of 21 CF centers in the United States over 10 years, 13% of the 986 patients studied had culture-positive NTM with 2.5% meeting American Thoracic Society criteria for NTM disease, being more common in older patients, with Mycobacterium avium complex being the most common.[91] However, recent data suggest an increase in the Mycobacterium abscessus prevalence. M abscessus may be associated with more severe clinical disease.[20] Its colonies are either rough or smooth depending on the expression of glycopeptidolipid; the smooth form (glycopeptidolipid present) creates biofilm, favoring colonization with less pathogenicity, whereas the rough form produces little glycopeptidolipid, yet infects human monocytes and may cause persistent infection. When in biofilm, M abscessus is less susceptible to antibiotics. The clinical significance of a positive NTM culture is uncertain, because most patients with CF are coinfected with other organisms and different NTM species may be isolated over time. It may be difficult to distinguish "colonizer" NTM species from pathogenic species, and to distinguish repeat environmental infections from established infections (person-to-person NTM infection has not yet been reported). Also, as laboratory methods improve and taxonomy changes, previous benign species, such as *Mycobacterium fortuitum* or *Mycobacterium chelonae*, may now be identified as *M abscessus*. The usefulness of antibiotic susceptibility testing is uncertain, because clinical correlation is poor. NTM isolation should lead to the consideration of a diagnosis of CF (most likely nonclassic) in older patients, because a significant proportion of adults with bronchiectasis or pulmonary NTM infection may have previously undiagnosed CF.[92] Few studies have directly examined the impact of NTM on clinical outcomes in CF. An older study at the Leeds CF clinic followed NTM patients over 2 years and the NTM patients did not differ significantly in FEV_1, forced vital capacity, growth, or clinical well-being as well-matched non-NTM controls.[93] Analyzing all NTM species as a group masks the more virulent nature of some NTM species, such as *M abscessus*. A study from the University of North Carolina looked at 38 patients with NTM, and the subset with *M abscessus* had a significantly more rapid decline in FEV_1 compared with the non-*abscessus* species.[20]

Biofilm

Biofilm has attracted considerable interest from the CF community. Similar to other bacteria seen in CF, *P aeruginosa* forms biofilm in culture and can be seen in biofilm aggregates in expectorated sputum. Biofilms are communities of bacteria within an acellular matrix, usually attached to a surface, such as the CF respiratory epithelium. The microbes in biofilm are kept together by a self-produced biopolymeric matrix containing polysaccharides, proteins, and extracellular DNA originating from the microbes. The bacteria appear different in biofilm because the pattern of gene expression resembles planktonically growing bacteria and there is upregulation of genes, which are necessary for anaerobic growth.[94] Biofilms also contain other species of bacteria and host-derived products. Once in a biofilm, bacteria are difficult to eradicate because the biofilm offers shelter from the immune system and provides antibiotic resistance by multiple mechanisms. For example, antibiotics may bind to the extracellular matrix rather than the bacteria; they may be ineffective during the specific growth phase (dividing or dormant); or they may have reduced activity in areas of poor oxygenation or low pH. Biofilm-growing bacteria exhibit increased tolerance

against antibiotics, disinfectants, and innate and adaptive host immune mechanisms. The minimal inhibitory concentrations of antibiotics to biofilm-growing bacteria are up to 1000-fold higher than non–biofilm-producing bacteria. Biofilm also produces a gradient of oxygen, nutrients, and metabolites; thus the microbes protected by them are heterogeneous.

Fungi and Viruses

Fungal spores are common in the air and water and originate from rotting vegetation. *Aspergillus* sp, particularly *A fumigatus*, can cause allergic bronchopulmonary aspergillosis (ABPA) in patients with CF similar to patients with asthma.[95] ABPA is capable of causing short-term deterioration in lung function, although it is not clear whether ABPA is associated with irreversible long-term pulmonary decline in the CF population. Aspergillomas, although relatively rare in the CF population, have been documented, as has *Aspergillus* bronchitis. Other fungi may cause a syndrome of ABPA (allergic bronchopulmonary mycoses), such as *Scedosporium apiospermum* in patients with CF. *Candida* spp are frequently found in CF sputum, but are rarely pathogenic outside of transplant or immunosuppression. Respiratory viruses are common among the general population but their specific role in the CF population is not well studied. This is partly caused by the lack of sensitive techniques for detecting viruses until recently. It is thought that respiratory viruses may trigger an acute CF exacerbation, and play a role in the first acquisition or predisposition to chronic infection with bacterial pathogens. A 25-year Danish study showed that patients with CF were more likely to acquire *P aeruginosa* infection between October and March, the peak season for respiratory viruses.[96] Influenza may have a significant impact on lung function in patients with CF; annual vaccination is recommended and initiation of antiviral therapy with onset of flulike symptoms.

RECENT AND EMERGING THERAPIES AND NEW APPROACHES TO THE DELIVERY OF CARE IN CF

In parallel with the increase in knowledge in genetics and pathophysiology of the disease, new therapeutic approaches have been developed in recent years. The increase in life expectancy in the CF population has a multifactorial basis, mainly thought to relate initially to the development of pancreatic enzymes and antibiotics, and more recently to the development of a multifaceted approach to the management of CF.[97] Early in the 1990s, clinical studies showed that inhalation of recombinant human DNase resulted in improvement in lung function and imaging scores, and exacerbation frequency. This was quite exciting at the time because it was a relatively "targeted therapy."[1] After that, there have been many novel therapies in clinical development. This section reviews recently approved drugs and briefly addressing the many emerging novel therapies for CF.

Molecular Therapies

As early as 1989, when the genetic basis for the disease was first described, the possibility of gene-targeted therapy quickly emerged. However, early excitement was tempered with the reality of the challenges involved in successful gene transfer in CF. Initially, viral vectors using adenoviruses and adenoassociated viruses were tried but they were unsuccessful, with adverse events.[98] Trials with liposomal vectors were also ineffective.[99] The UK Cystic Fibrosis Gene Therapy Consortium is currently studying a plasmid-DNA and nonviral vector approach and has started phase 1 trials. Other new therapies affecting CFTR transcription, processing, or functioning are in the development pipeline. These molecules may be ingested orally, and range from agents that allow the ribosome to read through premature stop codons in CFTR mRNA, "correctors" that help CFTR fold properly, and "potentiators" that increase chloride channel activity at the cell surface. The most common CF mutation, ΔF508, is a class II mutation where misfolded CFTR is degraded before reaching the apical cell membrane. However, the misfolded protein retains enough function that if it were guided to the apical membrane it could show a clinical impact. VX-809 is a possible corrector that assists in the delivery of CFTR to the airway apical epithelium. Current phase II studies in homozygote ΔF508 patients show promise with significant improvement in sweat chloride levels. Ten percent of CF mutations are class I nonsense mutations that lead to premature termination of mRNA translation and result in an abridged, nonfunctional CFTR protein. PTC124 is a small molecule that allows ribosomal read through of premature stop codons and formation of a functional CFTR protein and this molecule was found safe and well tolerated in phase I trials. Phase II studies in adults with CF showed enhancement in Cl^- efflux and a large phase III study looking at FEV_1 is currently underway.[100] Class III mutations are associated with reduced opening of the CFTR channel with a reduction in Cl^- movement into the airway lumen and mutations. Potentiator therapy directed at these mutations increases the function of a correctly placed CFTR, and a current potentiator, VX-770, is currently in phase II studies in patients with G551D mutations ($\sim$ 4% of patients in the United States). These trials have shown improvement in nasal potential differences and, more importantly, lung function parameters.[101] At the time of writing, the clinical data for this compound (now known as ivacaftor) are very exciting, with improvements in lung function at two weeks that were sustained, with substantial improvements in the risk of pulmonary exacerbations, quality of life measures, weight, and concentrations of sweat chloride.[102] There are also interesting studies examining the combination of potentiators and correctors, specifically VX-770 and VX-809 in ΔF508 homozygote patients with CF (http://www.cff.org/research/ClinicalResearch/FAQs/CombinedVX-770-VX-809/).

Finally, phosphodiesterase inhibitors, such as sildenafil and vardenafil, have some efficacy in animal models in modulating CFTR.

Ion Transport Therapies

Defective Cl^- secretion and Na^+ hyperabsorption lead to airway dehydration with impairment of mucociliary transport. Airway hydration therapies include those that activate Cl^- secretion by non–CFTR-dependent pathways, inhibit Na^+ absorption, or by the addition of osmotic agents directly to the airway surface. These therapies alone or in combination should hypothetically enhance mucociliary clearance of bacteria, mucus, and inflammatory products, and it is hoped preserve lung function.[30] Osmotic agents may also increase ciliary beat frequency and enhance cough clearance. The best known and widely used of this class of therapy is inhaled hypertonic saline (7%).[103] Used twice daily, hypertonic saline has been shown to improve mucociliary clearance and lung function and is currently used in pediatric and adult patients with CF. Inhaled mannitol, another osmotic agent, was shown to improve FEV_1 over a 2-week period in phase II trials and is currently under study in CF and non-CF bronchiectasis.[104] Denufosol tetrasodium is a puridinine triphosphate derivative and $P2Y_2$ receptor agonist that activates alternate chloride channels in the respiratory epithelium. Initial studies using aerosolized denufosol showed significant differences in FEV_1 compared with placebo controls, but follow-up studies failed to show an improvement in the primary outcome of lung function and the compound has been dropped from further study.[105]

Antiinflammatory Therapies

Inflammation without overt infection occurs in CF lungs and is neutrophil predominant, with activation of numerous inflammatory cascades. There is no standard antiinflammatory regimen for patients with CF. Oral glucocorticoids were initially used, but adverse effects outweigh any potential benefits for chronic therapy, unless there is concurrent asthma or ABPA. Initial trials with ibuprofen showed an improvement in FEV_1 in children; however, repeat studies did not reproduce the benefit in FEV_1 and there was a risk for peptic ulcers and renal insufficiency, especially in combination with aminoglycosides. There are current trials looking at statins, hydroxychloroquine, and phosphodiesterase inhibitors. To counter the high levels of neutrophil elastase secreted by the active and abundant neutrophils, some groups are studying the effects of α_1-antitrypsin on lung function and airway inflammation. Data show some limited effect on sputum neutrophil elastase activity and inflammatory markers with inhaled α_1-antitrypsin. Antioxidants could also counter the oxidative damage caused by the immune system. Such agents are inhaled glutathione and oral N-acetylcysteine, which replenishes the antioxidant glutathione. Macrolides, mainly azithromycin, are used to reduce inflammation in patients with CF colonized with P aeruginosa and were shown to significantly reduce the number of respiratory exacerbations, the rate of FEV_1 decline, and the quality of life. Recent studies have also shown a reduction in exacerbations in non–P aeruginosa patients.

Antimicrobial Drugs

Treating infection in the CF airways is a standard therapy; oral and intravenous regimens are considered standard of care, and the advent of implantable devices has continued to improve to make this a safe, feasible option for hospital and at home.[106] Inhaled antibiotics offer an alternative method of delivery that delivers high concentrations of drug to the site of infection, while minimizing systemic exposure and toxicity, with the intent to serve as "preventive" therapies. Current inhaled agents target P aeruginosa, because it is the most common pathogenic microbe in the adult airway. Aerosolizing antibiotics is complicated because there are many considerations, such as drug stability, particle size, site, airway concentration, and total dose delivered, and ease of use and expense. There are new innovations in antibiotic formulations, such as dry powder formulations and lipid nanoparticle aerosols, and improvements in delivery devices. The first of this class to be formally studied and approved for use in CF was inhaled tobramycin (300 mg/mL). This drug was shown to improve FEV_1, decrease P aeruginosa density, and decrease hospitalization rates.

Inhaled aztreonam has been a more recent development, and initial trials have shown that patients with P aeruginosa with moderate to severe lung disease improved respiratory symptoms and FEV_1.[107] Another inhaled antibiotic, colistin, has long been available but has not been as well studied to date in formal double-blind controlled trials. Inhaled antibiotics also under study include amikacin, levofloxacin, ciprofloxacin, and a fosfomycin–tobramycin combination. Inhaled amikacin is a liposomal nanoparticle being developed as a once-daily medication that can penetrate into the bacterial biofilm. Recent phase II trials have shown a significant improvement in FEV_1, P aeruginosa density, and reduction in sputum production. Inhaled ciprofloxacin is being formulated as a dry powder, with obvious advantages in delivery and ease of use and portability. Recently, intermittent inhalation strategies (every other month) have been challenged and many centers have moved to continuous inhalation regimens consisting of aerosolized colomycin–tobramycin combinations, or tobramycin–aztreonam. Attempts to eradicate various organisms before they become chronically present in the airway have been the focus of attention in recent years, with a particular focus on P aeruginosa given the evidence for its adverse effects on outcomes. The ELITE study showed that a 28-day regimen of inhaled tobramycin 300 mg/ml is effective in treating early P aeruginosa infections.[108] Treatments aimed to eradicate MRSA should also be considered after first isolation.

Airway Clearance

Because airway clearance is an integral component of CF therapy, specific techniques and devices have been developed to promote mobilization of secretions, such as the active cycle of breathing techniques, autogenic drainage, positive expiratory pressure masks, the Flutter and Acapella valves, and high-frequency chest wall oscillation devices (eg, the Vest). None of these methodologies or devices is considered superior to the other, but daily airway clearance is strongly suggested for all patients. Aerobic exercise has numerous beneficial effects including augmenting airway clearance and cardiovascular fitness.

Miscellaneous

Nonpulmonary manifestations that can be problematic include gastrointestinal and nutritional issues. Destruction of acinar pancreatic tissue, pancreatic ductular obstruction, and lack of enzymatic activity lead to malabsorption (particularly of fats), diarrhea, and failure to thrive, and progressive lung disease further increases calorie requirements. Malnutrition is closely related to a decline in lung function and early infection with *P aeruginosa*. The use of replacement therapy with pancreatic enzymes with an emphasis on a calorific, high-protein diet with fat-soluble vitamin (ADEK) supplementation is important and helps lead to normal growth and better lung function. Pancreatic enzyme products (PEP) were initially exempted from Food and Drug Administration approval; thus there were more than 15 different products in a variety of formulations including microsphere, microcapsule, enteric-coated, and regular-release products. Recently, a review of PEPs was instituted, because some patients experienced treatment failures thought to relate to these differences. A mandate in all PEPs to seek formal new drug approval was issued, and in April 2010 several preparations of PEPs became unavailable.[109] CF-related diabetes becomes more common as patients grow older, and if poorly controlled may be associated with a rapid decline in lung function and recurrent infections. It is important to screen for the problem, because impaired glucose tolerance may occur before the development of overt diabetes. The management of CF-related diabetes is now recognized as quite different from other forms of diabetes; insulin is the preferred agent, and caloric restriction should not be instituted. Treatment with insulin enhances the nutritional state and may improve lung function and slow FEV_1 decline (see next section).[110] ABPA has prevalence up to 15% and increases with age, presumably with increased *Aspergillus* exposures. Although systemic steroids have been the mainstay of treatment for some time, antifungals may play a role.[95]

OUTCOMES RESEARCH AND QI

CF is as yet an incurable genetic disease, although survival for patients with CF has improved. Survival improvement has been correlated to the decade in which the patient was born; patients born in 2010 are now expected to have a median survival into their sixth decade of life.[97] Some of the improvements in survival are caused by an established network of centers in which CF-focused clinicians collaborate in clinical trials, engage in the translation of basic science advances into improved clinical practices, and review and improve the process of delivery of care at a team level. This section reviews the factors associated with predictors of outcomes in CF, and the improvements in CF care at the "system of care" level, which may have an impact on outcomes.

The factors that influence the expression of the phenotype of CF have already been reviewed in detail: genetic, environmental, social, and infectious. An example of the study of the genetic influences includes a study by Koch and colleagues[111] where data from the European registry were examined, and frequency and severity of the major clinical manifestations in patients with CF was compared among the different classes of mutations. Patients with class IV or V mutations had the best outcomes, whereas class I homozygotes had the poorest outcomes. A new international initiative, the CFTR2 project, will provide complete, advanced, and expert reviewed functional and clinical information on the CFTR mutations with important implications for diagnosis, prognosis, and therapy to patients and families, especially the CFTR mutation carriers (http://www.cftr2.org). The occurrence of pulmonary complications, including pneumothorax and massive hemoptysis, is a poor prognostic marker. Several studies have shown that pulmonary exacerbations negatively affect quality of life and are associated with significant cost.[112] A large observational study of more than 11,000 patients with CF showed that 42% had experienced a pulmonary exacerbation within a 6-month period.[113] Following from that observation, de Boer and colleagues[114] recently showed that patients with CF with frequent exacerbations have an accelerated decline in lung function and an increased 3-year risk of death or lung transplant. It also demonstrated that females, diabetics, and patients with poorer lung function at baseline are particularly at risk. Thus, interventions that reduce exacerbation rates are likely to have an impact on not only quality of life, but also survival. Onset of insulin-dependent diabetes is associated with worse lung function, poorer nutrition, and increased mortality compared with nondiabetic patients with CF. There may be a decline in lung function and body weight 2 to 6 years before the onset of overt insulin-requiring diabetes. Currently, there is still debate on the best time to start insulin therapy. It is also documented that there is an association between better nutritional status and lung function; data from the German CF registry found that low body mass index and low FEV_1 correlated with increased mortality.[115] Pain, also common in the CF population, interferes with activities and is associated with lower quality of life and an increased risk of exacerbation and death. Age at diagnosis, primarily through newborn screening, is emerging as a possible determinant of survival. It was first noticed that among sibling pairs, the younger sibling diagnosed at 1 year of age before symptom onset had better pulmonary function at 7 years of age than the older sibling diagnosed at an older age with symptoms. The Wisconsin study showed that early intervention improves nutritional outcomes and there was a slight trend toward improved survival in newborns diagnosed before 1 month of age compared with infants diagnosed at a later age.[116] All 50 states in the United States now screen for CF at birth and by 2007, more than 30% of new cases were being diagnosed using newborn screening.[117] Initial care can now focus on preventative measures, particularly nutritional intervention and supplementation, and a wealth of related data will likely emerge in the future.

Although outcomes for patients with CF in the intensive care unit have been shown to be reasonable, and despite advances in intensive care unit care, the survival of patients with CF requiring mechanical ventilation for respiratory failure remains low, particularly in older patients with end-stage lung disease who have a mortality of up to 82%.[118,119] Thus, there has been a focus of effort at improvement in these outcomes. For example, Hayes and Mansour[120] recently showed that a novel antibiotic strategy, using a continuous infusion of a β-lactam antibiotic combined with extended interval tobramycin, improved survival in intubated, critically ill patients with CF with end-stage lung disease and malnutrition. Although this study and other intensive care unit studies are small, the data illustrate that aggressive intervention may provide clinicians with some hope for improving outcomes in critically ill patients with CF who may face prolonged intubation.

With improvement in survival of women with CF, pregnancy has become commonplace. In prior decades relatively underreported, now pregnancy in CF can occur with good outcomes for mother and child. One such early study showed that pregnant women with CF had better nutritional status, more preserved FEV_1, and decreased mortality compared with women with CF who did not get pregnant. A study[121] recently demonstrated that most women tolerated pregnancy well without major complications despite having at least moderate lung impairment. Nonetheless, prepregnancy FEV_1 and body mass index were important predictors of outcomes. Thus, good outcomes can be achieved if the pregnancy is planned ahead and the mother's clinical status is optimized in advance.

Over the past 15 years, there has been growing interest in developing quantitative ways to measure subjective perceptions of patients by using rigorous standards of measurements and psychometric analysis. It is recommended now that health-related quality of life measures be included in clinical trials of new therapies because optimization of quality of life is as important as longevity. Patients have complex therapeutic regimens that must be balanced with school, work, and family and it is important to prioritize and select the most optimal and sustainable therapies. Adolescents often balance academic demands and peer pressure with time-consuming treatments and adherence declines. Anxiety and depressive symptoms are common in patients with CF, especially as they mature into adolescence. They are associated with poorer quality of life, low lung function, reduced physical functioning, and severity of chest symptoms.[122] Therefore, routine screening for symptoms of anxiety and depression is worthwhile and those identified with should be referred for appropriate therapy.

QI initiatives in the delivery of care to patients with CF have become common worldwide. This partly relates to standardizing clinician and team member education, and adherence to practice guidelines. QI using a clinical microsystem approach provides CF centers the ability to make significant positive impacts on the health of their patients. The Lewis Walker Cystic Fibrosis Center at Akron Children's Hospital used the QI process, from the initial team-building phase, through the assessment of care process, standardization of care, and developing a culture of continuous improvement, to improve the pulmonary health (decrease exacerbation frequency) of their patients with CF.[123] Challenges to the implementing of guidelines recommendations may vary by center. Building a robust team educated in the nuances of delivering quality care in a complex health system may be challenging; smaller centers may suffer from a lack of resources, personnel, and time to engage fully in these initiatives, whereas larger centers may have to deal with administrative issues, and difficulties in changing set practice patterns. Nonetheless, these are critical issues, and recent studies have borne out the early hypotheses that QI would have an impact on clinical outcomes, with an improvement in clinical practice, without necessarily losing individualization of medical care. The CFF's Learning and Leadership Collaborative is another initiative in which the CF community may participate, and registry analysis shows an increased rate of improvement in pulmonary and nutritional outcomes, suggesting that the time spent in QI is having an impact.[124] There are several examples of how the US CFF Patient Registry has been used by CF centers to motivate QI. In 1998, the Northern New England Cystic Fibrosis Consortium showed significant variation in its screening rates for CF-related diabetes (17% below the national average). After a 3-year QI initiative that involved feedback of data to clinicians, patient education about CF-related diabetes, and clinic system changes, to trigger annual diabetes measures, and data tracking, the Northern New England

Cystic Fibrosis Consortium reduced variation in its centers to 4% above the national average.[125] In another example, the Children's Memorial Hospital in Chicago was able to reduce rates of nutritional failure by documenting nutritional status at every clinic visit, and targeting those patients at the highest risk for nutritional failure with a customized self-management plan (http://www.childrensmemorial.org/documents/cfcnews_winter04.pdf). The CF community has become a leader in the area of QI, resulting in opportunities for other fields to follow in the area of delivery of care.[126]

ACKNOWLEDGMENTS

The authors thank Scott Donaldson, MD, for helpful comments on the manuscript.

REFERENCES

1. Boucher RC, Knowles MR, Yankaskas JR. Cystic fibrosis. In: Mason RJ, Martin T, King T, et al, editors. Murray and Nadel's textbook of respiratory medicine. 5th edition. Philadelphia: Elsevier; 2010. p. 985–1022.
2. Cohen-Cymberknoh M, Shoseyov D, Kerem E. Managing cystic fibrosis strategies that increase life expectancy and improve quality of life. Am J Respir Crit Care Med 2011;183:1463–71.
3. Cystic Fibrosis Foundation Patient Registry. 2010 Annual Report to the Center Directors. Cystic fibrosis foundation annual data report 2010. 2011. p. 2–3. Available at: http://www.cff.org. Accessed February 22, 2012.
4. Cutting GR. Modifier genes in mendelian disorders: the example of cystic fibrosis. Ann N Y Acad Sci 2010;1214:57–69.
5. Rogan MP, Stoltz DA, Hornick DB. Cystic fibrosis transmembrane conductance regulator intracellular processing, trafficking, and opportunities for mutation-specific treatment. Chest 2011;139:1480–90.
6. Noone PG, Pue CA, Zhou Z, et al. Lung disease associated with the IVS8 5T allele of the CFTR gene. Am J Respir Crit Care Med 2000;162:1919–24.
7. Li W, Sun L, Corey M, et al. Understanding the population structure of North American patients with cystic fibrosis. Clin Genet 2011;79:136–46.
8. Vanscoy LL, Blackman SM, Collaco JM, et al. Heritability of lung disease severity in cystic fibrosis. Am J Respir Crit Care Med 2007;175:1036–43.
9. Wright FA, Strug LJ, Doshi VK, et al. Genome-wide association and linkage identify modifier loci of lung disease severity in cystic fibrosis at 11p13 and 20q13.2. Nat Genet 2011;43:539–46.
10. Blohmke CJ, Park J, Hirschfeld AF, et al. TLR5 as an anti-inflammatory target and modifier gene in cystic fibrosis. J Immunol 2010;185:7731–8.
11. Bartlett JR, Friedman KJ, Ling SC, et al. Genetic modifiers of liver disease in cystic fibrosis. JAMA 2009;302:1076–83.
12. Dorfman R, Taylor C, Lin F, et al. Modulatory effect of the SLC9A3 gene on susceptibility to infections and pulmonary function in children with cystic fibrosis. Pediatr Pulmonol 2011;46:385–92.
13. Blackman SM, Hsu S, Ritter SE, et al. A susceptibility gene for type 2 diabetes confers substantial risk for diabetes complicating cystic fibrosis. Diabetologia 2009;52:1858–65.
14. Pittman JE, Calloway EH, Kiser M, et al. Age of Pseudomonas aeruginosa acquisition and subsequent severity of cystic fibrosis lung disease. Pediatr Pulmonol 2011;46:497–504.
15. Dasenbrook EC, Checkley W, Merlo CA, et al. Association between respiratory tract methicillin-resistant Staphylococcus aureus and survival in cystic fibrosis. JAMA 2010;303:2386–92.
16. Dasenbrook EC, Merlo CA, Diener-West M, et al. Persistent methicillin-resistant Staphylococcus aureus and rate of FEV1 decline in cystic fibrosis. Am J Respir Crit Care Med 2008;178:814–21.
17. Jones AM, Dodd ME, Govan JR, et al. Burkholderia cenocepacia and Burkholderia multivorans: influence on survival in cystic fibrosis. Thorax 2004; 59:948–51.
18. Razvi S, Quittell L, Sewall A, et al. Respiratory microbiology of patients with cystic fibrosis in the United States, 1995 to 2005. Chest 2009;136:1554–60.
19. Kunst H, Wickremasinghe M, Wells A, et al. Nontuberculous mycobacterial disease and Aspergillus-related lung disease in bronchiectasis. Eur Respir J 2006;28:352–7.
20. Esther CR, Esserman DA, Gilligan P, et al. Chronic Mycobacterium abscessus infection and lung function decline in cystic fibrosis. J Cyst Fibros 2010;9:117–23.
21. Wolfenden LL, Schechter MS. Genetic and non-genetic determinants of outcomes in cystic fibrosis. Paediatr Respir Rev 2009;10:32–6.
22. Schechter MS. Non-genetic influences on cystic fibrosis lung disease: the role of sociodemographic characteristics, environmental exposures, and healthcare interventions. Semin Respir Crit Care Med 2003;24:639–52.
23. Tippets BM, Shoff SM, Lin F, et al. CF newborn screening in Wisconsin: comparison of pulmonary outcomes during the first six years of life between children diagnosed during the randomized clinical trial (1985-1994) and the Routine Program (1994-2003). Abstract at the NACF meeting, 2009. Pediatr Pulmonol 2009;351.
24. Sanders D, Lai HJ, Rock M, et al. Infants with CF diagnosed in IRT/DNA states are treated earlier than those diagnosed in IRT/IRT states. Abstract at the NACF meeting, 2009. Pediatr Pulmonol 2010;389.

25. Quittner AL, Schechter MS, Rasouliyan L, et al. Impact of socioeconomic status, race, and ethnicity on quality of life in patients with cystic fibrosis in the United States. Chest 2010;137:642–50.

26. Knowles MR, Durie PR. What is cystic fibrosis? N Engl J Med 2002;347:439–42.

27. Smith JJ, Travis SM, Welsh MJ. Cystic fibrosis airway epithelia fail to kill bacteria because of abnormal airway surface liquid. Cell 1996;85:229–36.

28. Matsui H, Grubb BR, Tarran R, et al. Evidence for periciliary liquid layer depletion, not abnormal ion composition, in the pathogenesis of cystic fibrosis airways disease. Cell 1998;95:1–20.

29. Boucher RC. Airway surface dehydration in cystic fibrosis: pathogenesis and therapy. Annu Rev Med 2007;58:157–70.

30. Donaldson SH, Boucher RC. Sodium channels and cystic fibrosis. Chest 2007;132:1631–6.

31. Clunes MT, Boucher RC. Cystic fibrosis: the mechanisms of pathogenesis of an inherited lung disorder. Drug Discov Today Dis Mech 2007;4:63–72.

32. Ferrera L, Caputo A, Galietta LJ. TMEM16A protein: a new identity for Ca(2+)-dependent Cl(-) channels. Physiology 2010;25:357–63.

33. Voynow JA, Rubin BK. Mucins, mucus, and sputum. Chest 2009;135:505–12.

34. Chen JH, Stoltz DA, Karp PH, et al. Loss of anion transport without increased sodium absorption characterizes newborn porcine cystic fibrosis airway epithelia. Cell 2010;143:911–23.

35. Ribeiro CM, Boucher RC. Role of endoplasmic reticulum stress in cystic fibrosis-related airway inflammatory responses. Proc Am Thorac Soc 2010;7:387–94.

36. Wilke M, Buijs-Offerman RM, Aarbiou J, et al. Mouse models of cystic fibrosis: phenotypic analysis and research applications. J Cyst Fibros 2011;10:S152–71.

37. Keiser NW, Engelhardt JF. New animal models of cystic fibrosis: what are they teaching us? Curr Opin Pulm Med 2011;17:478–83.

38. Zhou Z, Duerr J, Johannesson B, et al. The beta ENaC-overexpressing mouse as a model of cystic fibrosis lung disease. J Cyst Fibros 2011;10:S172–82.

39. Rogers CS, Stoltz DA, Meyerholz DK, et al. Disruption of the CFTR gene produces a model of cystic fibrosis in newborn pigs. Science 2008;321:1837–41.

40. Stoltz DA, Meyerholz DK, Pezzulo AA, et al. Cystic fibrosis pigs develop lung disease and exhibit defective bacterial eradication at birth. Sci Transl Med 2010;2:29–31.

41. Meyerholz DK, Stoltz DA, Namati E, et al. Loss of cystic fibrosis transmembrane conductance regulator function produces abnormalities in tracheal development in neonatal pigs and young children. Am J Respir Crit Care Med 2010;182:1251–61.

42. Sun XS, Sui HS, Fisher JT, et al. Disease phenotype of a ferret CFTR-knockout model of cystic fibrosis. J Clin Invest 2010;120:3149–60.

43. Kerem E, Bistritzer T, Hanukoglu A, et al. Pulmonary epithelial sodium-channel dysfunction and excess airway liquid in pseudohypoaldosteronism. N Engl J Med 1999;341:156–62.

44. Pillarisetti N, Williamson E, Linnane B, et al. Infection, inflammation, and lung function decline in infants with cystic fibrosis. Am J Respir Crit Care Med 2011;184:75–81.

45. Wojewodka G, De Sanctis JB, Radzioch D. Ceramide in cystic fibrosis: a potential new target for therapeutic intervention. J Lipids 2011;2011:1–12.

46. Debray D, Kelly D, Houwen R, et al. Best practice guidance for the diagnosis and management of cystic fibrosis-associated liver disease. J Cyst Fibros 2011;10:S29–36.

47. Freudenberg F, Leonard MR, Liu SA, et al. Pathophysiological preconditions promoting mixed "black" pigment plus cholesterol gallstones in a Delta F508 mouse model of cystic fibrosis. Am J Physiol Gastrointest Liver Physiol 2010;299:G205–14.

48. Meyerholz DK, Stoltz DA, Pezzulo AA, et al. Pathology of gastrointestinal organs in a porcine model of cystic fibrosis. Am J Pathol 2010;176:1377–89.

49. Rowland M, Gallagher CG, O'Laoide R, et al. Outcome in cystic fibrosis liver disease. Am J Gastroenterol 2011;106:104–9.

50. Chryssostalis A, Hubert D, Coste J, et al. Liver disease in adult patients with cystic fibrosis: a frequent and independent prognostic factor associated with death or lung transplantation. J Hepatol 2011;55(6):1377–82.

51. Wouthuyzen-Bakker M, Bodewes FA, Verkade HJ. Persistent fat malabsorption in cystic fibrosis; lessons from patients and mice. J Cyst Fibros 2011;10:150–8.

52. Cohn JA, Noone PG, Jowell PS. Idiopathic pancreatitis related to CFTR: complex inheritance and identification of a modifier gene. J Investig Med 2002;50:247S–55S.

53. Ooi CY, Dorfman R, Cipolli M, et al. Type of CFTR mutation determines risk of pancreatitis in patients with cystic fibrosis. Gastroenterology 2011;140:153–61.

54. Chamnan P, Shine BS, Haworth CS, et al. Diabetes as a determinant of mortality in cystic fibrosis. Diabetes Care 2010;33:311–6.

55. van der Doef HP, Kokke FT, Beek FJ, et al. Constipation in pediatric cystic fibrosis patients: an underestimated medical condition. J Cyst Fibros 2010;9:59–63.

56. Colombo C, Ellemunter H, Houwen R, et al. Guidelines for the diagnosis and management of distal intestinal obstruction syndrome in cystic fibrosis patients. J Cyst Fibros 2011;10:S24–8.

57. Werlin SL, Benuri-Silbiger I, Kerem E, et al. Evidence of intestinal inflammation in patients with cystic fibrosis. J Pediatr Gastroenterol Nutr 2010;51:304–8.

58. Millar FA, Simmonds NJ, Hodson ME. Trends in pathogens colonising the respiratory tract of adult patients with cystic fibrosis, 1985-2005. J Cyst Fibros 2009;8:386–91.

59. Rosenfeld M, Gibson RL, McNamara S, et al. Early pulmonary infection, inflammation, and clinical outcomes in infants with cystic fibrosis. Pediatr Pulmonol 2001;32:356–66.

60. Rosenfeld M, Emerson J, Accurso F, et al. Diagnostic accuracy of oropharyngeal cultures in infants and young children with cystic fibrosis. Pediatr Pulmonol 1999;28:321–8.

61. Gibson RL, Burns JL, Ramsey BW. Pathophysiology and management of pulmonary infections in cystic fibrosis. Am J Respir Crit Care Med 2003; 168:918–51.

62. Bittar F, Richet H, Dubus JC, et al. Molecular detection of multiple emerging pathogens in sputa from cystic fibrosis patients. Plos One 2008;3:e2908.

63. Sibley CD, Parkins MD, Rabin HR, et al. A polymicrobial perspective of pulmonary infections exposes an enigmatic pathogen in cystic fibrosis patients. Proc Natl Acad Sci U S A 2008; 105:15070–5.

64. Rogers GB, Hoffman LR, Whiteley M, et al. Revealing the dynamics of polymicrobial infections: implications for antibiotic therapy. Trends Microbiol 2010;18:357–64.

65. Harris JK, De Groote MA, Sagel SD, et al. Molecular identification of bacteria in bronchoalveolar lavage fluid from children with cystic fibrosis. Proc Natl Acad Sci U S A 2007;104:20529–33.

66. Stuart B, Lin JH, Mogayzel PJ. Early eradication of pseudomonas aeruginosa in patients with cystic fibrosis. Paediatr Respir Rev 2010;11:177–84.

67. Juhas M, Eberl L, Tummler B. Quorum sensing: the power of cooperation in the world of pseudomonas. Environ Microbiol 2005;7:459–71.

68. Cigana C, Curcuru L, Leone MR, et al. Pseudomonas aeruginosa exploits lipid A and muropeptides modification as a strategy to lower innate immunity during cystic fibrosis lung infection. Plos One 2009;4:e8439.

69. Foweraker JE, Laughton CR, Brown DF, et al. Phenotypic variability of Pseudomonas aeruginosa in sputa from patients with acute infective exacerbation of cystic fibrosis and its impact on the validity of antimicrobial susceptibility testing. J Antimicrob Chemother 2005;55:921–7.

70. Smith AL, Fiel SB, Mayer-Hamblett N, et al. Susceptibility testing of Pseudomonas aeruginosa isolates and clinical response to parenteral antibiotic administration: lack of association in cystic fibrosis. Chest 2003;123:1495–502.

71. Govan JR, Deretic V. Microbial pathogenesis in cystic fibrosis: mucoid Pseudomonas aeruginosa and Burkholderia cepacia. Microbiol Rev 1996;60: 539–74.

72. Taccetti G, Campana S, Festini F, et al. Early eradication therapy against Pseudomonas aeruginosa in cystic fibrosis patients. Eur Respir J 2005;26:458–61.

73. Govan JR, Brown AR, Jones AM. Evolving epidemiology of Pseudomonas aeruginosa and the Burkholderia cepacia complex in cystic fibrosis lung infection. Future Microbiol 2007;2:153–64.

74. Liou TG, Adler FR, Fitzsimmons SC, et al. Predictive 5-year survivorship model of cystic fibrosis. Am J Epidemiol 2001;153:345–52.

75. Aris RM, Routh JC, Lipuma JJ, et al. Lung transplantation for cystic fibrosis patients with Burkholderia cepacia complex. Survival linked to genomovar type. Am J Respir Crit Care Med 2001;164:2102–6.

76. Hadjiliadis D. Special considerations for patients with cystic fibrosis undergoing lung transplantation. Chest 2007;131:1224–31.

77. Murray S, Charbeneau J, Marshall BC, et al. Impact of Burkholderia infection on lung transplantation in cystic fibrosis. Am J Respir Crit Care Med 2008; 178:363–71.

78. Kahl BC, Duebbers A, Lubritz G, et al. Population dynamics of persistent Staphylococcus aureus isolated from the airways of cystic fibrosis patients during a 6-year prospective study. J Clin Microbiol 2003;41:4424–7.

79. Vergison A, Denis O, Deplano A, et al. National survey of molecular epidemiology of Staphylococcus aureus colonization in Belgian cystic fibrosis patients. J Antimicrob Chemother 2007;59:893–9.

80. Navarro J, Rainisio M, Harms HK, et al. Factors associated with poor pulmonary function: cross-sectional analysis of data from the ERCF. Eur Respir J 2001;18:298–305.

81. Huang NN, Schidlow DV, Szatrowski TH, et al. Clinical-features, survival rate, and prognostic factors in young-adults with cystic-fibrosis. Am J Med 1987; 82:871–9.

82. Roman F, Canton R, Perez-Vazquez M, et al. Dynamics of long-term colonization of respiratory tract by Haemophilus influenzae in cystic fibrosis patients shows a marked increase in hypermutable strains. J Clin Microbiol 2004;42:1450–9.

83. Rayner RJ, Hiller EJ, Ispahani P, et al. Haemophilus infection in cystic-fibrosis. Arch Dis Child 1990;65: 255–8.

84. De Baets F, Schelstraete P, Van Daele S, et al. Achromobacter xylosoxidans in cystic fibrosis: prevalence and clinical relevance. J Cyst Fibros 2007;6:75–8.

85. Wellinghausen N, Kothe J, Wirths B, et al. Superiority of molecular techniques for identification of gram-negative, oxidase-positive rods, including morphologically nontypical Pseudomonas aeruginosa,

from patients with cystic fibrosis. J Clin Microbiol 2005;43:4070–5.

86. Rogers GB, Carroll MP, Stressmann FA, et al. Cystic fibrosis lung infections: from ecological insights to clinical benefit. Abstract at the NACF meeting, 2009. Pediatr Pulmonol 2010;189–91.

87. Tunney M, Moriarty F, Field T, et al. Detection of anaerobic bacteria in sputum from cystic fibrosis patients with an acute pulmonary exacerbation. Abstract at the NACF meeting, 2009. Pediatr Pulmonol 2007;311–2.

88. Ulrich M, Beer I, Braitmaier P, et al. Relative contribution of *Prevotella intermedia* and *Pseudomonas aeruginosa* to lung pathology in airways of patients with cystic fibrosis. Thorax 2010;65:978–84.

89. Tunney MM, Klem ER, Fodor AA, et al. Use of culture and molecular analysis to determine the effect of antibiotic treatment on microbial community diversity and abundance during exacerbation in patients with cystic fibrosis. Thorax 2011;66:579–84.

90. Worlitzsch D, Rintelen C, Bohm K, et al. Antibiotic-resistant obligate anaerobes during exacerbations of cystic fibrosis patients. Clin Microbiol Infect 2009;15:454–60.

91. Olivier KN, Weber DJ, Wallace RJ Jr, et al. Nontuberculous mycobacteria: I. Multicenter prevalence study in cystic fibrosis. Am J Respir Crit Care Med 2003;167:828–34.

92. Rodman DM, Polis JM, Heltshe SL, et al. Late diagnosis defines a unique population of long-term survivors of cystic fibrosis. Am J Respir Crit Care Med 2005;171:621–6.

93. Torrens JK, Dawkins P, Conway SP, et al. Nontuberculous mycobacteria in cystic fibrosis. Thorax 1998;53:182–5.

94. Lee B, Schjerling CK, Kirkby N, et al. Mucoid *Pseudomonas aeruginosa* isolates maintain the biofilm formation capacity and the gene expression profiles during the chronic lung infection of CF patients. APMIS 2011;119:263–74.

95. Stevens DA, Moss RB, Kurup VP, et al. Allergic bronchopulmonary aspergillosis in cystic fibrosis: state of the art: Cystic Fibrosis Foundation Consensus Conference (vol 37, pg S225, 2003). Clin Infect Dis 2004;38:158.

96. Kistler A, Avila PC, Rouskin S, et al. Pan-viral screening of respiratory tract infections in adults with and without asthma reveals unexpected human coronavirus and human rhinovirus diversity. J Infect Dis 2007;196:817–25.

97. Cystic Fibrosis Foundation Patient Registry. 2009 Annual Report to the Center Directors. Cystic fibrosis foundation annual data report 2009. 2010. p. 2–3. Available at: http://www.cff.org.

98. Griesenbach U, Alton EW. Current status and future directions of gene and cell therapy for cystic fibrosis. BioDrugs 2011;25:77–88.

99. Noone PG, Hohneker KW, Zhou Z, et al. Safety and biological efficacy of a lipid-CFTR complex for gene transfer in the nasal epithelium of adult patients with cystic fibrosis. Mol Ther 2000;1:105–14.

100. Kerem E, Hirawat S, Armoni S, et al. Effectiveness of PTC124 treatment of cystic fibrosis caused by nonsense mutations: a prospective phase II trial. Lancet 2008;372:719–27.

101. Clancy JP, Rowe SM, Durie PR, et al. Comparison of NPD parameters in a phase IIA study to optimize detection of CFTR modulator bioactivity in clinical trials. Abstract at the NACF meeting, 2009. Pediatr Pulmonol 2010;301.

102. Ramsey BW, Davies J, McElvaney NG, et al. A CFTR potentiator in patients with cystic fibrosis and the G551D mutation. N Engl J Med 2011;365(18):1663–72.

103. Donaldson SH, Bennett WD, Zeman KL, et al. Mucus clearance and lung function in cystic fibrosis with hypertonic saline. N Engl J Med 2006;354:241–50.

104. Daviskas E, Anderson SD, Jaques A, et al. Inhaled mannitol improves the hydration and surface properties of sputum in patients with cystic fibrosis. Chest 2010;137:861–8.

105. Accurso FJ, Moss RB, Wilmott RW, et al. Denufosol tetrasodium in patients with cystic fibrosis and normal to mildly impaired lung function. Am J Respir Crit Care Med 2011;183:627–34.

106. Batacchi S, Zagli G, Peris A, et al. Totally implantable vascular access devices in adult patients for cystic fibrosis management. Am J Respir Crit Care Med 2011;183:133–4.

107. Retsch-Bogart GZ, Quittner AL, Gibson RL, et al. Efficacy and safety of inhaled aztreonam lysine for airway pseudomonas in cystic fibrosis. Chest 2009;135:1223–32.

108. Ratjen F, Munck A, Kho P, et al. Treatment of early *Pseudomonas aeruginosa* infection in patients with cystic fibrosis: the ELITE trial. Thorax 2010;65:286–91.

109. Giuliano CA, Dehoorne-Smith ML, Kale-Pradhan PB. Pancreatic enzyme products: digesting the changes. Ann Pharmacother 2011;45:658–66.

110. Mohan K, Israel KL, Miller H, et al. Long-term effect of insulin treatment in cystic fibrosis-related diabetes. Respiration 2008;76:181–6.

111. Koch C, Cuppens H, Rainisio M, et al. European Epidemiologic Registry of Cystic Fibrosis (ERCF): comparison of major disease manifestations between patients with different classes of mutations. Pediatr Pulmonol 2001;31:1–12.

112. Goldbeck L, Zerrer S, Schmitz TG. Monitoring quality of life in outpatients with cystic fibrosis: feasibility and longitudinal results. J Cyst Fibros 2007;6:171–8.

113. Goss CH, Burns JL. Exacerbations in cystic fibrosis center dot 1: epidemiology and pathogenesis. Thorax 2007;62:360–7.

114. de Boer K, Vandemheen KL, Tullis E, et al. Exacerbation frequency and clinical outcomes in adult patients with cystic fibrosis. Thorax 2011;66: 680–5.

115. Pedreira CC, Robert RG, Dalton V, et al. Association of body composition and lung function in children with cystic fibrosis. Pediatr Pulmonol 2005;39: 276–80.

116. Farrell PM, Kosorok MR, Laxova A, et al. Nutritional benefits of neonatal screening for cystic fibrosis. N Engl J Med 1997;337:963–9.

117. Tluczek A, Becker T, Laxova A, et al. Relationships among health-related quality of life, pulmonary health, and newborn screening for cystic fibrosis. Chest 2011;140:170–7.

118. Sood N, Paradowski LJ, Yankaskas JR. Outcomes of intensive care unit care in adults with cystic fibrosis. Am J Respir Crit Care Med 2001;163: 335–8.

119. Slieker MG, van Gestel JP, Heijerman HG, et al. Outcome of assisted ventilation for acute respiratory failure in cystic fibrosis. Intensive Care Med 2006;32:754–8.

120. Hayes D, Mansour H. Improved outcomes of patients with end-stage cystic fibrosis requiring invasive mechanical ventilation for acute respiratory failure. Lung 2011;189:409–15.

121. Lau EM, Barnes DJ, Moriarty C, et al. Pregnancy outcomes in the current era of cystic fibrosis care: a 15-year experience. Aust N Z J Obstet Gynaecol 2011;51:220–4.

122. Quittner AL, Barker DH, Snell C, et al. Prevalence and impact of depression in cystic fibrosis. Curr Opin Pulm Med 2008;14:582–8.

123. Kraynack NC, McBride JT. Improving care at cystic fibrosis centers through quality improvement. Semin Respir Crit Care Med 2009;30:547–58.

124. Marshall BC, Penland CM, Hazle L, et al. Cystic Fibrosis Foundation: achieving the mission. Respir Care 2009;54:788–95.

125. Quinton HB, O'Connor GT. Current issues in quality improvement in cystic fibrosis. Clin Chest Med 2007;28:459–72.

126. Quon BS, Goss CH. A story of success: continuous quality improvement in cystic fibrosis care in the USA. Thorax 2011;66(12):1106–8.

Evaluating Success of Therapy for Bronchiectasis
What End Points to Use?

Maeve P. Smith, MB ChB, MRCP[a],*, Adam T. Hill, MB ChB, MD, FRCPE[a,b]

KEYWORDS

- Bronchiectasis • Treatment • End points

KEY POINTS

- There are currently few clinical or laboratory markers specifically validated to assess response to treatment in bronchiectasis.
- Studies to date suggest that sputum volume and color, sputum bacteriology, exercise capacity, health-related quality-of-life indices, and exacerbation frequency may be relevant and useful measures of treatment efficacy.
- Spirometry currently has little role in evaluating treatment success but is important for monitoring for adverse treatment effects.
- There is an urgent need to both validate current end points used in the assessment of treatment response and to establish other pertinent and reliable markers.

Treatment efficacy is typically measured by the ability to halt the pathogenesis of the disease. In chronic conditions, defining treatment efficacy necessitates encompassing the intent of treatment: to slow disease progression and to improve patients' health-related quality-of-life. Long-term treatment goals of bronchiectasis frequently include limiting the bacterial burden and inflammatory insult in the airways with the aim of improving symptoms, reducing exacerbation frequency and severity, and improving health-related quality-of-life.

At present, few clinical or laboratory markers specifically validated for bronchiectasis exist, and how best to assess the disease and its response to treatment is poorly understood. Treatment strategies used in long-term management of stable disease and strategies used for the management of acute exacerbations address different aspects of the disease and, as such, have different aims. Useful markers to assess the efficacy of such strategies will therefore vary. Early case reports of bronchiectasis relied predominantly on subjective nonquantitative measures such as "the foetor of the breath and sputum" to assess treatment success.[1] More recently, interventional studies have used a variety of clinical and laboratory parameters to monitor response to treatment, many of which have been selected based on their utility in other chronic respiratory disease processes, the reliability of which has recently been questioned.[2] Laboratory markers used in studies have included qualitative and quantitative sputum bacteriology as well as sputum and serum inflammatory measures. Clinical indices used include 24-hour sputum volume, sputum purulence, lung function (typically forced expiratory volume in

The authors have nothing to disclose.
a Department of Respiratory Medicine, Royal Infirmary of Edinburgh, 51 Little France Cresecent, Old Dalkeith Road, Edinburgh EH16 4SA, UK
b University of Edinburgh, Edinburgh, UK
* Corresponding author.
E-mail address: maevemurray@hotmail.com

Clin Chest Med 33 (2012) 329–349
doi:10.1016/j.ccm.2012.03.001
0272-5231/12/$ – see front matter © 2012 Elsevier Inc. All rights reserved.

1 second [FEV$_1$], forced vital capacity [FVC]), symptoms scores and, in longer-term studies, frequency and severity of exacerbations. Pertinent, reliable markers are urgently needed both to facilitate effective treatment of this chronic, debilitating condition and to ensure ongoing development and research of future therapies.

The aim of this article is to explore the utility of potential end points in evaluating therapies used in the long-term management of stable bronchiectasis.

MANAGEMENT STRATEGIES FOR CHRONIC BRONCHIECTASIS

The aims of management of bronchiectasis are to reduce symptoms (reduce cough frequency and severity, improve sputum volume and purulence, and reduce breathlessness, chest pain, and fatigue), reduce exacerbation frequency and severity, preserve lung function, and improve health-related quality-of-life. The impact of bronchiectasis on mortality is unclear, but studies have explored factors that may predict mortality, and these should be considered in the management of bronchiectasis.[3–5]

Interventional studies of stable bronchiectasis have evaluated a multitude of interventions such as the role of long-term antibiotics, long-term anti-inflammatories such as macrolides, physiotherapy and exercise training, inhaled corticosteroids, nebulized saline and β_2-agonists, as well as surgery. The markers used to define treatment success in these studies have varied, but typically include lung function, sputum bacteriology, sputum color, sputum volume, sputum inflammatory markers, serum inflammatory markers, health-related quality-of-life scores, exercise capacity, and exacerbation frequency. This review encompasses key interventional studies exploring the utility of the end points used to define treatment success.

TREATMENT END POINTS
Lung Function

Lung function, typically the FEV$_1$ and FVC, are frequently and reliably used as markers of treatment efficacy in the management of other chronic respiratory diseases such as cystic fibrosis and asthma. Many interventional studies in bronchiectasis also report the effect of treatment on these parameters (**Table 1**). Irrespective of the intervention studied, most of these studies have not observed any significant change in FEV$_1$ or FVC. The few studies that do report a statistical improvement achieve changes in FEV$_1$ and FVC that are of little clinical significance.[6–8] The most important significant change seen was perhaps

the significantly negative impact of treatment on lung function, suggesting that the role of lung function as an end point in interventional studies should be to monitor for potential adverse treatment effects rather than to assess treatment response.[9] The lack of response of lung function in the studies reported is initially surprising; it may be that the older median age of patients with bronchiectasis minimizes the opportunity for airways reversibility.

Different measures of lung function such as the mid-expiratory flows, total lung capacity, residual volume, and lung diffusion capacity may offer more utility as markers of treatment response, but to date have been used in a very limited number of studies. The lung diffusion capacity in a longitudinal study in 61 patients over a median of 7 years observed a progressive median decline of 2.4% of predicted value per year, and a separate study found it to be an independent predictor of mortality.[3,10] Respiratory muscle pressures in bronchiectasis have also recently been studied in 20 patients with clinically stable disease, with maximal inspiratory pressure demonstrated to have reliability.[11] The recent study of inspiratory muscle training by Liaw and colleagues[12] found a significant improvement in age-adjusted maximum inspiratory and expiratory pressures, suggesting that there may be a role for it as a clinical outcome measure, but further studies are needed. More recently, in other chronic inflammatory lung diseases such as cystic fibrosis and asthma, the assessment of small airway function as a measure of disease has been explored. The Lung Clearance Index (LCI) is derived from multiple breath washout (MBW) tests. MBW tests involve the washout of an inert tracer gas from the lungs during relaxed tidal breathing: with each successive breath of the washout there is a decrease in the peak concentration of the exhaled tracer.[13] In chronic inflammatory lung diseases, factors that may contribute to airway narrowing such as mucus retention, inflammation, and airway wall remodeling contribute to ventilation heterogeneity, and washout takes longer. The LCI represents the number of times the volume of gas in the lung at the start of the washout must be turned over to effectively wash out the inert tracer gas; with increasing disease severity, the LCI increases. The LCI has been proved to be more sensitive than spirometry in adults with cystic fibrosis, and has proven utility in pediatric patients with asthma and cystic fibrosis.[14,15] To date, the role of the LCI has not been explored in non–cystic fibrosis bronchiectasis. Further studies are needed to investigate the relevance of different aspects of lung function in bronchiectasis, to help assess its potential utility as a pertinent marker of treatment response.

Table 1
FEV$_1$ and FVC as end points to assess treatment of stable bronchiectasis

Authors, Year	Intervention Studied	Study Design	No. of Patients	Duration	Outcome	Significance (P, Unless Otherwise Stated)
Currie et al,[27] 1990	Oral antibiotic	Double-blind randomized controlled trial of amoxicillin 3 g twice daily vs placebo	32	8 mo	Median reduction in FEV$_1$: 50 mL (amoxicillin) 40 mL (placebo)	Between-group comparison NS
Orriols et al,[57] 1999	Nebulized antibiotic	Randomized controlled trial of nebulized ceftazidime 1 g twice daily and tobramycin 100 mg twice daily vs placebo	15	12 mo	Mean reduction in FEV$_1$: 104.3 mL (treatment) 63.1 mL (placebo) Mean reduction in FVC: 117.1 mL (treatment) 229.2 mL (placebo)	Between-group comparison NS Between-group comparison NS
Barker et al,[58] 2000	Nebulized antibiotic	Double-blind randomized controlled trial of tobramycin 300 mg twice daily vs placebo	74	28 d	Mean change in FEV$_1$% predicted: −2.2% (treatment) 1.5% (placebo) Mean change in FVC % predicted: −2.8% (treatment) 2.2% (placebo)	Between-group comparison NS Between-group comparison NS
Murray et al,[29] 2011	Nebulized antibiotic	Single-blind randomized controlled trial of gentamicin 80 mg twice daily vs 0.9% saline twice daily	57	12 mo	Median change in FEV$_1$% predicted: −2.9% (gentamicin) −1.9% (saline) Median change in FVC % predicted: −1.9% (gentamicin) 0.7% (saline)	Between-group comparison NS Between-group comparison NS
Tsang et al,[36] 1999	Macrolide therapy	Double-blind randomized controlled trial erythromycin 500 mg twice daily vs control	21	8 wk	Mean change in FEV$_1$: 140 mL (erythromycin) −50 mL (placebo) Mean increase in FVC: 120 mL (erythromycin) 0 mL (placebo)	Between-group comparison <.05 Between-group comparison NS
Thompson et al,[6] 2002	Physiotherapy	Randomized crossover trial of active cycle of breathing (ACBT) twice daily vs flutter twice daily	17	4 wk	Mean improvement in FEV$_1$: 80 mL with flutter vs ACBT Mean improvement in FVC: 110 mL with flutter vs ACBT	Between-group comparison .03 Between-group comparison NS

(continued on next page)

Table 1
(continued)

Authors, Year	Intervention Studied	Study Design	No. of Patients	Duration	Outcome	Significance (P, Unless Otherwise Stated)
Patterson et al,[59] 2004	Physiotherapy	Randomized crossover trial of ACBT vs Test of Incremental Respiratory Endurance (TIRE)	20	Single session	Mean improvement in FEV_1: 9 mL (ACBT), 30 mL (TIRE) Mean improvement in FVC: 6 mL (ACBT), 3 mL (TIRE)	Within-group comparison NS NS Within-group comparison NS NS
Murray et al,[31] 2009	Physiotherapy	Randomized crossover trial of physiotherapy twice daily vs no physiotherapy	20	3 mo	Median change in FEV_1: −10 mL (physiotherapy), −10 mL (no physiotherapy) Median change in FVC: −10 mL (physiotherapy), −60 mL (no physiotherapy)	Between-group comparison NS Between-group comparison NS
Kellett and Robert,[8] 2011	Nebulized hypertonic saline	Single-blind randomized crossover study of 7% saline once daily vs 0.9% saline once daily	32	3 mo	Mean change in FEV_1: 15.1% (7% saline), 1.8% (0.9% saline) Mean change in FVC: 11.2% (7% saline), 0.7% (0.9% saline)	Between-group comparison <.01 Between-group comparison <.01
Elborn et al,[7] 1992	Inhaled corticosteroid	Double-blind crossover study of 750 μg beclometasone twice daily vs placebo	20	6 wk	Mean difference in FEV_1 at end of beclometasone vs placebo: 110 mL Mean difference in FVC at end of beclometasone vs placebo: 20 mL	Between-group comparison .03 Between-group comparison NS
Tsang et al,[37] 1998	Inhaled corticosteroid	Double-blind placebo-controlled trial of fluticasone 500 μg twice daily vs placebo	24	4 wk	Mean change in FEV_1: 200 mL (fluticasone), 0 mL (placebo) Mean change in FVC: 100 mL (fluticasone), 0 mL (placebo)	Between-group comparison NS Between-group comparison NS

Study	Therapy	Study description	No.	Duration	Results	Comparison
Tsang et al,[30] 2005	Inhaled corticosteroid	Randomized controlled trial of 500 μg fluticasone twice daily vs placebo	86	52 wk	Mean difference in FEV$_1$% predicted between fluticasone and placebo at end of study: −0.02% Mean difference in FVC % predicted between fluticasone and placebo at end of study: 2.81%	Between-group comparison NS Between-group comparison NS
Martinez-Garcia et al,[60] 2006	Inhaled corticosteroid	Prospective, randomized, double-blind trial of fluticasone 500 μg daily vs 1000 μg daily vs no treatment	93	6 mo	Mean change in FEV$_1$: 64 mL (1000 μg fluticasone) −11 mL (500 μg fluticasone) −38 mL (control) Mean change in FVC: 25 mL (1000 μg fluticasone) −39 mL (500 μg fluticasone) −62 mL (control fluticasone)	Between-group comparison NS Between-group comparison NS
Martinez-Garcia et al,[61] 2012	Inhaled corticosteroid/ inhaled corticosteroid with long acting β$_2$-agonist	Randomized, controlled double-blind trial of 1600 μg budesonide daily vs 18 μg formoterol/640 μg budesonide daily	40	12 mo	Mean change in FEV$_1$: 37 mL (budesonide) 23 mL (budesonide/formoterol) Mean change in FVC: 60 mL (budesonide) 74 mL (budesonide/formoterol)	Between-group comparison NS Between-group comparison NS
Daviskas et al,[62] 2005	Inhaled mannitol	Open-label study of 400 mg daily mannitol	9	12 d	Mean change in % predicted FEV$_1$: 1% Mean change in % predicted FVC: 3.7%	Within-group comparison NS Within-group comparison NS
O'Donnell et al,[9] 1998	Inhaled rhDNase	Double-blind randomized controlled trial of 2.5 mg twice daily inhaled rhDNase	349	24 wk	Mean change in FEV$_1$% predicted: −3.6% (rhDNase) −1.7% (placebo) Mean change in FVC% predicted: −3.4% (rhDNase) 0.3% (placebo)	Between-group comparison ≤.05 Between-group comparison ≤.01

Abbreviation: NS, no statistically significant difference.

Sputum Bacteriology

The airways in bronchiectasis are frequently chronically infected with pathogenic bacteria.[16–18] Chronic airway infection is associated with increased airway inflammation, a poorer health-related quality-of-life, and more frequent exacerbations, and with chronic *Pseudomonas* infection there may be a more rapid decline in lung function.[19–23] Interventional studies have therefore used sputum bacterial clearance as an important marker of treatment efficacy. The impact of treatment on both qualitative and quantitative bacteriology has been used to assess response to treatment including nebulized antibiotic therapy, macrolide therapy, physiotherapy, and inhaled corticosteroid treatment (**Table 2**). Qualitative bacteriology reports the presence or absence of pathogens in sputum and is the most frequent technique used by laboratories to measure airways infection. Quantitative bacteriology provides an accurate assessment of bacterial density in the infected airways, and in patients with chronic infection unlikely to achieve complete eradication of pathogens, quantitative bacteriology measuring any impact or reduction in density may be a more useful measure. The antibiotic studies in **Table 2** found significant improvements in quantitative bacteriology, but other interventions including macrolide therapy, physiotherapy, and inhaled corticosteroid therapy did not. The studies reported in **Table 2** provide evidence for using quantitative bacteriology as a treatment end point, although this is frequently available purely as a research tool, and further studies are needed to support its routine use in assessing bronchiectasis as opposed to the current standard of qualitative bacteriology.

Sputum Color

Sputum purulence reflects airway inflammation and is positively associated with bacterial infection.[24,25] Changes in sputum purulence have been used as measures of treatment response since the earliest observational reports of management of bronchiectasis and since the first randomized controlled trial of antibiotics.[26] Sputum purulence is a noninvasive, inexpensive, and pertinent marker that can be reliably measured and reported.[25] A sputum color chart specific to bronchiectasis describing the 3 typical gradations of sputum color, namely mucoid (clear), mucopurulent (pale yellow/pale green), and purulent (dark yellow/dark green), has been developed, with reliable interpretation of sputum color in stable disease demonstrated for both patient and clinician.[25] High-dose twice-daily long-term oral amoxicillin improved sputum purulence to a mean of 20% of baseline purulence;[27] nebulized twice-daily tobramycin over 12 weeks improved sputum purulence in 43.9% of patients,[28] and nebulized gentamicin also achieved a significant improvement, with 8.7% of treated patients expectorating purulent sputum at the end of 12 months of treatment compared with 66.7% at the start of treatment.[29] No macrolide, physiotherapy, exercise, or hypertonic saline studies formally reported sputum purulence as an end point. Twice-daily inhaled fluticasone, 500 µg over 1 year, had no significant impact on sputum purulence compared with placebo.[30] Overall, sputum purulence is a potentially useful treatment end point.

Sputum Volume

Sputum expectoration is the defining symptom of bronchiectasis, and is a pertinent and noninvasive potential marker of bronchiectasis. As such, sputum expectoration has been used to assess bronchiectasis and its response to treatment since the earliest reported case studies of the disease.[1] Sputum volume has been assessed using different means including: wet weight and volume; dry weight and volume; the volume collected during and or immediately following the intervention being studied; and the volume collected over a 24-hour period, or indeed the mean 24-hour volume collected over a 3-day period. **Table 3** highlights the utility of sputum volume as a measure of treatment response to various interventions. The studies included in **Table 3** typically report a reduction in sputum volume with the exception of one randomized crossover study that reported an increase in 24-hour sputum volume with physiotherapy.[31] It is widely acknowledged that the aim of chest physiotherapy is to enhance sputum expectoration; however, the longer-term effect of regular airway clearance in stable disease is unknown, and it may be that with frequent chest clearance the airways may become clearer and actual sputum volume decreases. Sputum volume relies on patient compliance for accurate collection, which may be difficult to achieve particularly in long-term studies of stable disease. The optimum method for measuring sputum volume requires further study to determine whether wet or dry weight or volume is best and to establish which measurement is reliable and repeatable, particularly when collections may include saliva in addition to sputum. The role of 24-hour sputum volume as a marker of treatment response requires further study.

Sputum Inflammatory Markers

Bronchiectasis is characterized by neutrophilic airway inflammation, and it has been hypothesized that direct measures of lung inflammation using markers in exhaled breath and sputum may be useful in assessing disease activity and response to treatment.[32–34] A limited number of interventional studies have explored the effect of treatment on various markers of neutrophilic airway inflammation including sputum neutrophil elastase, myeloperoxidase, and proinflammatory cytokines such as interleukin (IL)-1α, IL-8, tumor necrosis factor α (TNF-α), and leukotriene B4 (LTB4).[29,35–37] The effect of antibiotic therapy on sputum inflammatory indices was explored by Stockley and colleagues[35] in 1984, although the amoxicillin administered to the 15 patients in the open label study was for 14 days only. However, in the 67% of patients who clinically responded with macroscopic clearing of sputum purulence and eradication of the sputum pathogen, there was a significant reduction in sputum elastase and albumin leakage.[35] Long-term nebulized gentamicin over 1 year significantly reduces sputum myeloperoxidase and elastase concentrations compared with 0.9% saline.[29] Twice-daily erythromycin over 8 weeks did not have any significant effect on sputum IL-8, IL-1α, TNF-α, LTB4, or indeed on sputum leukocyte density, although the majority of patients in this study were infected with *Pseudomonas aeruginosa*.[36] Inhaled fluticasone over 8 weeks was found to significantly reduce sputum IL-1β, IL-8, and LTB-4 but had no effect on TNF-α.[37] The clinical utility of such markers as cost effective, reliable, and pertinent end points requires further work.

Other markers of airway inflammation that may have a role in assessing disease activity in bronchiectasis that have been studied in other chronic inflammatory respiratory diseases include exhaled hydrogen peroxide and exhaled nitric oxide. Loukides and colleagues[38] found significantly higher levels of hydrogen peroxide in the exhaled breath condensate of patients with bronchiectasis compared with controls (0.87 ± 0.01 μM and 0.26 ± 0.04 μM, respectively; $P<.001$). Although not an interventional study, the same investigators observed that there was no significant difference in the concentration of hydrogen peroxide present in patients receiving treatment with inhaled corticosteroids compared with those who were not on regular inhaled corticosteroids.[38,39] Shoemark and colleagues[40] found higher levels of peripheral airway nitric oxide in patients with bronchiectasis compared with controls, with levels of fractional exhaled nitric oxide (FeNO) correlating with severity of bronchiectasis according to lung function, health-related quality-of-life, and radiological extent of disease. Its role as a marker of response to treatment, however, is less clear, as no difference was found in levels of FeNO following treatment of an acute exacerbation in 20 patients.[40] There have been no formal validation studies of any such markers, and their use in interventional studies as markers of treatment response at present is limited.

Further work is needed to identify markers that are responsive to changes in disease activity.

Serum Inflammatory Markers

A limited number of interventional studies have explored the impact of treatment on serum inflammatory markers such as leukocyte count (WCC), C-reactive protein (CRP), erythrocyte sedimentation rate (ESR), and procalcitonin. In 1990, Currie and colleagues[27] found no significant effect on ESR or WCC following 8 months' treatment with high-dose amoxicillin compared with placebo. Similarly, a randomized controlled trial of nebulized gentamicin compared with nebulized saline over 12 months found no significant change in WCC, CRP, or ESR at the end of treatment.[29] It may be, however, that a response would have been found if highly selective CRP had been used. Procalcitonin, the peptide precursor to the hormone calcitonin, is a useful marker of severity in pneumonia and other sepsis syndromes. However, a study of its utility in exacerbations of bronchiectasis found that it is unlikely to be useful, as serum levels were generally low. In patients requiring inpatient management, there was no correlation between serum procalcitonin and other inflammatory markers.[41] The correlation between airway inflammation and systemic inflammation has previously been shown to be poor, and it may be that in stable disease such systemic markers have little or no role in evaluating treatment success.[19] Systemic markers are more likely to have a role in assessing interventions in the management of acute exacerbations of bronchiectasis that are typically accompanied by a systemic inflammatory response, although further studies, for example using highly selective CRP in stable disease, are needed.[42]

Health-Related Quality-of-life Indices

Improving patients' health-related quality-of-life is a major goal of management. Studies have frequently used symptoms as a guide to treatment efficacy, with the earliest interventional studies relying on patients reporting changes in their symptoms—a useful guide to treatment response but one that was difficult to quantify and use for comparison between studies. The development of health-related quality-of-life questionnaires that target symptoms specific to the condition offer

Table 2
Sputum bacteriology as an end point to assess treatment of stable bronchiectasis

Authors, Year	Intervention Studied	Study Design	No. of Patients	Duration	Outcome	Significance (P, Unless Otherwise Stated)
Barker et al,[58] 2000	Nebulized antibiotic	Double-blind randomized controlled trial of tobramycin 300 mg twice daily vs placebo	74	28 d	Mean change in bacterial density: $-4.54 \log_{10}$ cfu/mL (tobramycin) $0.02 \log_{10}$ cfu/mL (placebo)	Between-group comparison $<.01$
Couch[63] 2001	Nebulized antibiotic	Randomized controlled trial of tobramycin 300 mg twice daily vs placebo	74	4 wk	Mean change in bacterial density: $-4.5 \log_{10}$ cfu/mL (tobramycin) $0.22 \log_{10}$ cfu/mL (placebo)	Between-group comparison $<.05$
Scheinberg and Shore,[28] 2005	Nebulized antibiotic	Open-label pilot study of tobramycin 300 mg twice daily (14 d on, 14 d off)	41	12 wk	% Patients with qualitative bacterial eradication at end of study: 22%	Not reported
Murray et al,[29] 2011	Nebulized antibiotic	Single-blind randomized controlled trial of gentamicin 80 mg twice daily vs 0.9% saline twice daily	57	12 mo	Median change in bacterial density: $-5.06 \log_{10}$ cfu/mL (gentamicin) $-0.21 \log_{10}$ cfu/mL (saline)	Between-group comparison $<.0001$
Tsang et al,[36] 1999	Macrolide therapy	Double-blind randomized controlled trial of erythromycin 500 mg twice daily vs control	21	8 wk	Mean change in bacterial density: 1.91×10^7 cfu/mL (erythromycin) -5.81×10^7 cfu/mL (control)	Between-group comparison NS
Murray et al,[31] 2009	Physiotherapy	Randomized crossover trial of physiotherapy twice daily vs no physiotherapy	20	3 mo	Median change in bacterial density: -1×10^3 cfu/mL (physiotherapy) 1×10^3 cfu/mL (no physiotherapy)	Between-group comparison NS

						Between-group comparison
Tsang et al,[37] 1998	Inhaled corticosteroid	Double-blind placebo controlled trial of fluticasone 500 μg twice daily vs placebo	24	4 wk	Median change in bacterial density: 7.7 × 10⁷ cfu/mL (fluticasone) −1.4 × 10⁷ cfu/mL (placebo)	Between-group comparison NS
Martinez-Garcia et al,[60] 2006	Inhaled corticosteroid	Prospective, randomized, double-blind trial of fluticasone 500 μg daily vs 1000 μg daily vs no treatment	93	6 mo	% Change in patients colonized with *Haemophilus influenzae:* 7% (1000 μg fluticasone) 7% (500 μg fluticasone) −6% (control) % Change in patients colonized with *Pseudomonas aeruginosa:* 0% (1000 μg fluticasone) −3% (500 μg fluticasone) 3% (control)	Between-group comparison NS Between-group comparison NS
Martinez-Garcia et al,[61] 2012	Inhaled corticosteroid/ inhaled corticosteroid with long acting β2-agonist	Randomized, controlled double-blind trial of 1600 μg budesonide once daily vs 18 μg formoterol/640 μg budesonide once daily	40	12 mo	% Change in %patients colonized with *H influenzae:* 0% (budesonide) −5% (budesonide/formeterol) % Change in patients colonized with *P aeruginosa:* 0% (budesonide) 0% (budesonide/formeterol)	Between-group comparison NS Between-group comparison NS

Abbreviation: NS, no statistically significant difference.

Table 3
Sputum volume as an end point to assess treatment of stable bronchiectasis

Authors, Year	Intervention Studied	Study Design	No. of Patients	Duration	Outcome	Significance (P, Unless Otherwise Stated)
Currie et al,[27] 1990	Oral antibiotic	Double-blind randomized controlled trial of amoxicillin 3 g twice daily vs placebo	32	8 mo	% of mean pretreatment 24-h volume at end of study: 42% (amoxicillin) 81% (placebo)	Between-group comparison .04
Murray et al,[29] 2011	Nebulized antibiotic	Single-blind randomized controlled trial of gentamicin 80 mg twice daily vs 0.9% saline twice daily	57	12 mo	Median change in 24-h sputum volume at end of study: −7.5 mL (gentamicin) −1.5 mL (saline)	Between-group comparison NS
Tsang et al,[36] 1999	Macrolide therapy	Double-blind randomized controlled trial of erythromycin 500 mg twice daily vs control	21	8 wk	Mean change in 24-h sputum volume at end of study: −9.9 mL (erythromycin) −3.5 mL (control)	Within-group comparison <.05 NS
Patterson et al,[59] 2004	Physiotherapy	Randomized crossover trial of active cycle of breathing (ACBT) vs Test of Incremental Respiratory Endurance (TIRE)	20	Single session	Mean sputum weight expectorated during & 30 min posttreatment: 8.98 g (ACBT) 6.53 g (TIRE)	Between-group comparison .02
Eaton et al,[64] 2007	Physiotherapy	Randomized prospective study single sessions of: flutter, ACBT, & ACBT with postural drainage (PD)	30	Single session	Total wet weight of sputum expectorated during & 30 min posttreatment: 5.6 g (flutter) 5.6 g (ACBT) 11.2 g (ACBT & PD) Flutter vs ACBT Flutter vs ACBT & PD ACBT vs ACBT & PD	Between-group comparison NS <.001 <.001
Murray et al,[31] 2009	Physiotherapy	Randomized crossover trial of physiotherapy twice daily vs no physiotherapy	20	3 mo	Median change in 24-h sputum volume: 2 mL (physiotherapy) −1 mL (no physiotherapy)	Between-group comparison .02

Source	Therapy	Study design	No. of patients	Duration	Results	Comparison
Newall et al,[65] 2005	Pulmonary rehabilitation (PR)	Randomized controlled trial of PR vs PR with inspiratory muscle training (IMT) vs control	32	8 wk	Mean change in 24-h sputum volume: −2.6 mL (PR) −4.2 mL (PR and IMT) −0.9 mL (control)	Within-group comparison NS NS NS
Elborn et al,[7] 1992	Inhaled corticosteroid	Double-blind crossover study of 750 μg beclometasone twice daily vs placebo	20	6 wk	Mean 24-h sputum volume at end of study: 22.3 g (beclometasone) 27.3 g (control)	Between-group comparison <.003
Tsang et al,[37] 1998	Inhaled corticosteroid	Double-blind placebo-controlled trial of fluticasone 500 μg twice daily vs placebo	24	4 wk	Median change in 24-h sputum volume: 3.1 mL (fluticasone) −1.9 mL (placebo)	Within-group comparison NS NS
Tsang et al,[30] 2005	Inhaled corticosteroid	Randomized controlled trial of 500 μg fluticasone twice daily vs placebo	86	52 wk	% Patients with an improvement in 24-h sputum volume at end of study: 65.1% (fluticasone) 41.9% (placebo)	Between-group comparison <.05
Martinez-Garcia et al,[60] 2006	Inhaled corticosteroid	Prospective, randomized, double-blind trial of fluticasone 500 μg daily vs 1000 μg daily vs no treatment	93	6 mo	% Patients with >50% reduction in 24-h sputum volume: 48.3% (1000 μg fluticasone) 37.9% (500 μg fluticasone) 10.7% (control)	Between-group comparison 1000 μg vs 500 μg .03 1000 μg vs control .009

Abbreviation: NS, no statistically significant difference.

Table 4
Health-related quality-of-life scores as an end point to assess treatment of stable bronchiectasis

Authors, Year	Intervention Studied	Study Design	No. of Patients	Duration	Outcome	Significance (P, Unless Otherwise Stated)
Scheinberg and Shore,[28] 2005	Nebulized antibiotic	Open-label pilot study of tobramycin 300 mg twice daily (14 d on, 14 d off)	41	12 wk	Improvement in Pulmonary total symptom severity score: 1.5 units	Within-group comparison .006
					Improvement in SGRQ total score: −9.8 units	<.001
Murray et al,[29] 2011	Nebulized antibiotic	Single-blind randomized controlled trial of gentamicin 80 mg twice daily vs 0.9% saline twice daily	57	12 mo	% Patients with ≥1.3-unit improvement in total LCQ score: 81.4% (gentamicin) 20% (saline)	Between-group comparison <.01
					% Patients with ≥4-unit improvement in total SGRQ score: 87.5% (gentamicin) 19.2% (saline)	Between-group comparison <.004
Thompson et al,[6] 2002	Physiotherapy	Randomized crossover trial of active cycle of breathing twice daily vs flutter twice daily	17	4 wk	Mean difference in Chronic Respiratory Disease Questionnaire Total Score at end of treatment with flutter and acapella: −0.09 units	Between-group comparison NS
Mutalithas et al,[66] 2008	Physiotherapy	Prospective open label study of bronchopulmonary hygiene physical therapy	53	4 wk	Mean improvement in Cough Visual Analogue Scale: 15.8 mm	Within-group comparison <.0001
					Mean improvement in LCQ total score: 3.1 units	Within-group comparison <.001
Murray et al,[31] 2009	Physiotherapy	Randomized crossover trial of physiotherapy twice daily vs no physiotherapy	20	3 mo	Median change in LCQ total score: 1.3 units (physiotherapy) 0 units (no physiotherapy)	Between-group comparison .002
					Median change in SGRQ total score: −7.8 units (physiotherapy) −0.7 units (no physiotherapy)	Between-group comparison .005
Kellett and Robert,[8] 2011	Nebulized hypertonic saline	Single-blind randomized crossover study of 7% saline once daily vs 0.9% saline once daily	32	3 mo	Mean change in total SGRQ score at end of study: −6.0 units (7% saline) −1.2 units (0.9% saline)	Between-group comparison <.05

Study	Therapy	Description	N	Duration	Outcome	Comparison	p-value
Ong et al,[67] 2011	Pulmonary rehabilitation (PR)	Retrospective review of 6–8 wk of PR	95	6–8 wk	Mean improvement in Chronic Respiratory Disease Questionnaire at end of PR: 14.0 (11.3–16.7)	Within-group comparison	<.05
Newall et al,[65] 2005	Pulmonary rehabilitation	Randomized controlled trial of PR vs PR with inspiratory muscle training (IMT) vs control	32	8 wk	Mean change in total SGRQ score: −7.7 units (PR & IMT), 2.3 units (PR), Data not reported (control group)	Between-group comparison PR & IMT vs control, PR vs control	.05, NS
Elborn et al,[7] 1992	Inhaled corticosteroid	Double-blind crossover study of 750 μg beclometasone twice daily vs placebo	20	6 wk	Mean improvement in Visual Analog Score in beclometasone compared with placebo: Cough: 5 mm, Wheeze: 2 mm, Dyspnea: 4 mm	Between-group comparison	.02, NS, NS
Martinez-Garcia et al,[60] 2006	Inhaled corticosteroid	Prospective, randomized double-blind trial of fluticasone 500 μg daily vs 1000 μg daily vs no treatment	93	6 mo	% Patients with clinically significant improvement in SGRQ total score: 51.7% (1000 μg fluticasone), 34.4% (500 μg fluticasone), 7.4% (control)	Between-group comparison 1000 μg fluticasone vs 500 μg fluticasone & control	.009
Martinez-Garcia et al,[61] 2012	Inhaled corticosteroid/inhaled corticosteroid with long acting β₂-agonist	Randomized controlled double-blind trial of 1600 μg budesonide daily vs 18 μg formoterol/640 μg budesonide daily	40	12 mo	Change in total SGRQ score: −5.3 units (budesonide/formeterol), Data not reported (budesonide)	Within-group comparison	.006, NS
Daviskas et al,[62] 2005	Inhaled mannitol	Open-label study of 400 mg daily mannitol	9	12 d	Mean change in SGRQ total score: −12.4 units	Within-group comparison	<.01

a unique integration of physical and psychosocial morbidity, unlike other clinical parameters, and allow the clinician to directly quantify the effect of disease on patients' daily life. There are 2 health-related quality-of-life questionnaires validated for use in bronchiectasis: the St George's Respiratory Questionnaire (SGRQ) and the Leicester Cough Questionnaire (LCQ).[43,44] The St George's Respiratory Questionnaire is a 50-item self-administered health-related quality-of-life questionnaire assessing the impact of multiple chronic respiratory symptoms on health-related quality-of-life, originally intended for use in chronic obstructive pulmonary disease (COPD).[45] It consists of 3 components, namely symptoms (8 items), activity (16 items), and impacts (26 items), and assesses the impact of symptoms over the preceding 4 weeks. The total score ranges from 0 to 100, with a higher score indicating a poorer health-related quality-of-life. In bronchiectasis it has been shown to have repeatability over a 2-week period with an intra-class correlation coefficient of 0.97. Responsiveness of the SGRQ was validated by assessing change in score in comparison with parameters such as the level achieved in the shuttle walk test, Medical Research Council dyspnea score, and Short-Form 36 health-related quality-of-life score over a 6-month period. The minimum clinically important difference for change is 4 units. The LCQ is a 19 item self-completed quality-of-life measure of chronic cough.[46] It has 3 domains: physical (8 items), psychological (7 items), and social (4 items). The total severity score ranges from 3 to 21, with a lower score indicating greater impairment of health status because of cough. It assesses the impact of symptoms over the preceding 2 weeks, and the minimum clinically important difference for change is 1.3 units. Other indices of health-related quality-of-life have been used in interventional studies in bronchiectasis, including visual analog scales and other chronic respiratory disease questionnaires such as the Chronic Respiratory Disease Questionnaire.[47] More recently, preliminary results have been published validating a health-related quality-of-life questionnaire specific to non–cystic fibrosis bronchiectasis, the Quality of Life questionnaire in Bronchiectasis (QOL-B).[48,49] This questionnaire consists of 37 items in 8 domains including Respiratory Symptoms, Physical Functioning, Vitality, Role Functioning, Health Perceptions, Emotional Functioning, Social Functioning, and Treatment Burden. **Table 4** demonstrates that health-related quality-of-life scores in bronchiectasis are highly responsive to change irrespective of the intervention being studied, and as such have an important role in evaluating response to treatment.

Exercise Capacity

Exercise capacity is influenced by several factors including both respiratory health and systemic health. Lung function, bronchial secretions, respiratory muscle strength, and general health status (including nutrition and the impact of any comorbidity) may all influence performance, and increasing the distance completed in the test may reflect either direct or indirect improvements in these aspects of health. The incremental shuttle walk test is a means of assessing exercise capacity and although not validated for use in bronchiectasis, it has been proved in patients with COPD to provide an objective measure of disability and can be used for direct comparison of patients' performances.[50] The 6-minute walking test (6MWT) is another frequently used exercise test that has been demonstrated to be strongly associated with health-related quality-of-life in bronchiectasis and radiologic extent of disease (defined by the generations of bronchial divisions affected), but again has not been validated for use as a parameter of treatment response.[51] It measures the distance that a patient can walk at their own intensity over a 6-minute period on a hard, flat surface. It is thought to be a reflection of patients' functional capacity for exercise rather than maximal exercise capacity. In a study of 27 patients with bronchiectasis the 6MWT has been shown to positively correlate with FVC and generations of affected bronchopulmonary divisions, and negatively correlate with health-related quality-of-life as measured by the SGRQ.[52] Exercise capacity has been used as a treatment end point predominantly in physiotherapy and exercise studies (**Table 5**). The studies highlighted in **Table 5** demonstrate exercise capacity to be a responsive measure to intervention. It is of particular interest that these studies found no parallel improvement in spirometry (FEV_1 and FVC). This finding suggests that exercise capacity reflects systemic factors as well as respiratory factors, and provides potential support for exercise capacity as an independent measure of treatment response and evidence for its validation as a treatment end point.

Exacerbation Frequency

Exacerbations are a stimulus to the vicious cycle of infection and inflammation in the already damaged bronchiectatic airways, and have an adverse impact on health-related quality-of-life. Reducing their frequency is a major goal of management.[53–55] Exacerbations are a significant source of morbidity, and reducing frequency is typically a major goal of management. The studies that

Table 5
Exercise capacity as an end point to assess treatment of stable bronchiectasis

Authors, Year	Intervention Studied	Study Design	No. of Patients	Duration	Outcome	Significance (P Unless Otherwise Stated)
Murray et al,[29] 2011	Nebulized antibiotic	Single-blind randomized controlled trial of gentamicin 80 mg twice daily vs 0.9% saline twice daily	57	12 mo	Median improvement in distance achieved in ISWT: 160 m (gentamicin) 70 m (saline)	Between-group comparison .03
Murray et al,[31] 2009	Physiotherapy	Randomized crossover trial of physiotherapy twice daily vs no physiotherapy	20	3 mo	Median change in distance achieved in ISWT: 40 m (physiotherapy) 0 m (no physiotherapy)	Between-group comparison .001
Ong et al,[67] 2011	Pulmonary rehabilitation	Retrospective review of 6–8 wk of pulmonary rehabilitation	95	6–8 wk	Mean change in 6MWD: 53.4 m	Within-group comparison <.05
Liaw et al,[12] 2011	Inspiratory muscle training (IMT)	Prospective single-blind randomized controlled trial of 30-min sessions 5 d/wk vs control	26	8 wk	Change in 6MWD: 61.3 m (IMT) Change in 6MWW 2864.5 m/kg (IMT)	Within-group comparison .021 Within-group comparison .022
Newall et al,[65] 2005	Pulmonary rehabilitation	Randomized controlled trial of pulmonary rehabilitation vs pulmonary rehabilitation with IMT vs control	32	8 wk	Mean improvement in distance achieved in ISWT: 96.7 m (pulmonary rehabilitation) 124.5 m (pulmonary rehabilitation & IMT) 11.0 m (control) PR vs control PR & IMT vs control	Between-group comparison <.01 <.01

Abbreviations: ISWT, Incremental Shuttle Walk Test; NS, no statistically significant difference; 6MWD, 6-minute walking distance; 6MWW, 6-minute walking work.

Table 6
Exacerbations as an end point to assess treatment of stable bronchiectasis

Authors, Year	Intervention Studied	Study Design	No. of Patients	Duration	Outcome	Significance (P, Unless Otherwise Stated)
Currie et al,[27] 1990	Oral antibiotic	Double-blind randomized controlled trial of amoxicillin 3 g twice daily vs placebo	32	8 mo	Median no. of exacerbations: 2 (amoxicillin) 4 (placebo)	Between-group comparison NS
Orriols et al,[57] 1999	Nebulized antibiotic	Randomized controlled trial of nebulized ceftazidime 1 g twice daily and tobramycin 100 mg twice daily vs placebo	15	12 mo	Mean no. of admissions: 0.6 (treatment) 2.5 (placebo) Mean number of days of admission: 13.1 (treatment) 57.9 (placebo)	Between-group comparison <.05 Between-group comparison <.05
Barker et al,[58] 2000	Nebulized antibiotic	Double-blind randomized controlled trial of tobramycin 300 mg twice daily vs placebo	74	28 d	No. of patients hospitalized with an exacerbation: 5 (tobramycin) 1 (placebo)	Between-group comparison NS
Drobnic et al,[68] 2005	Nebulized antibiotic	Double-blind randomized crossover trial of 300 mg tobramycin twice daily	30	6 mo	Mean no. of admissions with an exacerbation: 0.15 (tobramycin) 0.75 (placebo) Mean no. of admission days with an exacerbation: 2.05 (tobramycin) 12.65(placebo)	Between-group comparison <.047 Between-group comparison <.047
Murray et al,[29] 2011	Nebulized antibiotic	Single-blind randomized controlled trial of gentamicin 80 mg twice daily vs 0.9% saline twice daily	57	12 mo	Median no. of exacerbations: 0 (gentamicin) 1.5 (saline) Median no. of days to first exacerbation: 120 (gentamicin) 61.5 (saline)	Between-group comparison <.0001 Between-group comparison .02

Study	Therapy	Description	No.	Duration	Outcome	Comparison
Davies and Wilson,[69] 2004	Macrolide therapy	Open-label study 250 mg azithromycin thrice weekly	39	4 mo	Exacerbation frequency (oral antibiotics/month): 0.71 (pretreatment) 0.13 (with treatment) / Exacerbation frequency (intravenous antibiotics/month) 0.8 (pretreatment) 0.03 (with treatment)	Within-group comparison <.01 / Within-group comparison <.01
Serisier and Martin,[70] 2011	Macrolide therapy	Uncontrolled study 250 mg erythromycin daily	24	12 mo	Median no. of exacerbations: 4 (12 mo prestudy) 2 (during study) / Median no. of days of antibiotic use/year: 44 (12 mo prestudy) 21 (during study)	Within-group comparison <.001 / Within-group comparison <.001
Murray et al,[31] 2009	Physiotherapy	Randomized crossover trial of physiotherapy twice daily vs no physiotherapy	20	3 mo	No. of exacerbations: 5 (physiotherapy) 7 (no physiotherapy)	Between-group comparison NS
Kellett and Robert,[8] 2011	Nebulized hypertonic saline	Single-blind randomized crossover study of 7% saline once daily vs 0.9% saline once daily	32	3 mo	Prospective annualized antibiotic use/year: 2.4 (7% saline) 5.4 (0.9% saline) / Prospective annualized exacerbtions/year: 2.1 (7% saline) 4.9 (0.9% saline)	Between-group comparison <.05 / Between-group comparison <.05
Tsang et al,[37] 1998	Inhaled corticosteroid	Double-blind placebo-controlled trial of fluticasone 500 μg twice daily vs placebo	24	4 wk	Data not reported for: No. of exacerbations requiring oral antibiotics or oral steroids / No. of emergency visits / No. of admissions	Between-group comparison NS / Between-group comparison NS / Between-group comparison NS
Tsang et al,[30] 2005	Inhaled corticosteroid	Randomized controlled trial of 500 μg fluticasone twice daily vs placebo	86	52 wk	No. of exacerbations: 96 (fluticasone) 117 (placebo)	Between-group comparison NS

(continued on next page)

Table 6
(continued)

Authors, Year	Intervention Studied	Study Design	No. of Patients	Duration	Outcome	Significance (*P*, Unless Otherwise Stated)
Martinez-Garcia et al,[60] 2006	Inhaled corticosteroid	Prospective, randomized, double-blind trial of fluticasone 500 μg daily vs 1000 μg daily vs no treatment	93	6 mo	Mean no. of exacerbations in 1000-μg fluticasone group: 1.2 (with treatment) 1.4 (pretreatment) Data not reported for 500-μg fluticasone or control group	Within-group comparison NS Between-groups comparison NS
Martinez-Garcia et al,[61] 2012	Inhaled corticosteroid/ inhaled corticosteroid with long acting β2-agonist	Randomized controlled double-blind trial of 1600 μg budesonide daily vs 18 μg formeterol/640 μg budesonide daily	40	12 mo	No. of exacerbations: 7 (budesonide) 4 (budesonide/formeterol)	Between-group comparison NS
O'Donnell et al,[9] 1998	Inhaled rhDNase	Double-blind randomized controlled trial of 2.5 mg twice daily inhaled rhDNase	349	24 wk	Total exacerbation rate: 0.95 (rhDNase) 0.71 (placebo) No. of days of antibiotic use: 56.9 (rhDNase) 44.1 (placebo) Hospitalization rate: 0.39 (rhDNase) 0.21 (placebo)	Between-group comparison Relative risk 1.35 Between-group comparison $\leq$.05 Between-group comparison Relative risk 1.85

Abbreviation: NS, no statistically significant difference.

have used exacerbations as a treatment end point (**Table 6**) have presented the effect of the intervention using various means including the number of exacerbations, number of hospital admissions, number of days of hospital admissions, number of emergency visits, need for oral antibiotics, need for intravenous antibiotics, or need for oral corticosteroids. Using exacerbations as an end point to assess treatment success relies on the accurate and repeatable diagnosis of an exacerbation, as well as the duration of and the number of patients in the study, to adequately assess exacerbation frequency. The recent British Thoracic Society Guideline has defined an exacerbation as a persistent (more than 24 hours) deterioration in respiratory symptoms (increased cough, increased sputum volume, increased sputum purulence, breathlessness, or wheeze) with or without systemic disturbance.[56] However, there is little guidance to assess exacerbation severity or indeed evidence for the optimal duration of treatment of an exacerbation, making comparisons of exacerbation frequency, severity, and treatment between studies and interventions difficult. Interventional studies also need to be of adequate duration to accurately reflect any impact on exacerbation frequency. More studies of longer duration are necessary to accurately evaluate exacerbation frequency as a marker of successful treatment response, and further studies defining exacerbation severity and management are necessary before exacerbation frequency can be usefully and reliably adopted as a measure of successful treatment response.

SUMMARY

Bronchiectasis is responsible for significant morbidity and frequent utilization of health care resources. Over the past few decades it has become increasingly recognized that effective, evidence-based treatment strategies are necessary. To effectively assess a treatment strategy, clear and validated end points are needed. For a parameter to be useful in disease management, it is must be pertinent to the condition, noninvasive, inexpensive, easily accessible, reliable, and responsive to change. There are few such markers currently available for non–cystic fibrosis bronchiectasis, and much work is needed to allow any progress to be made in the development and implementation of potential therapies. Interventional studies to date suggest that sputum volume and color, sputum bacteriology, exercise capacity, health-related quality-of-life indices, and exacerbation frequency may be relevant and useful measures of treatment efficacy. Spirometry currently has

little role in evaluating treatment success but is important for monitoring for adverse treatment effects. There is an urgent need to both validate current end points used in the assessment of treatment response and establish other pertinent and reliable markers.

REFERENCES

1. Grainger-Stewart T. On the treatment of bronchiectasis. Br Med J 1893;1:1147–8.
2. Athanazio RA, Rached SZ, Rohde C, et al. Should the bronchiectasis treatment given to cystic fibrosis patients be extrapolated to those with bronchiectasis from other causes? J Bras Pneumol 2010; 36(4):425–31.
3. Loebinger MR, Wells AU, Hansell DM, et al. Mortality in bronchiectasis: a long-term study assessing the factors influencing survival. Eur Respir J 2009; 34(4):843–9.
4. Finklea JD, Khan G, Thomas S, et al. Predictors of mortality in hospitalized patients with acute exacerbation of bronchiectasis. Respir Med 2010;104(6): 816–21.
5. Roberts HJ, Hubbard R. Trends in bronchiectasis mortality in England and Wales. Respir Med 2010; 104(7):981–5.
6. Thompson CS, Harrison S, Ashley J, et al. Randomised crossover study of the Flutter device and the active cycle of breathing technique in non-cystic fibrosis bronchiectasis. Thorax 2002;57(5):446–8.
7. Elborn JS, Johnston B, Allen F, et al. Inhaled steroids in patients with bronchiectasis. Respir Med 1992; 86(2):121–4.
8. Kellett F, Robert NM. Nebulised 7% hypertonic saline improves lung function and quality of life in bronchiectasis. Respir Med 2011;105(12):1831–5.
9. O'Donnell AE, Barker AF, Ilowite JS, et al. Treatment of idiopathic bronchiectasis with aerosolized recombinant human DNase I. rhDNase Study Group. Chest 1998;113(5):1329–34.
10. King PT, Holdsworth SR, Freezer NJ, et al. Lung diffusing capacity in adult bronchiectasis: a longitudinal study. Respir Care 2010;55(12):1686–92.
11. Moran F, Piper A, Elborn JS, et al. Respiratory muscle pressures in non-CF bronchiectasis: repeatability and reliability. Chron Respir Dis 2010;7(3):165–71.
12. Liaw MY, Wang YH, Tsai YC, et al. Inspiratory muscle training in bronchiectasis patients: a prospective randomized controlled study. Clin Rehabil 2011;25(6): 524–36.
13. Robinson PD, Goldman MD, Gustafsson PM. Inert gas washout: theoretical background and clinical utility in respiratory disease. Respiration 2009;78(3): 339–55.
14. Horsley AR, Gustafsson PM, Macleod KA, et al. Lung clearance index is a sensitive, repeatable

and practical measure of airways disease in adults with cystic fibrosis. Thorax 2008;63(2):135–40.

15. Gustafsson PM. Peripheral airway involvement in CF and asthma compared by inert gas washout. Pediatr Pulmonol 2007;42(2):168–76.

16. Pasteur MC, Helliwell SM, Houghton SJ, et al. An investigation into causative factors in patients with bronchiectasis. Am J Respir Crit Care Med 2000; 162(4 Pt 1):1277–84.

17. Angrill J, Agusti C, de Celis R, et al. Bacterial colonisation in patients with bronchiectasis: microbiological pattern and risk factors. Thorax 2002;57(1): 15–9.

18. King PT, Holdsworth SR, Freezer NJ, et al. Microbiologic follow-up study in adult bronchiectasis. Respir Med 2007;101(8):1633–8.

19. Angrill J, Agusti C, De Celis R, et al. Bronchial inflammation and colonization in patients with clinically stable bronchiectasis. Am J Respir Crit Care Med 2001;164(9):1628–32.

20. Hill AT, Campbell EJ, Hill SL, et al. Association between airway bacterial load and markers of airway inflammation in patients with stable chronic bronchitis. Am J Med 2000;109(4):288–95.

21. Wilson CB, Jones PW, O'Leary CJ, et al. Effect of sputum bacteriology on the quality of life of patients with bronchiectasis. Eur Respir J 1997;10(8):1754–60.

22. Ho PL, Chan KN, Ip MS, et al. The effect of Pseudomonas aeruginosa infection on clinical parameters in steady-state bronchiectasis. Chest 1998;114(6): 1594–8.

23. Davies G, Wells AU, Doffman S, et al. The effect of Pseudomonas aeruginosa on pulmonary function in patients with bronchiectasis. Eur Respir J 2006;28(5): 974–9.

24. Stockley RA, Bayley D, Hill SL, et al. Assessment of airway neutrophils by sputum colour: correlation with airways inflammation. Thorax 2001;56(5):366–72.

25. Murray MP, Pentland JL, Turnbull K, et al. Sputum colour: a useful clinical tool in non-cystic fibrosis bronchiectasis. Eur Respir J 2009;34(2):361–4.

26. Prolonged antibiotic treatment of severe bronchiectasis; a report by a subcommittee of the Antibiotics Clinical Trials (non-tuberculous) Committee of the Medical Research Council. Br Med J 1957;2(5039): 255–9.

27. Currie DC, Garbett ND, Chan KL, et al. Double-blind randomized study of prolonged higher-dose oral amoxycillin in purulent bronchiectasis. Q J Med 1990;76(280):799–816.

28. Scheinberg P, Shore E. A pilot study of the safety and efficacy of tobramycin solution for inhalation in patients with severe bronchiectasis. Chest 2005;127(4):1420–6.

29. Murray MP, Govan JR, Doherty CJ, et al. A randomized controlled trial of nebulized gentamicin in non-cystic fibrosis bronchiectasis. Am J Respir Crit Care Med 2011;183(4):491–9.

30. Tsang KW, Tan KC, Ho PL, et al. Inhaled fluticasone in bronchiectasis: a 12 month study. Thorax 2005; 60(3):239–43.

31. Murray MP, Pentland JL, Hill AT. A randomised crossover trial of chest physiotherapy in non-cystic fibrosis bronchiectasis. Eur Respir J 2009;34(5): 1086–92.

32. Stockley RA, Hill SL, Morrison HM, et al. Elastolytic activity of sputum and its relation to purulence and to lung function in patients with bronchiectasis. Thorax 1984;39(6):408–13.

33. Currie DC, Saverymuttu SH, Peters AM, et al. Indium-111-labelled granulocyte accumulation in respiratory tract of patients with bronchiectasis. Lancet 1987;1(8546):1335–9.

34. Gaga M, Bentley AM, Humbert M, et al. Increases in CD4+ T lymphocytes, macrophages, neutrophils and interleukin 8 positive cells in the airways of patients with bronchiectasis. Thorax 1998;53(8):685–91.

35. Stockley RA, Hill SL, Morrison HM. Effect of antibiotic treatment on sputum elastase in bronchiectatic outpatients in a stable clinical state. Thorax 1984; 39(6):414–9.

36. Tsang KW, Ho PI, Chan KN, et al. A pilot study of low-dose erythromycin in bronchiectasis. Eur Respir J 1999;13(2):361–4.

37. Tsang KW, Ho PL, Lam WK, et al. Inhaled fluticasone reduces sputum inflammatory indices in severe bronchiectasis. Am J Respir Crit Care Med 1998; 158(3):723–7.

38. Loukides S, Bouros D, Papatheodorou G, et al. Exhaled H(2)O(2) in steady-state bronchiectasis: relationship with cellular composition in induced sputum, spirometry, and extent and severity of disease. Chest 2002;121(1):81–7.

39. Loukides S, Horvath I, Wodehouse T, et al. Elevated levels of expired breath hydrogen peroxide in bronchiectasis. Am J Respir Crit Care Med 1998;158(3): 991–4.

40. Shoemark A, Devaraj A, Meister M, et al. Elevated peripheral airway nitric oxide in bronchiectasis reflects disease severity. Respir Med 2011;105(6): 885–91.

41. Loebinger MR, Shoemark A, Berry M, et al. Procalcitonin in stable and unstable patients with bronchiectasis. Chron Respir Dis 2008;5(3):155–60.

42. Murray MP, Turnbull K, Macquarrie S, et al. Assessing response to treatment of exacerbations of bronchiectasis in adults. Eur Respir J 2009;33(2):312–8.

43. Wilson CB, Jones PW, O'Leary CJ, et al. Validation of the St. George's Respiratory Questionnaire in bronchiectasis. Am J Respir Crit Care Med 1997;156(2 Pt 1): 536–41.

44. Murray MP, Turnbull K, MacQuarrie S, et al. Validation of the Leicester Cough Questionnaire in non-cystic fibrosis bronchiectasis. Eur Respir J 2009; 34(1):125–31.

45. Jones PW, Quirk FH, Baveystock CM, et al. A self-complete measure of health status for chronic airflow limitation. The St. George's Respiratory Questionnaire. Am Rev Respir Dis 1992;145(6):1321–7.

46. Birring SS, Prudon B, Carr AJ, et al. Development of a symptom specific health status measure for patients with chronic cough: Leicester Cough Questionnaire (LCQ). Thorax 2003;58(4):339–43.

47. Guyatt GH, Berman LB, Townsend M, et al. A measure of quality of life for clinical trials in chronic lung disease. Thorax 1987;42(10):773–8.

48. Quittner AL, Salathe M, Gotfried M, et al. National validation of a patient-reported outcome measure for bronchiectasis: psychometric results on the QOL-B. Am J Respir Crit Care Med 2010;181:A5793.

49. Quittner AL, Marciel K, Kimberg C, et al. Content validity of a disease-specific patient reported outcome for bronchiectasis. Chest 2011;140:453A.

50. Singh SJ, Morgan MD, Scott S, et al. Development of a shuttle walking test of disability in patients with chronic airways obstruction. Thorax 1992;47(12):1019–24.

51. ATS statement: guidelines for the six-minute walk test. Am J Respir Crit Care Med 2002;166(1):111–7.

52. Lee AL, Button BM, Ellis S, et al. Clinical determinants of the 6-Minute Walk Test in bronchiectasis. Respir Med 2009;103(5):780–5.

53. Martinez-Garcia MA, Soler-Cataluna JJ, Perpina-Tordera M, et al. Factors associated with lung function decline in adult patients with stable non-cystic fibrosis bronchiectasis. Chest 2007;132(5):1565–72.

54. Martinez-Garcia MA, Perpina-Tordera M, Roman-Sanchez P, et al. Quality-of-life determinants in patients with clinically stable bronchiectasis. Chest 2005;128(2):739–45.

55. Courtney JM, Kelly MG, Watt A, et al. Quality of life and inflammation in exacerbations of bronchiectasis. Chron Respir Dis 2008;5(3):161–8.

56. Pasteur MC, Bilton D, Hill AT. British Thoracic Society guideline for non-CF bronchiectasis. Thorax 2010;65(Suppl 1):i1–58.

57. Orriols R, Roig J, Ferrer J, et al. Inhaled antibiotic therapy in non-cystic fibrosis patients with bronchiectasis and chronic bronchial infection by Pseudomonas aeruginosa. Respir Med 1999;93(7):476–80.

58. Barker AF, Couch L, Fiel SB, et al. Tobramycin solution for inhalation reduces sputum Pseudomonas aeruginosa density in bronchiectasis. Am J Respir Crit Care Med 2000;162(2 Pt 1):481–5.

59. Patterson JE, Bradley JM, Elborn JS. Airway clearance in bronchiectasis: a randomized crossover trial of active cycle of breathing techniques (incorporating postural drainage and vibration) versus test of incremental respiratory endurance. Chron Respir Dis 2004;1(3):127–30.

60. Martinez-Garcia MA, Perpina-Tordera M, Roman-Sanchez P, et al. Inhaled steroids improve quality of life in patients with steady-state bronchiectasis. Respir Med 2006;100(9):1623–32.

61. Martinez-Garcia MA, Soler-Cataluna JJ, Catalan-Serra P, et al. Clinical efficacy and safety of budesonide-formoterol in non-cystic fibrosis bronchiectasis. Chest 2012;141(2):461–8.

62. Daviskas E, Anderson SD, Gomes K, et al. Inhaled mannitol for the treatment of mucociliary dysfunction in patients with bronchiectasis: effect on lung function, health status and sputum. Respirology 2005;10(1):46–56.

63. Couch LA. Treatment with tobramycin solution for inhalation in bronchiectasis patients with Pseudomonas aeruginosa. Chest 2001;120(Suppl 3):114S–7S.

64. Eaton T, Young P, Zeng I, et al. A randomized evaluation of the acute efficacy, acceptability and tolerability of flutter and active cycle of breathing with and without postural drainage in non-cystic fibrosis bronchiectasis. Chron Respir Dis 2007;4(1):23–30.

65. Newall C, Stockley RA, Hill SL. Exercise training and inspiratory muscle training in patients with bronchiectasis. Thorax 2005;60(11):943–8.

66. Mutalithas K, Watkin G, Willig B, et al. Improvement in health status following bronchopulmonary hygiene physical therapy in patients with bronchiectasis. Respir Med 2008;102(8):1140–4.

67. Ong HK, Lee AL, Hill CJ, et al. Effects of pulmonary rehabilitation in bronchiectasis: a retrospective study. Chron Respir Dis 2011;8(1):21–30.

68. Drobnic ME, Sune P, Montoro JB, et al. Inhaled tobramycin in non-cystic fibrosis patients with bronchiectasis and chronic bronchial infection with Pseudomonas aeruginosa. Ann Pharmacother 2005;39(1):39–44.

69. Davies G, Wilson R. Prophylactic antibiotic treatment of bronchiectasis with azithromycin. Thorax 2004;59(6):540–1.

70. Serisier DJ, Martin ML. Long-term, low-dose erythromycin in bronchiectasis subjects with frequent infective exacerbations. Respir Med 2011;105(6):946–9.

Chest Physiotherapy Techniques in Bronchiectasis

Lizzie J. Flude, BSc, MCSP[a],*, Penny Agent, MCSP, DMS[a],
Diana Bilton, MD, FRCP[b]

KEYWORDS

- Chest physiotherapy • Physiotherapy • Airway clearance techniques • Bronchiectasis

KEY POINTS

- All patients with bronchiectasis should be assessed and taught an Airway Clearance Technique (ACT) by a specialist Respiratory Physiotherapist.
- Respiratory Physiotherapists managing Bronchiectasis need to be proficient in a range of techniques as patients will present with a diversity of symptoms, severity of disease and competance in techniques.
- ACT's in bronchiectasis offer similar effectiveness with Active Cycle of Breathing Technique (ACBT) and Gravity Assisted Positioning (GAP) perhaps being the most effective although the least preferred.

Bronchiectasis is a persistent and progressive condition characterized by destruction of the bronchial wall and airway dilatation as shown on computed tomography (CT) scan in association with clinical symptoms of cough and production of sputum.[1] The pathophysiology of bronchiectasis causes patients to enter a vicious circle of airway infection and inflammation (**Fig. 1**). Furthermore, part of this core principle is the ability of infecting bacteria or the individual's own inflammatory response to perturb usual mucociliary function. Impaired clearance in turn facilitates bacterial persistence, thus potentiating the vicious cycle. In this context, the rationale for promoting improved airway clearance is so that purulent secretions harboring bacteria and potent neutrophil-derived damaging proteases can be removed from the airways. Thus a variety of airway clearance techniques (ACTs) have developed over time (**Table 1**).

Evidence for such techniques from randomized trials with appropriate controls are lacking. They have also failed to show long-term benefit in improvement in lung function or reductions in exacerbations. A UK survey in 2002[2] showed that 87% of physiotherapists believe that more disease-specific research is required, a point also highlighted in recent UK guidelines.[3] Moreover, the clinical applications of these techniques are often extrapolated from other research not specific to bronchiectasis (eg, cystic fibrosis [CF] and chronic obstructive pulmonary disease [COPD]). Although understandable, such extrapolation should be performed with caution and the physiologic differences in the conditions considered carefully. Despite this lack of trial evidence, it is apparent that patients feel better once they can manage the clearance of secretions rather than being troubled by uncontrolled cough.

Expert clinical opinion recommends that ACTs are important in this population to enhance mucociliary clearance, improve ventilation, manage breathlessness, and reduce cough frequency.[4]

The authors have nothing to disclose.
[a] Physiotherapy Department, The Royal Brompton and Harefield NHS Foundation Trust, Royal Brompton Hospital, Sydney Street, London SW3 6NP, UK
[b] Department of Respiratory Medicine, The Royal Brompton and Harefield NHS Foundation Trust, Royal Brompton Hospital, Sydney Street, London SW3 6NP, UK
* Corresponding author.
E-mail address: l.flude@rbht.nhs.uk

Clin Chest Med 33 (2012) 351–361
doi:10.1016/j.ccm.2012.02.009
0272-5231/12/$ – see front matter © 2012 Elsevier Inc. All rights reserved.

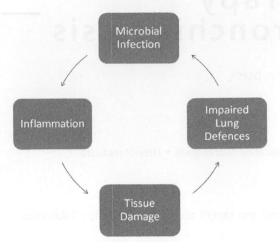

Fig. 1. The vicious cycle of inflammation and infection. (*Adapted from* Cole PJ. A new look at the pathogenesis and management of persistent bronchial sepsis; a vicious circle hypothesis and its logical therapeutic connotations. In: Davies RJ, editor. Strategies for the management of Chronic Bronchial Sepsis. Oxford: The Medicine Publishing Foundation; 1984. p. 2.)

Clinical practice seems to support this opinion, because separate surveys of UK and Australian physiotherapists managing bronchiectasis have shown ACT to be frequently used in this population.[2,5]

This article describes the spectrum of ACT available in the context of modern respiratory physiotherapy practice that aims to augment physiologic mechanisms of clearance and improve symptom-management. The useful end points that have been used to assess ACT are also described.

INDEPENDENT TECHNIQUES
Active Cycle of Breathing Technique

Active Cycle of Breathing Technique (ACBT) is a repetitive cycle consisting of 3 distinct components: breathing control (BC), thoracic expansion exercises (TEE), and the forced expiration technique (FET). The cycle and length of each component are flexible and can be adapted to individual need (**Fig. 2**).

BC
BC is relaxed tidal breathing using the lower chest and performed at the patient's own rate. It is an integral part of the cycle, aiming to minimize any increase in airflow obstruction, especially after the more dynamic parts of the cycle.

TEE
TEE are dynamic and are performed by taking deep slow inspirations through the nose (if possible), followed by an inspiratory pause with an open glottis, and subsequently relaxed expiration. This procedure is repeated 4 or more times and aims to mobilize the secretions. Physiologically, this part of the cycle depends on collateral

Table 1	
A summary of the variety of techniques available for use in bronchiectasis	
Independent techniques	Active cycle of breathing techniques Autogenic drainage

Device-dependent techniques	Positive expiratory pressure
	Oscillating positive expiratory pressure
	    Intrathoracic: Flutter, Acapella
	    Extrathoracic: high-frequency chest wall oscillations
	Intermittent positive pressure breathing
	Noninvasive ventilation
	Test of incremental respiratory endurance

Assistive components to techniques	Manual techniques
	    Chest percussion/clapping
	    Chest wall vibrations
	    Overpressure
	Gravity-assisted positioning
	Modified postural drainage

Adjuncts to assist techniques	Humidification
	Nebulized therapy
	    β_2 agonists
	    Mucolytics
	    Saline (0.9%)
	    Hypertonic saline 7%
	    Mannitol

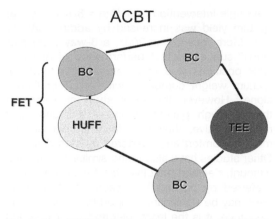

Fig. 2. The ACBT. (*Adapted from* Pryor JA, Prasad SA. Physiotherapy techniques. In: Physiotherapy for respiratory and cardiac problems–adults and pediatrics. 4th edition. Oxford: Churchill Livingstone; 2008. p. 138.)

ventilation and interdependence to help enhance ventilation and facilitate mobilization of secretions.

FET

The FET is a principle component of the ACBT and is defined as a combination of 1 or 2 forced expirations (huffs) interspersed with periods of BC.[6] It is also commonly used in conjunction with other device-dependent techniques. Forced expiratory maneuvers produce dynamic compression and collapse of the airways downstream of the equal pressure point.[7] The forced expirations should create a controlled acceleration of airflow through an open glottis, ensuring airway collapse is minimized but shearing forces are optimized. The lung volume can be varied depending on which segment to target. FET from high lung volumes helps to clear secretions, whereas FET from low lung volumes helps to mobilize secretions. The FET aims to move the mobilized secretions to the proximal airways to be cleared, which then may subsequently require a cough.

ACBT can also be modified by repeating the TEE section more than once, each time following with BC, and it may be used in conjunction with other techniques such as gravity-assisted positioning (GAP), oscillating positive expiratory pressure (OPEP), positive expiratory pressure (PEP), intermittent positive pressure breathing (IPPB), and manual techniques (MT).

Much of the research in bronchiectasis uses ACBT within its methodology, giving frequent information about its effectiveness. Eaton and colleagues[8] used sputum wet weight to compare a single intervention of ACBT, with ACBT and GAP and an OPEP device, the Flutter (Clement Clarke International, Harlow, UK). Although sputum wet weight was similar between ACBT and the Flutter,

ACBT and GAP was the most effective. However, when subjectively rated by the patients, ACBT alone was the least preferred. A further single-intervention study that used sputum weight to compare ACBT with Acapella (Henley's Medical Supplies, Welwyn Garden City, UK), an alternative OPEP device,[9] showed that ACBT was as effective as OPEP. Another study compared ACBT with test of incremental respiratory endurance (TIRE) and showed ACBT to be more effective.[10]

In the United Kingdom, ACBT seems to be the most common technique taught by physiotherapists treating patients who have bronchiectasis.[2,5] However, no studies have shown that this technique is more or less effective than any other ACT.[11]

Autogenic Drainage

Autogenic drainage (AD) is a 3-phase breathing regime using high expiratory flow rates at varying lung volumes to facilitate mucus clearance.[12,13] The breathing regime begins at low lung volumes, moving up through medium and high volumes, aiming to maximize expiratory flow velocity to produce shearing forces and move secretions.[14,15] Inspiration should be low flow with an inspiratory pause and open glottis. Expiration should be higher flow, although aiming to minimize airway collapse.[12] It is often described as an exaggerated sigh. In AD, we are aiming to ensure the equal pressure point is moved more distally and produces greater expiratory airflows in the smaller airways than in FET (**Fig. 3**). The patient repeats multiple breaths at each level until the mucus is moved to the next level, and the patient learns to feel and hear the mucus to enable movement through each of the stages.

There is minimal evidence for this technique in bronchiectasis, limited to 1 pilot study,[16] although clinically it is becoming an increasingly popular alternative independent technique to ACBT. The results of this pilot study suggested that AD is an effective technique, because more sputum was produced compared with a control. Airway resistance was measured by the interrupter technique, but no differences were found with this tool. However, the investigators were uncertain if this tool is sensitive or specific enough to assess changes in AD. Guidelines agree that AD should be considered if other techniques are deemed less effective,[3] but significantly more research is required to assess its effectiveness.

ASSISTIVE COMPONENTS TO INDEPENDENT ACTs
Gravity-assisted Positioning

Within physiotherapy, there has been a long history of use of GAP (since the 1950s). It has

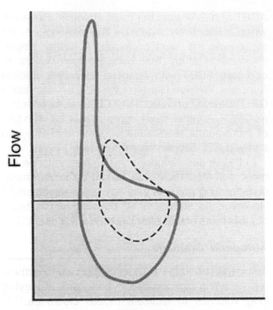

Fig. 3. The flow/volume loop achieved in AD (*dotted line*) verses a forced expiration. (*Adapted from* Pryor JA, Prasad SA. Physiotherapy techniques. In: Physiotherapy for respiratory and cardiac problems – adults and paediatrics. 4th edition. Oxford (United Kingdom): Churchill Livingstone; 2008. p. 142.)

been the mainstay of practice since the 1980s, but because it is passive and relies solely on the effects of gravity and changes in regional ventilation with positioning, it cannot be used alone as an ACT. The patient positions themselves to drain specific lobes within the lungs, using gravity to enhance movement of secretions. For the lower and middle zones of the lung, this technique often includes a head-down tip (**Fig. 4**). It is often used in conjunction with other techniques including ACBT, with or without MT and with IPPB. Evidence has suggested that the performance of ACTs in GAP positions may help enhance sputum clearance.[3]

A single-intervention study[16] (n = 8) showed that sputum yield was increased by adding GAP to FET. More recently, in 2007, a 3-way crossover study[8] suggested that performance of ACBT in GAP positions was more effective in terms of sputum weight compared with ACBT or Flutter alone.[8] However, the same study also showed that although patients found ACBT and GAP more effective, they also found it caused the most discomfort and interfered most in daily life. Other studies have also found similar results, and although deemed effective, the technique is less preferred by patients.[17] It seems that although GAP may be significantly important in maximizing clearance, it is the least tolerated technique and causes the most discomfort. Current guidelines suggest that GAP should be taught if tolerated and adherence is not impaired.[3]

Modified Postural Drainage

Modified postural drainage (MPD) uses similar specific lobar drainage positions as in GAP, but eliminates any head-down tip, thus using gravity-neutral positions (**Fig. 5**). Cecins and colleagues[18] assessed the effectiveness of modified positions without a head-down tip and showed no significant difference in MPD versus GAP, because results of sputum weight did not vary more than 15%. However, these results should be interpreted with caution because only 4 of 20 patients had bronchiectasis; the others had CF. Differences in sputum rheology and anatomic distribution of disease between conditions could mean that these results have limited validity in bronchiectasis. Furthermore, recent evidence for contraindications to GAP, including gastroesophageal reflux disease (GORD), has reduced the use of GAP. However, Chen and colleagues[19] found that the frequency and duration of GORD were not affected by GAP in patients with bronchiectasis. Current guidelines suggest using modified positions if they reduce discomfort associated with GAP.[3] A patient-specific approach is required to monitoring symptoms of reflux.

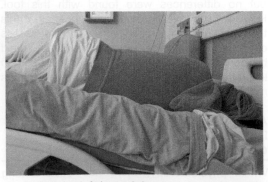

Fig. 4. GAP for left lower lobe, with head-down tilt.

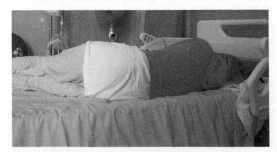

Fig. 5. MPD for left lower lobe, without head-down tilt.

Manual Techniques

MT are usually applied by an assistant during airway clearance and include techniques such as percussion/chest clapping, chest wall vibrations (shakes or vibrations) and overpressure.[6] Percussion uses a cupped, 1-handed or 2-handed technique over the chest wall. Chest wall vibrations produce oscillating pressures in the direction of chest wall movement. A shake usually describes a technique with a larger and slower movement, whereas a vibration describes a smaller, more rapid movement. Percussion should be performed during TEEs. Percussion aims to translate shearing forces within the airways to mobilize secretions. Chest wall vibrations may also be performed during TEE, but only during expiration and sometimes on FET/ cough. This strategy is to produce compression, oscillating airflows, and shearing forces during expiration as well as to enhance elastic recoil and help bias expiratory airflow.[20] Overpressure is used during FET/cough, again in the direction of chest wall movement, but providing a constant pressure. Overpressure may also be used to help bias expiratory airflow as well as to improve expiratory airflow through reduction of mechanical effort. Overpressure also causes thoracic cage compression, which is helpful in facilitating lower lung volume breathing during AD.[3]

There is little evidence of the effectiveness of MTs. Evidence suggests a trend toward an increased rate of clearance with percussion and chest compression.[21–23]

DEVICE-DEPENDENT TECHNIQUES
Positive Expiratory Pressure

PEP uses a set resistance that is applied throughout expiration to enhance the mobilization of secretions. The effect is produced by using either a mask or a mouthpiece attachment (**Figs. 6** and **7**) and induces a temporary increase in functional residual capacity. Furthermore, it augments interdependence between alveoli, facilitates collateral ventilation, and encourages the recruitment of closed airways.[24,25] Moreover, it may splint airways open, aiding expiratory airflow, because airways are often prone to collapse during active expiration as a result of increased intrathoracic pressure. The pressure gradient created across the mucus plug helps to push the secretions centrally to the larger airways. Users perform 5 to 20 tidal volume breaths with active expiration. It is now standard clinical practice to combine the use of PEP with the FET. It can be also be combined with ACBT during the TEE component. Evidence suggests that a pressure of 10 to 20 cm H_2O should be used.[26]

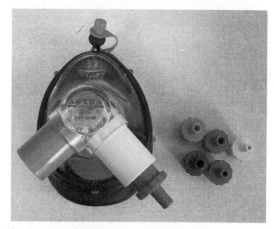

Fig. 6. A PEP device with mask attachment (Astra PEP, Astra Tech, Stonehouse, UK).

The sole evidence for PEP bronchiectasis is from a small pilot study (n = 8) using sputum transportability to assess effectiveness.[27] No changes were found after use of the PEP. However, the sample size was small and the outcome measure may not have been sensitive to sputum velocity and its relative viscoelasticity.[3]

Oscillating Expiratory Pressure

OPEP devices alter expiratory airflow and can be either intrathoracic, as in the Flutter or Acapella, which are placed directly in the mouth to provide resistance during exhalation, or extrathoracic, as in high-frequency chest wall oscillation (HFCWO) devices, which are applied externally to the chest wall by an inflatable vest or cuirass.

Intrathoracic devices (eg, Flutter and Acapella)

Intrathoracic devices have a similar mechanism of action to PEP; however, they produce an oscillating expiratory resistance. As with the PEP, patients actively breathe out through the device, followed by the FET. Clinically, OPEP may also be added during the TEE component of ACBT, when combining these 2 techniques. Examples of OPEP are the Flutter and Acapella (**Figs. 8** and **9**). The oscillating flow causes shearing forces within the airway, which may reduce sputum viscoelasticity.[28,29]

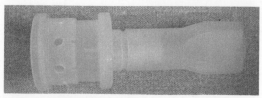

Fig. 7. A PEP device with mouthpiece attachment (Pari PEP, Pari Medical, West Byfleet, UK).

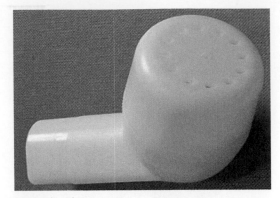

Fig. 8. The Flutter.

Several interventional studies (mainly using Acapella and Flutter) have used OPEP devices in non-CF bronchiectasis. A 4-week crossover study evaluated Flutter with FET and GAP compared with ACBT with GAP.[17] Flutter was shown to be as effective as ACBT in the context of sputum weight. However, most patients (11 of 17) expressed a preference for Flutter, alongside having statistically significant improvement in quality of life (QoL) as measured by the Chronic Respiratory Questionnaire. This study should be commended for aiming to look at longer term intervention as well as including an assessment of QoL, the use of sputum weight collected by patients at home remains a controversial end point, which as yet does not have proven validity in bronchiectasis studies. A single-intervention study using Flutter, compared with ACBT alone and ACBT with GAP, also showed that Flutter was as effective as ACBT and was preferred by patients. Most recently, the efficacy of Flutter was assessed using sputum weight and impulse oscillometry.[30] This was a small crossover study (n = 8) but showed the OPEP cleared more sputum and also diminished airways resistance as measured by impulse oscillometry. However, these results should be interpreted with caution because little is understood about the use of impulse oscillometry in bronchiectasis.

Although Acapella is a newer device and is popular in clinical practice, its use has been studied in the bronchiectasis population. Patterson and

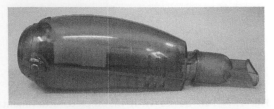

Fig. 9. The Acapella.

colleagues[9] compared Acapella (used with ACBT and GAP) with ACBT and GAP alone. This single-intervention study showed this device to be as effective as ACBT/GAP when measured by sputum weight, treatment duration, spirometry, and oxygen saturations. The same device was also compared with ACBT but during an exacerbation and was shown to be as effective as ACBT and safe to use during an exacerbation.[31] In a further single-intervention study,[10] Acapella was compared with a TIRE device (Test of Incrmental Respiratory Endurance), a type of inspiratory muscle trainer (IMT). Acapella was shown to clear more sputum and was preferred by patients.

A 3-month crossover study compared Acapella with no physiotherapy.[32] This study gives us unique information because most studies compare 2 different techniques. Sputum weight results although significant ($P>.05$) are clinically disappointing at only 1 g of difference between Acapella and no ACT. Significant differences were seen in patient-reported outcomes with the Leicester Cough Questionnaire (LCQ) and St Georges Respiratory Questionnaire in favor of Acapella compared with no ACT.

Extrathoracic devices eg, High Frequency Cest Wall Oscillation

In HFCWO, extrathoracic oscillations are generated by the application of an inflatable vest, wrap, or cuirass attached to a machine that delivers the oscillations to the chest wall at preset frequencies and intensities according to comfort and effect (**Fig. 10**). HFCWO uses the principles of 2-phased gas liquid flow to mobilize the secretions within the airway.[33] However, evidence suggests that it should be used with caution in those patients with small airway disease,[34] because they may be more prone to airway collapse. Therefore all patients should be assessed by a physiotherapist before starting this technique and reviewed for its effectiveness. In the United Kingdom, it is often used to compliment ACBT and is always used with FET.

Test of Incremental Respiratory Endurance

Traditionally, TIRE is used as a device for inspiratory muscle training, but because it creates resistance during inspiration and gives the user biofeedback on maximizing inspiration, it has been suggested as a possible ACT in bronchiectasis.[10] This randomized crossover study in 20 patients with stable bronchiectasis compared a single session of ACBT (with vibrations and GAP) with a single session of TIRE. However, sputum weight expectorated during and up to 30 minutes after treatment was significantly greater

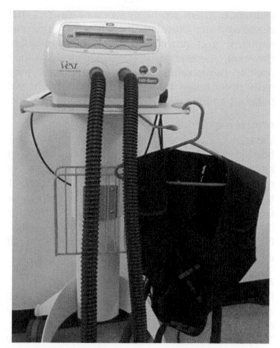

Fig. 10. An HFCWO device: the Vest (Hill-Rom, Ashby de la Zouch, UK).

with ACBT than with TIRE. This technique is not widely used in clinical practice.

Intermittent Positive Pressure Breathing

In the United Kingdom, IPPB is commonly created by using a Bird Ventilator Device (**Fig. 11**). This technique provides an inspiratory airflow created by an air/oxygen mix or pure air, driven via a pressure system. Speed of inspiratory flow, maximum

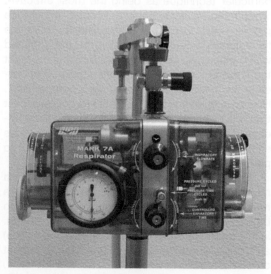

Fig. 11. IPPB: the BIRD ventilator.

inspiratory pressure (cm H_2O), and sensitivity of trigger can be preset. The device also allows nebulization to occur during use. IPPB is often used alongside other techniques including FET, ACBT, and GAP.[6] It aims to reduce work of breathing,[35] augment tidal volume, and mobilize secretions.[36] Most of this evidence is from patients with COPD; however, it is reasonable to extrapolate to bronchiectasis in these patients. Using IPPB aims to reduce the mechanical load that the patient undertakes during TEEs and to leave them better able to perform ACTs.[3]

NONINVASIVE VENTILATION

The use of noninvasive ventilation (NIV) to support ACT is also suggested, because it has been shown to reduce fatigue and dyspnea during ACT in patients with CF.[37,38] Evidence suggests that using NIV for ACT is also safe because oxygen saturations, small airway function, and maximal inspiratory pressure are maintained and respiratory rate is reduced.[38] Patients have reported that it is easier to clear secretions and therefore prefer NIV. In the absence of bronchiectasis disease-specific research, it may be appropriate to extrapolate such findings. Guidelines suggest that IPPB and NIV may be used to support patients who find ACT difficult[3] (most likely those patients with the most severe disease or who are suffering from an exacerbation) to promote tidal volumes and reduce work of breathing.

ADJUNCTS TO ACT
Nebulized β₂ Agonists

Using nebulized terbutaline is believed to maximize airway caliber through stimulation of β_2 receptors and enhance expiratory airflow and regional ventilation. Two different crossover studies have shown that if a predose of nebulized terbutaline was used before physiotherapy, then this yielded more sputum[39] and also improved radiolabeled clearance.[40] Therefore nebulizing a β_2 agonist before physiotherapy should be considered to enable better clearance of secretions through these effects.

Mucoactive and Mucolytic Agents

Infection and inflammation may reduce the height of the airway surface liquid (ASL) This ASL provides an important role in enabling the mucus to move upstream within the airway and to maximize the function of the cilia. Thus a low ASL can impair mucociliary clearance. There are 2 hyperosmolar agents that are potentially mucoactive: hypertonic saline (HTS) and mannitol. However, 0.9% normal saline may have mucoactive properties.

Evidence suggests that increased sputum yield and radiolabeled clearance was improved if 0.9% normal saline was nebulized before physiotherapy.[41] It is believed that nebulization helps to humidify the airways, enhancing ciliary function and increasing the efficiency of the cough mechanism.[3,41]

Furthermore, evidence has suggested that HTS may increase the salinity of sputum, thereby altering its rheology, enabling it to be better cleared by the cilia.[42] It may also help to increase the height of the ASL, improving sputum transportability.[43] As an irritant to the airways, it may also increase cough frequency.[44] Higher concentrations have an increased effect on mucociliary clearance, but may cause unwanted bronchoconstriction, and therefore HTS between 6% and 7% is usually prescribed, to combine what is effective and what is most tolerated.[45] Before using HTS, individuals must undergo a bronchoconstriction trial to assess airway response.[1] Predosing with a bronchodilator before the HTS should also be considered.[1,3,45]

Kellet and colleagues[39] randomized patients into performing ACBT either alone, with nebulized terbutaline before ACT, nebulized normal saline before ACT or nebulized HTS (7%) before ACT. Sputum yield and ease of expectoration were improved with all nebulized therapy, however, the greatest effect was seen with HTS. More recently, a longer-term crossover study was performed with patients completing either isotonic saline or HTS before physiotherapy. This study showed improvements in health-related QoL in both groups when compared with baseline.[46]

Mannitol may also improve mucociliary clearance in bronchiectasis. Because mannitol is a hyperosmolar agent, it is believed to create a driving force for water efflux within the airway, thus improving the viscosity of dehydrated mucus within the airway of someone with bronchiectasis.[47] A recent study[48] looked at regional lung clearance after using differing doses of mannitol. This study suggested that with increased doses of mannitol (up to 400 mg), regional lung clearance was improved. It also showed that this clearance was enhanced by the addition of voluntary coughing, which may suggest a role for mannitol to be used before physiotherapy. However, large-scale randomized trials are ongoing, and therefore this treatment is not used in current practice.

Other humidification devices

It is our understanding that current practice in the United Kingdom and Australia often includes the use of humidification devices to improve clearance. There are many types of devices that aid airway humidification, including the ultrasonic nebulizer and nasal heated high oxygenation. However, there is no current evidence for their use in bronchiectasis, but experientially they have been noted to improve expectoration and patient comfort while clearing secretions.

Ultrasonic nebulizers

Ultrasonic nebulizers use high-frequency vibrations (more than around 20,000 Hz) via a vibrating electric plate (piezoelectric) to turn liquid into a fine mist. This technique generates water particles of 1 to 6 μm. They are often used to nebulize water or 0.9% normal saline and may be used before or during physiotherapy to aid clearance by humidifying the airways and to aid mobilization of secretions.

Nasal heated high flow oxygenation

Nasal heated high flow oxygenation enables delivery of high flow of oxygen and air via specially designed nasal cannulae and other interfaces. They aim to match the patient's inspiratory flow and are therefore often used in patients with increased respiratory rates. In some patients, they may help to humidify the airways and aid clearance. However, this observation is based on clinical experience only.

DISCUSSION

When considering the evidence for ACTs in people with bronchiectasis, it is difficult to make conclusions as to the single most effective technique. Parallel data within CF can support this evidence.[49,50] A long-term 1-year follow-up study[51] comparing 5 different ACTs in CF highlighted no particular technique as being the most effective. Systematic reviews have described adherence problems with GAP in CF[49] and patient preference for adjuncts[52] Such data should be extrapolated with caution, as previously described, but highlight the importance of patient preference and adherence in choosing the most appropriate ACT. However, evidence in bronchiectasis does suggest that the inclusion of GAP and FET improves efficacy of techniques and therefore these techniques should be considered when choosing which ACT to perform.[3]

The criticisms of sputum weight as a valid and reliable outcome measure challenge the inferences made from results of many studies on ACTs in bronchiectasis.[50] However, other methods (eg, lung clearance index or radiolabeled clearance) are not without their problems. More robust outcome measures are needed to validate ACT. Establishment of a standard outcome measure may enable comparisons of data. It continues to be important to review patient-reported outcomes, including information on preference, adherence, and QoL with standardized tools.

More recently studies have attempted to link the objective benefits of ACT with QoL.[53,54] Plugging of secretions while causing airway inflammation and infection also heightens cough reflex sensitivity.[55,56] Patients with bronchiectasis have shown that increased cough is related to reduction in QoL.[54] It has been suggested therefore that measurements of cough severity and related QoL would measure the efficacy of ACT. The LCQ measures QoL as affected by cough[55] and is a robust and validated measure that is feasible in the clinical setting.

As well as choosing the correct outcome measure, adequate methodology needs to be applied to future physiotherapy studies, especially when developing longer-term studies of the efficacy of our techniques. Perhaps most significantly studies need to consider health economics within their research questions, helping to quantify benefits of ACT to stakeholders and patients.

SUMMARY

There is evidence to support the effectiveness of ACT in bronchiectasis. ACTs in bronchiectasis offer similar effectiveness, with ACBT and GAP perhaps being both the most effective although the least preferred. Current understanding suggests that we should balance effectiveness with adherence when deciding on a technique for each individual patient. In the United Kingdom, British Thoracic Society guidelines[1,3] advise that patients with a daily productive cough or evidence of mucus plugging on high-resolution CT should be taught ACT. It is recommended that patients without daily production of sputum should be taught methods for use during exacerbations.[1,3] Clinical practice may differ internationally; however, physiotherapists managing bronchiectasis need to be proficient in a range of techniques because patients present with a diversity of symptoms, disease state, and competence in techniques. It is therefore essential that patients are assessed by a specialist respiratory physiotherapist with an understanding of these ACTs who uses their experience and clinical reasoning to assess and teach the most relevant and effective technique.

REFERENCES

1. Pasteur MC, Bilton D, Hill AT. Guidelines for non CF bronchiectasis. Thorax 2010;65(Suppl):i6–8, i26–33.

2. O'Neill B, Bradley JM, McArdle N, et al. The current physiotherapy management of patients with bronchiectasis: a UK survey. Int J Clin Pract 2002; 56(1):34–5.

3. Bott J, Blumenthal S, Buxton M, et al. Physiotherapy management of the medical respiratory patient: the adult spontaneously breathing patient. Thorax 2009; 64(Suppl 1):i25–31.

4. Sheehan RE, Wells AU, Copley SJ, et al. A comparison of serial computed tomography and functional change in bronchiectasis. Eur Respir J 2002; 20:581–7.

5. Lee A, Button B, Denehy L. Current Australian and New Zealand physiotherapy practice in the management of patients with bronchiectasis and chronic obstructive pulmonary disease. New Zeal J Physiother 2008;36(2):49–58.

6. Pryor JA, Prasad SA. Physiotherapy techniques. In: Physiotherapy for respiratory and cardiac problems–adults and paediatrics. 4th edition. Oxford (UK): Churchill Livingstone; 2008. p. 134–217.

7. West JB. Respiratory physiology–the essentials. 7th edition. Baltimore (MD): Williams & Wilkins; 2007.

8. Eaton T, Young P, Zeng I, et al. A randomized evaluation of the acute efficacy, acceptability and tolerability of flutter and active cycle of breathing with and without postural drainage in noncystic fibrosis bronchiectasis. Chron Respir Dis 2007;4(1):23–30.

9. Patterson JE, Bradley JM, Hewitt O, et al. Airway clearance in bronchiectasis: a randomized crossover trial of active cycle of breathing techniques versus Acapella. Respiration 2005;72(3):239–42.

10. Patterson JE, Bradley JM, Elborn JS. Airway clearance in bronchiectasis: a randomized crossover trial of active cycle of breathing techniques (incorporating postural drainage and vibration) versus test of incremental respiratory endurance. Chron Respir Dis 2004;1(3):127–30.

11. Pryor JA. Physiotherapy for airway clearance in adults. Eur Respir J 1999;14(6):1418–24.

12. Dab I, Alexander F. The mechanism of autogenic drainage studied with flow volume curves. Monogr Paediatr 1979;10:50–3.

13. Schöni MH. Autogenic drainage: a modern approach to physiotherapy in cystic fibrosis. J R Soc Med 1989;82(Suppl 16):32–7.

14. David A. Autogenic drainage– the German approach. In: Pryor JA, editor. Respiratory care. London: Churchill Livingstone; 1991. p. 65–78.

15. Lapin CD. Airway physiology, autogenic drainage, and active cycle of breathing. Respir Care 2002; 47(7):778–85.

16. Sutton PP, Parker PA, Webber BA, et al. Assessment of the forced expiration technique, postural drainage and directed coughing in chest physiotherapy. Eur J Respir Dis 1983;64:62–8.

17. Thompson CS, Harrison S, Ashley J, et al. Randomised crossover study of the Flutter device and the active cycle of breathing technique in non-cystic fibrosis bronchiectasis. Thorax 2002;57(5):446–8.

18. Cecins NM, Jenkins SC, Pengelley J, et al. The active cycle of breathing techniques–to tip or not to tip? Respir Med 1999;93:660–5.

19. Chen HC, Liu CY, Cheng HF, et al. [Chest physiotherapy does not exacerbate gastroesophageal reflux in patients with chronic bronchitis and bronchiectasis]. Changgeng Yi Xue Za Zhi 1998;21(4):409–14.

20. McCarren B, Alison JA, Herbert RD. Manual vibration increased flow rate via increased intrapleural pressure in healthy adults: an experimental study. Aust J Physiother 2006;52:267–71.

21. Gallon A. Evaluation of chest percussion in the treatment of patients with copious sputum production. Respir Med 1991;85:45–51.

22. Sutton PP, Lopez Vidriero MT, Pavia D, et al. Assessment of percussion, vibratory-shaking and breathing exercises in chest physiotherapy. Eur J Respir Dis 1985;66:147–52.

23. Mazzocco MC, Owens GR, Kirilloff LH, et al. Chest percussion and postural drainage in patients with bronchiectasis. Chest 1985;88:360–3.

24. Andersen JB, Qvist J, Kann T. Recruiting collapsed lung through collateral channels with positive end-expiratory pressure. Scand J Respir Dis 1979;60:260–6.

25. Groth S, Stavanger G, Dirksen H, et al. Positive expiratory pressure (PEP-mask) physiotherapy improves ventilation and reduces volume of trapped gas in cystic fibrosis. Clin Respir Physiol 1985;21:339–43.

26. Falk M, Kelstrup M, Andersen JB, et al. Improving the ketchup bottle method with positive expiratory pressure (PEP), in cystic fibrosis. Eur J Respir Dis 1984;65:423–32.

27. Valante AM, Gastaldi AC, Cravo SL, et al. The effect of two techniques on the characteristics and transport of sputum in a patient with bronchiectasis, a pilot study. Physiotherapy 2004;90:158–64.

28. Dasgupta B, Brown NE, King M. Effects of sputum oscillations and RhDNase in vitro: a combined approach to treat cystic fibrosis lung disease. Pediatr Pulmonol 1998;26(4):250–5.

29. App EM, Kieselmann R, Reinhardt D, et al. Sputum rheology changes in cystic fibrosis lung disease following two different types of physiotherapy: flutter vs autogenic drainage. Chest 1998;114:171–7.

30. Figueiredo PH, Zin WA, Guimaraes FS. Flutter valve improves respiratory mechanics and sputum production in patients with bronchiectasis. Physiother Res Int 2010. [Epub ahead of print].

31. Patterson JE, Hewitt O, Kent L, et al. Acapella versus 'usual airway clearance' during acute exacerbation in bronchiectasis: a randomized crossover trial. Chron Respir Dis 2007;4(2):67–74.

32. Perry RJ, Man GC, Jine RL. Effects of positive end expiratory pressure on oscillated flow rate during high frequency chest compression. Chest 1998;113:1028–33.

33. Zucker T, Skjodt NM, Jones RL. Effects of high frequency chest wall oscillation on pleural pressure and oscillated flow. Biomed Instrum Technol 2008;42(6):485–91.

34. Ayres SM, Kozam RL, Lucas DS. The effects of intermittent positive expiratory pressure on intrathoracic pressure, pulmonary mechanics, pulmonary mechanics, and the work of breathing. Am Rev Respir Dis 1963;87:370–9.

35. IPPB Trial Group. Intermittent positive pressure breathing of chronic obstructive pulmonary disease–a clinical trial. Ann Intern Med 1983;99:612–20.

36. Moran F, Bradley J. Non-invasive ventilation for cystic fibrosis. Cochrane Database Syst Rev 2003;2:CD002769.

37. Holland AE, Denehy L, Ntoumenopoulos G. Non-invasive ventilation assists chest physiotherapy in adults with acute exacerbations of cystic fibrosis. Thorax 2003;58:880–4.

38. Sutton PP, Gemmell HG, Innes N, et al. Use of nebulised saline and nebulised terbutaline as an adjunct to chest physiotherapy. Thorax 1988;43:57–60.

39. Kellett F, Redfern J, Niven RM. Evaluation of nebulised hypertonic saline (7%) as an adjunct to physiotherapy in patients with stable bronchiectasis. Respir Med 2005;99(1):27–31.

40. Conway JH, Fleming JS, Perring S, et al. Humidification as an adjunct to chest physiotherapy in aiding tracheo-bronchial clearance in patients with bronchiectasis. Respir Med 1992;86(2):109–14.

41. Wills P, Greenstone M. Inhaled hyperosmolar agents for bronchiectasis. Cochrane Database Syst Rev 2006;2:CD002996.

42. Tarran B, Grubb BR, Gatzy JT, et al. The relative roles of passive surface forces and active ion transport in the modulation of airway surface liquid volume and composition. J Gen Physiol 2001;118:223–36.

43. Donaldson SH, Bennett WD, Zeman KL, et al. Mucus clearance and lung function in cystic fibrosis with hypertonic saline. N Engl J Med 2006;354:241–50.

44. Robinson M, Regnis JA, Bailey DL, et al. Effect of hypertonic saline, amiloride, and cough on mucociliary clearance in patients with cystic fibrosis. Am J Respir Crit Care Med 1996;153:1503–9.

45. Robinson M, Hemming AL, Regnis JA, et al. Effect of increasing doses of hypertonic saline on mucociliary clearance in patients with cystic fibrosis. Thorax 1997;52:900–3.

46. Nicolson CH, Stirling RG, Borg B, et al. The long term effect of inhaled hypertonic saline (6%) in non cystic fibrosis bronchiectasis. Am J Respir Crit Care Med 2010;181:A3183.

47. Daviskas E, Anderson SD, Eberl S, et al. Effect of increasing doses of mannitol on mucus clearance in patients with bronchiectasis. Eur Respir J 2008; 31(4):765–72.

48. Daviskas E, Anderson SD, Young IH. Effect of mannitol and repetitive coughing on the sputum properties in bronchiectasis. Respir Med 2010;104(3):371–7.

49. Main E, Prasad A, van de Schans CP. Conventional chest physiotherapy compared to other airway clearance techniques for cystic fibrosis. Cochrane Database Syst Rev 2005;1:CD002011.

50. van der Schans CP, Prasad A, Main E. Chest physiotherapy compared to no chest physiotherapy for cystic fibrosis. Cochrane Database Syst Rev 2000;2:CD001401.

51. Pryor JA, Tannenbaum E, Scott SF, et al. Beyond postural drainage and percussion: airway clearance in people with cystic fibrosis. J Cyst Fibros 2010;9:187–92.

52. Elkins M, Jones A, van der Schans CP. Positive expiratory pressure physiotherapy for airway clearance in people with cystic fibrosis. Cochrane Database Syst Rev 2006;2:CD003147.

53. Dentice R. Airway clearance physiotherapy improves quality of life in patients with bronchiectasis. Aust J Physiother 2009;55(4):285.

54. Lavery K, O'Neill B, Elborn JS, et al. Self-management in bronchiectasis: the patients' perspective. Eur Respir J 2007;29(3):541–7.

55. Murray MP, Turnbull K, MacQuarrie S, et al. Validation of the Leicester Cough Questionnaire in non-cystic fibrosis bronchiectasis. Eur Respir J 2009; 34(1):125–31.

56. Mutalithas K, Watkin G, Willig B, et al. Improvement in health status following bronchopulmonary hygiene physical therapy in patients with bronchiectasis. Respir Med 2008;102(8):1140–4.

Pharmacologic Agents for Mucus Clearance in Bronchiectasis

Girish B. Nair, MD[a], Jonathan S. Ilowite, MD[b],*

KEYWORDS

- Hyperosmolar agents • Mucociliary clearance • Bronchiectasis • Hypertonic saline
- Inhaled mannitol

KEY POINTS

- Clinicians should be aware that there are presently no medications approved by the US Food and Drug Administration (FDA) to improve mucus clearance in patients with bronchiectasis.
- Inhaled mannitol and hypertonic saline have both been extensively studied for use in patients with cystic fibrosis (CF) and are presently being studied in patients with non-CF bronchiectasis.
- Recombinant human DNase (rhDNase) has been studied in non-CF bronchiectasis and has been found to be ineffective.

Bronchiectasis is a heterogeneous condition that causes destruction and permanent dilatation of the airways, resulting in excessive sputum production. Diagnosis is based on clinical history and characteristic radiographic patterns. The prevalence in United States is approximately 1 in 3000 patients.[1] Even though it is a common disease; it is underappreciated, because of lack of recognition and similarity in symptoms to other chronic lung diseases.[2]

In patients with bronchiectasis, there is hypertrophy of the mucus-secreting glands, with increased mucus production. This is compounded by the normal mucociliary system being impaired, causing ineffective clearance of secretions. The airways become colonized by different bacterial pathogens, causing repeated infection, inflammation, and progressive obstruction of the airways.[2]

Management is traditionally focused on prevention and treatment of exacerbation with antibiotics and relieving airway obstruction with bronchodilators. Recently, encouraging results with use of hyperosmolar (HO) agents to facilitate mucus clearance has prompted more interest in this area. This article focuses on the pathophysiology of mucus hypersecretion in bronchiectasis and current evidence on the different pharmacologic agents available for clearance of airway mucus.

MUCOCILIARY SYSTEM

Mucociliary clearance (MCC) is an important part of the innate defense mechanism within the lung.[3] The cilia, periciliary layer, and mucus constitute the normal mucociliary system.[4] The airways are normally lined by a layer of protective mucus gel that traps inhaled toxins and transports them out of the lungs by coordinated ciliary beating and cough. In the airways, mucus is produced from the ciliated epithelium, goblet cells, and submucosal glands lining the bronchial wall (**Fig. 1**).

Normal mucus is made of mainly water (97%) and 3% of other constituents (mucins, nonmucin proteins, salts, lipids, and cellular debris).[5] Mucin

---

Financial disclosure: GB Nair has nothing to disclose. J Ilowite is participating in a multicentre clinical research study of inhaled mannitol in patients with bronchiectasis sponsored by Pharmaxis (Melbourne, Australia).
[a] Winthrop University Hospital, Mineola, NY, USA
[b] SUNY Stony Brook, Stony Brook, NY, USA
* Winthrop Pulmonary Associates, 222 Station Plaza North, Suite 400, Mineola, NY 11501.
E-mail address: jilowite@winthrop.org

Clin Chest Med 33 (2012) 363–370
doi:10.1016/j.ccm.2012.02.008
0272-5231/12/$ – see front matter © 2012 Elsevier Inc. All rights reserved.

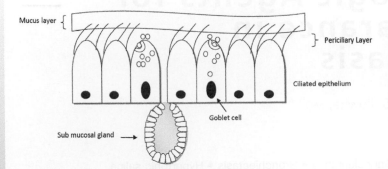

Mucus layer

Periciliary Layer

Ciliated epithelium

Goblet cell

Sub mucosal gland

Fig. 1. The normal mucociliary system consists of the ciliated columnar epithelium, periciliary layer, and the mucus layer. Mucus is produced from the submucous glands and goblet cells interposed with the ciliated epithelium. Normal transport of mucus from peripheral airways requires coordinated ciliary beating, plus the interaction between the mucus layer and the periciliary layer.

glycoproteins constitute the major macromolecules in the secreted mucus. The secreted mucins form disulfide bonds, resulting in polymers (MUC5AC and MUC5B) with characteristic biophysical and adhesive properties.[6] The adjacent mucins with regions rich in serine and threonine residues are linked by their hydroxyl side groups to sugar chains, increasing the number of entanglements. The glycan side chains incorporate large amounts of liquid, which allows mucus to act as a viscoelastic lubricant. The secreted mucus has antiinflammatory, antimicrobial properties.

Active ion transport by Na and Cl ions regulates the airway surface liquid volume. Feedback exists between the periciliary layer and airway epithelium to govern the rate of ion transport and volume absorption. The mucus layer acts as a reservoir by accepting and donating liquid to and from the periciliary layer, to optimize mucus transport.[7] An optimal ratio between viscous and elastic properties of the mucus gel is necessary for MCC.[8] The interaction between mucus layer, periciliary layer, and effective ciliary movement, coupled with cough reflex, helps protect the normal airways.

PATHOGENESIS

The normal clearance of the mucociliary system is dysfunctional in bronchiectasis. There is hypertrophy of the submucosal glands, with metaplasia and hyperplasia of the goblet cells, resulting in excessive secretion of mucus into the airway.[4] There is uncoupling of the ionic transport between the periciliary layer and epithelium. The loss of hydration results in an adhesive mucus layer. With persistent inflammation, there is loss of ciliated epithelial cells and hence transport of the excessive mucus is affected.

In patients with bronchiectasis, there is chronic inflammation with resultant overproduction of mucin glycoproteins mixed with other large polymers including DNA, filamentous actin, biofilms,

and proteoglycans.[6] The solid component of the mucus layer increases and this inhibits the motility of neutrophils within the mucus.[9] The inflammatory cells recruited for combating infection diminish in number, either through apoptosis or by necrosis, releasing proinflammatory mediators that further damage epithelium and release DNA and filamentous actin from the cytoskelton.[10] Along with mucus, inflammatory cells, and bacteria, this forms sputum.

Change in the viscoelastic properties of the secreted mucus, along with increased and persistent mucus production and mucociliary dysfunction, causes pooling of mucus within the airway. This pooling promotes bacterial colonization and recurrent exacerbation. In addition, the increased secretions and decreased drainage cause mucus plugs and airway obstruction. In such situations, clearance is primarily dependent on the efficiency of the cough reflex, which requires patients to generate high expiratory flow rates. In patients with advanced airway disease and flow limitation, the cough reflex is ineffective in clearing secretions, which adds to the vicious cycle.[11]

AGENTS FOR ENHANCED MUCUS CLEARANCE

Treatment of bronchiectasis is focused in part on enhancing clearance and decreasing production of mucus through pharmacologic and physical measures. The pharmacologic agents target ciliary dysfunction by stimulating ciliary activity, improving the rheology by optimizing the viscoelastic properties of the secreted mucus, and improving the interaction between cilia and mucus. Cough clearance is optimized when the secretions have high viscosity and low tenacity (the product of adhesivity and cohesivity).[10] Various agents are used in clinical practice to improve the characteristics of the secretions and stimulate cough clearance (**Box 1**).

Box 1
Mucoactive agents for enhanced MCC

HO agents: inhaled mannitol, hypertonic saline (HS)

Mucolytics agents: acetylcysteine, inhaled deoxyribonuclease I (DNase)

Mucokinetic agents: β-adrenoreceptor agonists

Other agents: erdosteine, guafenesin

HO Agents

The 2 most commonly investigated HO agents for mucus clearance are inhaled mannitol and HS (Table 1). HS is ionic and charged, whereas mannitol is nonionic. Other sugar entities like dextran, lactose, and heparin can produce similar mucus clearance to mannitol.[4]

Mechanism of action

The mechanism of action of HO agents is not known. They reduce the number of entanglements formed by the mucin polymers, thereby improving the viscoelasticity of the secreted mucus.[12] Dehydrated mucus is adhesive in the airway lumen. The HO agents increase the hydration in the airway mucus and periciliary layer, thereby altering the surface tension of the mucus, which may help with MCC.[4] Unlike the mucolytic agents, they do not break the disulfide bonds and denature the mucus, but break the hydrogen bonds between adjacent mucins. There is release of histamine, acetylcholine, and neuropeptides from the airway epithelium when challenged with HO agents, which in turn increases the ciliary beat frequency and improves airway hydration.[13–15] Thus multiple factors, which include change in rheology of mucus, increased hydration of the periciliary layer, and alterations to cilia activity, improve mucociliary and cough clearance.

Mannitol

The bronchial mucus clearance effects of inhaled mannitol have been studied in healthy subjects, patients with CF and bronchiectasis, and asthmatic patients. Phase III clinical trials are underway for inhaled dry powder mannitol (IDPM) to be used for MCC in patients with bronchiectasis. It was recently FDA approved to be used for the assessment of bronchial hyperresponsiveness in patients 6 years of age and older who do not have clinically apparent asthma. Mannitol has various other clinical applications. It remains in the extracellular compartment and raises the osmolarity, and is therefore used as an intravenous osmotic diuretic, and also to decrease intracranial and intraocular tension. It is also used in the oral form to prepare the bowel before colonoscopy.

Physical properties

Mannitol has the formula $C_6H_8(OH)_6$ and is a nonionic sugar alcohol, with a molecular weight of 182.17 g/mol and a density of 1.52 g/mL. It resists moisture absorption at high humidity. In powdered form, it has good flow ability and low permeability index. Hence, is a suitable inhalation agent and can sustain the osmotic effect in the airway for a longer period compared with HS.[16]

Delivery

IDPM has been commercialized for medical use (Pharmaxis, Sydney, Australia). Using a spray-drying technique, mannitol is converted into a dry powder aerosol. IDPM is usually packaged in gelatin capsule that can be easily crushed.

Various inhalers have been used, broadly classified into high and low inspiratory resistance. Almost all the devices have a mouthpiece, holding and piercing chamber for the capsule, and a spinning chamber with a mesh to maximize the powder

Table 1
Comparison between inhaled mannitol and HS

	Mannitol	HS
Physical properties	Nonionic sugar alcohol	Solution of sodium chloride
Dose	300–400 mg; inhaled	Usually 7% HS by nebulizer
Mechanism of action	Improving the rheology of mucus, increased hydration of the periciliary layer	Same
Half-life/duration of effect	4.7 ± 1.0 h; up to 24 h	Much shorter
Use	MCC, bronchial hyperresponsiveness in asthma	MCC
Side effects	Cough, bronchoconstriction	Cough, bronchoconstriction, salty taste

reduction into the respirable range. The common principle of the inhalers remains the same. As a result of the negative pressure created by the patient inhaling through the mouthpiece, they use the incoming air to carry a dose of the dry powder mannitol (released from the crushed capsule) with centrifugal spinning action, which gets filtered at the mesh.

Pharmacokinetics

The absorption profiles of mannitol by inhalation and oral routes are similar. The mean terminal elimination half-life of mannitol for inhalation was 4.7 ± 1.0 hours and was comparable across all routes of administration.

Dosing

Daviskas and colleagues[17] studied increasing dosages of mannitol and voluntary cough on 14 patients from Australia with stable bronchiectasis. They found increased MCC over 45 and 75 minutes with 160 mg, 320 mg, and 480 mg of inhaled mannitol. The clearance was measured using a radioaerosol technique and dynamic imaging with a double-head γ camera. Total clearance over 75 minutes, after mannitol administration and voluntary coughs, was $36.1\% \pm 5.5\%$, $40.9\% \pm 5.6\%$, and $46.0\% \pm 5.2\%$) with 160, 320, and 480 mg mannitol, respectively. Most of the clinical studies used a dose range between 300 and 400 mg of IDPM.

Mucus clearance

Increased hydration reduces the viscosity of the mucus and the surface tension of the sputum, facilitating airway clearance. IDPM increases MCC in healthy subjects and those with asthma.[18] The effect of 300 mg of inhaled mannitol on 11 patients with bronchiectasis was studied by Daviskas and colleagues[19] in 1999 using a radioaerosol technique. All patients were nonsmokers and had airway obstruction at baseline. The investigators measured only the clearance in the whole right lung, comparing that with the baseline and controls, when the patients did cough and inspiratory maneuvers alone. Mannitol significantly increased MCC over the 75 minutes from the start of the intervention compared with control and baseline. Mean clearance with mannitol was almost double in the right lung compared with control ($34.0\% \pm 5.0\%$ vs $17.4\% \pm 3.8\%$). Regional analysis showed increased clearance within the central and intermediate regions.

In another study, the 24-hour mucus retention was reduced on the days when patients had IDPM, but the clearance was not statistically different 24 hours later compared with baseline without IDPM.[20] This led the investigators to

suggest more frequent inhalation for a continued beneficial effect of IDPM. The MCC effect of a combination of IDPM with β2 agonists (terbutaline) was studied in 9 healthy subjects and 11 patients with mild asthma in a crossover study. Pretreatment with terbutaline delayed the MCC caused by IDPM and enhanced MCC when terbutaline was administered after mannitol. The total clearance at 140 minutes produced by terbutaline plus mannitol was unchanged overall irrespective of the timing of terbutaline.[21]

In a study of the physical properties of sputum collected from 14 patients with bronchiectasis with increasing doses of mannitol and repetitive cough, the investigators found that IDPM in combination with cough resulted in a statistically significant reduction in the surface tension, solid content, viscosity, and elasticity compared with controls with no IDPM or cough, and the effect was not dose dependent.[22]

Lung function and quality of life

Patients with bronchiectasis often have poor quality of life because of recurrent exacerbations and poor lung function.[23] An improvement in forced expiratory volume in 1 second (FEV_1) related to specific therapies is rarely seen in patients with bronchiectasis and hence is generally not useful for assessing a response to treatment.[16] The administration of 400 mg of mannitol once daily for 12 consecutive days was studied in 9 subjects with stable bronchiectasis. Mannitol significantly improved the health status over 12 days; assessed using the St George's Respiratory Questionnaire, this improvement was maintained for 6 to 10 days after cessation of treatment. The lung function remained unchanged with spirometry, the percent predicted scores at baseline, 12 days after continuous daily treatment, and 7 days after treatment cessation being FEV_1 $82.0\% \pm 18.8\%$, $83.0\% \pm 18.8\%$, and $84.7\% \pm 19.3\%$. Mannitol reduced the tenacity and increased the hydration of mucus acutely and improved cough clearance.[24] The main limitations of the study were the lack of blinding of the investigators and the lack of control groups.

Inhaled mannitol in patients with CF

Bilton and colleagues[25] recently reported the results from a double-blind, randomized, phase III study of the safety and efficacy of 400 mg IDPM twice a day for 26 weeks in patients with CF. The study had 2 phases: a double-blind 26-week efficacy and safety phase and a 26-week open-label extension phase. They included 324 patients with CF with FEV_1 greater than 30%, and age more than 6 years. A significant improvement in FEV_1

was seen over 26 weeks compared with controls (Δ 92.9 mL; 95% CI, 43.07, 142.70; P<.001) and this was evident by 6 weeks (Δ 77.7 mL; 95% CI, 33.75, 121.66; P<.001). The favorable effect was irrespective of concomitant rhDNase use. Those patients maintained on IDPM had less frequent exacerbations and the favorable effect on FEV_1 lasted for up to 52 weeks in the open-label arm.

Side effects
IDPM can provoke cough and bronchospasm soon after inhalation. It is used as a bronchoprovocation agent in many countries.[26] This effect can be mitigated by the use of a bronchodilator before use of inhaled mannitol. Nevertheless, there are patients who are unable to tolerate the medication secondary to severe coughing or bronchospasm. In the study by Bilton and colleagues,[25] a bronchoprovocation test with mannitol eliminated 12% of the patients secondary to bronchospasm.[25] Other common side effects reported are pharyngolaryngeal pain and hemoptysis. Concern has been raised regarding the denaturing of the airway defensins, part of the normal innate protective mechanism against invading microorganisms. Studies in patients with CF have not shown considerable change in bacterial load in patients inhaling hypertonic agents compared with normal saline.[4]

HS

HS has been studied in several chronic lung diseases as a means of mobilizing secretions. It may have 2 effects to improve MCC or cough clearance in patients with excess secretions: it may improve the viscoelastic properties of mucus to aid in clearance, or the osmotic gradient created by HS may increase the periciliary fluid layer and aid mucus transport.

Two landmark studies in patients with CF have shown the usefulness of HS in these patients. In one study, 7% HS or control normal saline was administered to 164 patients with stable CF twice daily for 48 weeks. The primary end point (rate of change of slope in FEV_1, and forced expiratory flow at 25%–75% of forced vital capacity) did not differ significantly between the 2 groups. The absolute difference in FEV_1 was significant at the end of the study; however, with the HS group having a greater improvement in FEV_1 of 68 mL (95% CI 3–132 mL). The HS group also had significantly fewer pulmonary exacerbations and a significantly higher percentage of patients without exacerbations.[27] In the other study, 7% HS was administered to 24 patients with CF 4 times daily with or without pretreatment with amiloride. Mucus clearance and lung function were measured during the 14-day baseline and treatment periods. The investigators concluded that inhalation of HS produced a sustained acceleration of mucus clearance and improved lung function.[28]

Studies in patients with non-CF bronchiectasis have been limited. The most recent Cochrane review of this subject found no papers worthy of analysis.[29] However, a small study did show benefit of HS when added to other mucus-clearing technologies.[30] In this study, 24 patients with bronchiectasis received each of 4 treatments on 4 separate days: active cycle breathing (ACB) alone; nebulized terbutaline followed by ACB; nebulized terbutaline, followed by isotonic saline (IS); then ACB and nebulized terbutaline, followed by 7% HS. For each group, sputum weight, ease of sputum mobilization by visual analog scale (VAS), and lung function were measured. Results are summarized in **Fig. 2**. Results favored the HS group

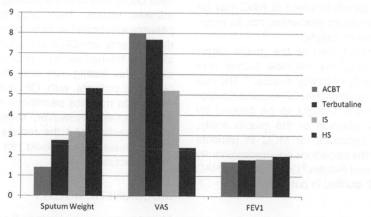

Fig. 2. Summary of results showing the benefit of HS added to other mucus-clearing technologies.[30] ACBT group received active cycle of breathing treatment; HS group received HS terbutaline, and ACBT; IS group received isotonic saline, terbutaline, and ACBT; terbutaline group received ACBT and terbutaline; VAS, visual analog scale (ease of expectorating mucus).

for all end points, with the results for sputum weight and VAS significantly better than for IS. For lung function, both IS and HS were significantly improved compared with ACB and terbutaline, but there was no significant difference in lung function.

MUCOLYTIC AGENTS

Mucolytics act by degrading the mucin polymers and other solid components (F-actin, DNA, fibrin), thereby reducing the viscosity of secreted mucus. Use of mucolytics in clearing secretions in patients with bronchiectasis is controversial. Although lowering viscosity could lead to improvements in MCC, it might have deleterious effects on cough clearance, which could in sum be harmful to the patient. The mucolytic agents that have been studied clinically are N-acetylcysteine (NAC) and dornase alpha.

NAC

The mechanism by which NAC may help with mucus clearance is ambiguous. Most of the studies reported have used the oral form. A meta-analysis of 8 double-blinded, randomized controlled trials of oral NAC showed decreased exacerbations with chronic bronchitis.[31] However, a more recent large randomized trial of NAC in chronic obstructive pulmonary disease (COPD) showed no benefit with the use of the medication.[32] Subgroup analysis of the study suggested that the exacerbation rate might be reduced with NAC in patients not treated with inhaled corticosteroids, and a post hoc analysis suggested a beneficial effect on hyperinflation. Oral NAC has low bioavailability in respiratory secretions, but it is deacetylated to cysteine, containing a thiol group, which accounts for its antioxidant properties.[10] Thus, any beneficial effect of NAC may be caused by its antioxidant properties, not its properties as a potential mucolytic.

Inhaled NAC depolymerizes the mucin oligomers by hydrolyzing the disulfide bonds and reduces the viscosity of airway mucus.[10] The use of inhaled NAC in patients with CF remains controversial. This action is thought to be caused by selective depolymerization of the mucin entity, which might be important for MCC in patients with CF, in whom the secretions are predominantly polymers of DNA and F-actin.[8] Oral or inhaled NAC has not been well studied in patients with non-CF bronchiectasis.

Dornase Alpha

Dornase alpha is produced by genetically engineered hamster ovary cells containing DNA encoded for the native human protein DNase. Purulent sputum has a high concentration of DNA, and the long strands of the molecule are thought to contribute to the viscous properties of CF sputum. By cleaving native DNA into nucleic acids, dornase alpha can greatly improve sputum rheology.

In patients with CF, regular administration of dornase alpha has been shown to improve lung function and decrease the frequency of exacerbations.[33] A pilot study in bronchiectasis suggested that sputum viscosity and other clinical parameters were unchanged with dornase alpha.[34]

A large, randomized study examined the effectiveness of dornase alpha in adult patients with bronchiectesis.[35] Three-hundred forty-nine patients were randomized to receive dornase alpha or placebo by aerosol twice daily for 24 weeks. The primary end point was the number of exacerbations during the 24-week period. In addition, hospitalizations, lung function, quality of life, use of steroids, and use of antibiotics were measured. The study found that exacerbations were more frequent in the group that received dornase alpha compared with placebo. In addition, hospitalizations, use of antibiotics, and use of steroids were more common in the dornase alpha group. Subjects treated with dornase alpha had a larger decrement in forced vital capacity compared with placebo. Quality of life measurements were comparable between both groups. The conclusion of the study was that dornase alpha has no demonstrated efficacy in patients with idiopathic bronchiectasis, and may be harmful in this group of patients. This finding is in contrast with the results seen in CF. The investigators postulated that patients with bronchiectasis might have more disease in their lower lobes, compared with patients with CF, which is predominantly an upper lobe disease, and thus bronchiectasis could lead to more pooling of secretions and adverse results. They also hypothesized that patients with bronchiectasis were older and weaker than patients with CF, and thus might not be able to clear the thinned secretions secondary to dornase alpha. This finding may have been compounded by more patients with CF using chest physiotherapy to mobilize secretions than patients with bronchiectasis. However, these hypotheses remain untested, and the results strongly suggest that dornase alpha should not be used in adult bronchiectasis.

MUCOKINETIC AGENTS

Mucokinetic agents such as β agonists and methylxanthene bronchodilators increase ciliary beat frequency and improve MCC. Both short-acting and long-acting β-adrenergic agonists have been shown to increase MCC acutely in patients with chronic bronchitis and asthma.[36,37] Recently Meyer and colleagues[38] reported an increased mucus clearance for up to 14 days in patients with mild to moderate COPD with inhaled formoterol (12 µg). However, these agents have not been well studied in patients with bronchiectasis, and their clinical usefulness in enhancing mucus clearance in bronchiectasis remains unknown.

OTHER AGENTS
Erdosteine

Erdosteine is a thiol derivative containing 2 sulfhydryl groups, metabolized to 3 active constituents. Its mechanism of action may be to improve sputum rheology and MCC and inhibit bacterial adhesion, although its predominant mechanism may be its antioxidant properties, not its direct effect on mucus. Erdosteine is not available in the United States. Although there has been significant interest in the use of erdosteine with patients with COPD and for prevention of lung toxicity associated with chemotherapy, there have been few studies on its use in patients with bronchiectasis.

In a 15-day, prospective pilot study from Italy, 30 consecutive, elderly patients with bronchiectasis were randomized to receive either a combination of erdosteine 225 mg oral twice a day and chest physiotherapy or chest physiotherapy alone.[39] The investigators found that both groups had significant improvement in 6-minute walk test and VAS of cough and dyspnea. However, the erdosteine group had also had a significant improvement in lung function measured as forced vital capacity and FEV_1. They also noted that the mucus volume produced was significantly greater in the erdosteine group. This pilot study was small and open label. The sputum qualities were not quantitatively measured and were subject to false interpretation. Nevertheless, considering the potential beneficial effect seen, further large clinical trials in patients with bronchiectasis are merited.

Guaifenesin

Guaifenesin is a widely used agent generally classified as an expectorant, and is a widely prescribed agent for many patients with difficulty in coughing up mucus, including patients with bronchiectasis. It is sold both over the counter and by prescription in the United States, alone or in combination with other products. In 2002, the FDA gave the rights to extended-release guaifenesin to 1 company, Adams Pharmaceuticals. In 2007, Adams Pharmaceuticals was acquired by Reckitt Benckiser, which continues to market extended release guaifenesin. In spite of its wide use, there is a paucity of data regarding its efficacy in any chronic or acute respiratory disease. Its mechanism of action is equally obscure. Originally thought to stimulate respiratory secretions, more recent studies suggest that it may reduce them.[40]

SUMMARY

There are no FDA-approved pharmacologic agents to enhance mucus clearance in non-CF bronchiectasis. Growing evidence supports the use of HO agents in CF, and studies with inhaled mannitol and HS in patients with bronchiectasis are ongoing at the time of writing. NAC has not been adequately studied in bronchiectasis, but may act more as an antioxidant than a mucolytic in other lung diseases. Although clearly beneficial to patients with CF, dornase alpha is not useful in patients with non-CF bronchiectasis, and may lead to more exacerbations and other adverse events. Mucokinetic agents such as β-agonists have the potential to improve MCC in normals and many disease states, but have not been adequately studied in patients with bronchiectasis.

REFERENCES

1. Weycker D, Edelsberg J, Oster G, et al. Prevalence and economic burden of bronchiectasis. Clin Pulm Med 2005;12:205–9.
2. Ilowite J, Spiegler P, Chawla S. Bronchiectasis: new findings in the pathogenesis and treatment of this disease. Curr Opin Infect Dis 2008;21:163–7.
3. Wanner A, Salathé M, O'Riordan TG. Mucociliary clearance in the airways. Am J Respir Crit Care Med 1996;154:1868–902.
4. Daviskas E, Anderson SD. Hyperosmolar agents and clearance of mucus in the diseased airway. J Aerosol Med 2006;19:100–9.
5. Fahy JV, Dickey BF. Airway mucus function and dysfunction. N Engl J Med 2010;363:2233–47.
6. Voynow JA, Rubin BK. Mucins, mucus, and sputum. Chest 2009;135:505–12.
7. Tarran R, Grubb BR, Gatzy JT, et al. The relative roles of passive surface forces and active ion transport in the modulation of airway surface liquid volume and composition. J Gen Physiol 2001;118:223–36.
8. Rubin BK. Mucolytics, expectorants, and mucokinetic medications. Respir Care 2007;52:859–65.
9. Matsui H, Verghese MW, Kesimer M, et al. Reduced three-dimensional motility in dehydrated airway mucus prevents neutrophil capture and killing bacteria on airway epithelial surfaces. J Immunol 2005;175:1090–9.
10. Rogers DF. Mucoactive agents for airway mucus hypersecretory diseases. Respir Care 2007;52:1176–93.
11. Foster WM. Mucociliary transport and cough in humans. Pulm Pharmacol Ther 2002;15:277–82.

12. King M. Mucoactive therapy: what the future holds for patients with cystic fibrosis. Pediatr Pulmonol 1997;24:122–3.

13. Silber G, Proud D, Warner J, et al. In vivo release of inflammatory mediators by hyperosmolar solutions. Am Rev Respir Dis 1988;137:606–12.

14. Jongejan RC, de Jongste JC, Raatgeep RC, et al. Effects of hyperosmolarity on human isolated central airways. Br J Pharmacol 1991;102:931–7.

15. Wong LB, Miller IF, Yeates DB. Pathways of substance P stimulation of canine tracheal ciliary beat frequency. J Appl Physiol 1991;70:267–73.

16. Metersky ML. New treatment options for bronchiectasis. Ther Adv Respir Dis 2010;4:93–9.

17. Daviskas E, Anderson SD, Eberl S, et al. Effect of increasing doses of mannitol on mucus clearance in patients with bronchiectasis. Eur Respir J 2008; 31:765–72.

18. Daviskas E, Anderson SD, Brannan JD, et al. Inhalation of dry-powder mannitol increases mucociliary clearance. Eur Respir J 1997;10:2449–54.

19. Daviskas E, Anderson SD, Eberl S, et al. Inhalation of dry powder mannitol improves clearance of mucus in patients with bronchiectasis. Am J Respir Crit Care Med 1999;159:1843–8.

20. Daviskas E, Anderson SD, Eberl S, et al. The 24-h effect of mannitol on the clearance of mucus in patients with bronchiectasis. Chest 2001;119:414–21.

21. Daviskas E, Anderson SD, Eberl S, et al. Effects of terbutaline in combination with mannitol on mucociliary clearance. Eur Respir J 2002;20:1423–9.

22. Daviskas E, Anderson SD, Young IH. Effect of mannitol and repetitive coughing on the sputum properties in bronchiectasis. Respir Med 2010;104:371–7.

23. Courtney JM, Kelly MG, Watt A, et al. Quality of life and inflammation in exacerbations of bronchiectasis. Chron Respir Dis 2008;5:161–8.

24. Daviskas E, Anderson SD, Gomes K, et al. Inhaled mannitol for the treatment of mucociliary dysfunction in patients with bronchiectasis: effect on lung function, health status and sputum. Respirology 2005; 10:46–56.

25. Bilton D, Robinson P, Cooper P, et al. Inhaled dry powder mannitol in cystic fibrosis: an efficacy and safety study. Eur Respir J 2011;38(5):1071–80.

26. Koskela HO, Hyvärinen L, Brannan JD, et al. Coughing during mannitol challenge is associated with asthma. Chest 2004;125:1985–92.

27. Elkins MR, Robinson M, Rose BR, et al. A controlled trial of long-term inhaled hypertonic saline in patients with cystic fibrosis. N Engl J Med 2006; 354:229–40.

28. Donaldson SH, Bennett WD, Zeman KL, et al. Mucus clearance and lung function in cystic fibrosis with hypertonic saline. N Engl J Med 2006;354:241–50.

29. Wills P, Greenstone M. Inhaled hyperosmolar agents for bronchiectasis. Cochrane Database Syst Rev 2006;2:CD002996.

30. Kellett F, Redfern J, Niven RM. Evaluation of nebulised hypertonic saline (7%) as an adjunct to physiotherapy in patients with stable bronchiectasis. Respir Med 2005;99:27–31.

31. Grandjean EM, Berthet P, Ruffmann R, et al. Efficacy of oral long-term N-acetylcysteine in chronic bronchopulmonary disease: a meta-analysis of published double-blind, placebo-controlled clinical trials. Clin Ther 2000;22:209–21.

32. Decramer M, Rutten-van Molken M, Dekhuijzen PN, et al. Effects of N-acetylcysteine on outcomes in chronic obstructive pulmonary disease: a randomized placebo-controlled trial. Lancet 2005;365: 1552–60.

33. Fuchs HJ, Borowitz DS, Christiansen DH, et al. Effect of aerosolized recombinant human DNase on exacerbations of respiratory symptoms and on pulmonary function in patients with cystic fibrosis. The Pulmozyme Study Group. N Engl J Med 1994; 331:637–42.

34. Wills PJ, Wodehouse T, Corkery K, et al. Short-term recombinant human DNase in bronchiectasis. Effect on clinical state and in vitro sputum transportability. Am J Respir Crit Care Med 1996;154:413–7.

35. O'Donnell AE, Barker AF, Ilowite JS, et al. Treatment of idiopathic bronchiectasis with aerosolized recombinant human DNase I. Chest 1998;113:1329–34.

36. Bennett WD. Effect of beta-adrenergic agonists on mucociliary clearance. J Allergy Clin Immunol 2002;110:291–7.

37. Bennett WD, Almond MA, Zeman KL, et al. Effect of salmeterol on mucociliary and cough clearance in chronic bronchitis. Pulm Pharmacol Ther 2006;19: 96–100.

38. Meyer T, Reitmeir P, Brand P, et al. Effects of formoterol and tiotropium bromide on mucus clearance in patients with COPD. Respir Med 2011; 105:900–6.

39. Crisafulli E, Coletti O, Costi S, et al. Effectiveness of erdosteine in elderly patients with bronchiectasis and hypersecretion: a 15-day, prospective, parallel, open-label, pilot study. Clin Ther 2007;29:2001–9.

40. Seagrave J, Albrecht H, Park YS, et al. Effect of guaifenesin on mucin production, rheology, and mucociliary transport in differentiated human airway epithelial cells. Exp Lung Res 2011;37:606–14.

The Use of Antiinflammatory Therapy and Macrolides in Bronchiectasis

Charles Feldman, MB BCh, DSc, PhD, FRCP, FCP (SA)

KEYWORDS

- Anti-inflammatory • Corticosteroids • Macrolides • Nonsteroidal antiinflammatory agents

KEY POINTS

- Airway inflammation is a major component of disease pathogenesis in bronchiectasis, suggesting that antiinflammatory therapies could be of benefit in treatment.
- There are very few evidence-based data on non–cystic fibrosis bronchiectasis for the various antiinflammatory treatment options, particularly in children.
- Although both inhaled and oral corticosteroids have long been used in patients with bronchiectasis, available data indicate that evidence for their benefit seems to be marginal.
- Macrolides seem to have benefit, particularly in patients with bronchiectasis and mucous hypersecretion, and their use is recommended in carefully selected patients.
- Potential rationale exists for the use of many other antiinflammatory agents, but data regarding their efficacy is lacking or inconclusive.

Bronchiectasis is an airway disease occurring most usually as a consequence of chronic airway infection and inflammation.[1] The major initiating event seems to be airway obstruction, primarily associated with infection, which is most commonly bacterial in nature, together with the associated airway inflammation.[2] As a consequence of the host inflammatory response, particularly in the setting of repeated insults, damage occurs to the ciliated epithelium lining the airways, perturbing the mucociliary clearance mechanism.[2] This leads to further airway obstruction, with retention of secretions, setting in motion what Professor Peter Cole called a vicious circle of chronic airway infection, with associated persistent airway inflammation.[3,4] This inflammation may ultimately lead to damage to the various components of the airway wall, including the muscles, cartilage, and vascular structures, causing chronic airway damage, resulting in the development of bronchiectasis.[2]

Much ongoing research has focused on understanding the inflammatory processes that occur in the airway of patients with bronchiectasis, providing a better understanding of the disease pathogenesis.[5] Several inflammatory cells, particularly neutrophils, which release their various enzymes, including elastase and matrix metalloproteases, together with various mediators, including cytokines, leukotrienes (LTs), reactive oxidants, and nitric oxide, act in concert to orchestrate the airway inflammation that ultimately leads to airway damage.[5–9] There are several treatment options recommended for the management of bronchiectasis. However, it has been suggested that because airway inflammation is a major component of disease pathogenesis, antiinflammatory and/or

Financial disclosure: CF has acted on the advisory board and/or received assistance for congress travel and/or received honoraria for lectures from pharmaceutical companies manufacturing or marketing macrolide antibiotics.
Division of Pulmonology, Department of Internal Medicine, Faculty of Health Sciences, Charlotte Maxeke Johannesburg Academic Hospital, University of the Witwatersrand, 7 York Road, Parktown 2193, Johannesburg, South Africa
E-mail address: charles.feldman@wits.ac.za

immunomodulatory therapies targeted against in-flammation could potentially be of benefit and, if successful, may be able to alter the natural history of the disease.[5,10–20] Surprisingly, for a disease that is increasingly recognized as being important globally, there are very few evidence-based data available for the various antiinflammatory treatment options, particularly in children, and much of the information regarding the various treatment options has been extrapolated from the management of cystic fibrosis (CF).[21] Furthermore, in contrast to many other conditions, guideline recommenda-tions for the assessment and management of such patients have been sorely lacking until more recently.[22]

This article addresses the use of antiinflammatory/immunomodulatory therapies in the management of patients with bronchiectasis and individually dis-cusses the use of corticosteroids, macrolides, and other potential antiinflammatory agents (**Box 1**). Although this article is devoted to the discussion of these agents in adults with non-CF bronchiectasis (because CF is discussed elsewhere), it is interesting to note that a recent publication has indicated that in pediatric patients with bronchiectasis there have been no significant studies evaluating the use of anti-inflammatory therapies, including inhaled or oral

---

Box 1
Antiinflammatory therapies that have been considered for use in patients with bronchiectasis

- Corticosteroids
  - Inhaled
  - Oral
- NSAIDs
  - Inhaled
  - Oral
- Macrolides
  - Erythromycin
  - Roxithromycin
  - Clarithromycin
  - Azithromycin
- Additional agents
  - Long-acting β-agonists
  - Long-acting anticholinergics
  - Methylxanthines
  - LT receptor antagonists
- Newer novel therapies

---

corticosteroids, LT receptor antagonists, or nonste-roidal antiinflammatory drugs (NSAIDs).[2,23]

CORTICOSTEROIDS

Corticosteroids are potent antiinflammatory agents, the effects of which are mediated through their activation of the glucocorticosteroid recep-tors that are present in virtually all cells of the body.[10] They have an impact on many of the cells and inflammatory mediators that play a role in the airway inflammation in patients with bronchiec-tasis.[10] The fact that they may have effects on airway inflammation in patients with bronchiec-tasis was demonstrated in a bronchial biopsy study of 12 patients (6 of whom were receiving inhaled corticosteroids) and 11 healthy controls. In the group receiving inhaled corticosteroids, there was less marked infiltration of the airway mucosa with T cells and interleukin (IL)-8–positive cells.[9]

Inhaled Corticosteroids

Several studies have investigated the clinical role of inhaled corticosteroids in patients with bronchiec-tasis (**Table 1**). Elborn and colleagues[24] studied the role of inhaled beclomethasone dipropionate (1500 μg/d) on symptoms, pulmonary function, and sputum production in a double-blind, placebo-controlled, crossover study of 20 patients with bron-chiectasis. The main findings were a decrease of 18% in daily sputum volumes ($P<.003$), a small but significant increase in morning peak flow rate and forced expiratory volume in the first second of expi-ration (FEV_1) (both $P<.03$) but with a clinically un-important absolute change, and an improvement in symptom score for cough ($P<.02$) in those in the corticosteroid arm. Tsang and coworkers[25,26] undertook 2 separate studies on inhaled corticoste-roid. The first was a double-blind placebo-controlled study of 24 patients to evaluate the effects of inhaled fluticasone (500 μg twice daily) over 4 weeks when compared with placebo.[25] There was a significant decrease in sputum leukocyte density and IL-1β, IL-8, and LT-B4 levels after treatment ($P<.05$). There was one exacerbation in the fluticasone group and 3 exacerbations in the placebo group, but no signifi-cant changes in spirometry in the treatment group. There were also no significant adverse reactions in either group. The second was a larger double-blind study conducted over 52 weeks using the same fluticasone dose, which documented a signifi-cant improvement in the 24-hour sputum volume (odds ratio [OR], 2.5; 95% confidence interval [CI], 1.1–6.0; $P = .03$) but no difference in the exacerba-tion frequency, FEV_1, forced vital capacity (FVC), or sputum purulence score in the treatment group

Table 1
Studies documenting the effects of inhaled corticosteroids in patients with non-CF bronchiectasis

References	Inhaled Corticosteroid Type (Dose and Duration)	Patient Population (Number Included/ Completed or Evaluated)	Type of Study	Significant Positive Finding
Elborn et al,[24] 1992	Beclomethasone dipropionate (1500 μg/d)	Adults (20 cases)	Double blind, placebo controlled, crossover	Daily sputum production decreased by 18%, increased morning peak flow and FEV_1, improved symptom score for cough
Tsang et al,[25] 1998	Fluticasone (500 μg bid × 4 wk)	Adults (24 cases)	Double blind, placebo controlled	Decreased sputum leukocyte density and IL-1β, IL-8, and LT-B4 levels
Tsang et al,[26] 2005	Fluticasone (500 μg bid × 52 wk)	Adults (73 cases)	Double blind, placebo controlled	Improved 24-h sputum volume and exacerbation frequency in subgroup with Pseudomonas aeruginosa infection
Martinez-Garcia et al,[28] 2006	Fluticasone (250 μg or 500 μg bid × 6 mo)	Adults (93 cases)	Prospective, randomized, double blind (for effective dose)	Improved dyspnea points, sputum production, days without cough, and short-acting β2-agonist use and improved health-related quality of life in the high-dose inhaled corticosteroid group only
Guran et al,[29] 2008	Inhaled corticosteroid withdrawal × 12 wk	Children (27 cases)	Withdrawal of inhaled corticosteroids	Increased bronchial hyperreactivity, decreased neutrophil apoptosis

compared with the placebo group.[26] However, significantly more patients, infected with *Pseudomonas aeruginosa*, who were receiving fluticasone, showed improvement in their 24-hour sputum volume (OR, 13.5; 95% CI, 1.8–100.2; $P = .03$) and exacerbation frequency (OR, 13.3; 95% CI, 1.8–100.2; $P = .01$) compared with those in the placebo group. Logistic regression models documented a significantly better response in sputum volume with fluticasone in subgroups of patients who had a 24-hour sputum volume less than 30 mL ($P = .04$), exacerbation frequency of 2 or more per year ($P = .04$), and a sputum purulence score greater than 5 ($P = .03$). The same investigator group[27] reported a single case of a 60-year-old woman, with bilateral idiopathic bronchiectasis, whose symptoms, including sputum, rapidly disappeared after the initiation of inhaled budesonide, with repeated computed tomography (CT) of the chest showing partial resolution of the bronchial dilatation and resolution of small airway sepsis after 40 months.

A further prospective, randomized, double-blind study of 93 patients with CT confirmed bronchiectasis using fluticasone proprionate (FP), 250 μg twice daily, 500 μg twice daily, or no treatment, was conducted over 6 months.[28] The group treated with the FP dose of 1000 μg had significant improvement in dyspnea (1.03 [2.1]–12.4 [2.2] points; $P = .01–.04$), sputum production ($P = .001$), days without cough ($P = .02$), and short-acting β_2-agonist use ($P = .01$) from the first month, without change in lung function, number of exacerbations, or sputum microbiological profile. Furthermore, an improvement of health-related quality of life was seen in this group after 3 months of treatment (45.4 [14.2] vs 40.5 [13.9]; $P = .01$). The number of adverse events was also greater in this group, although they were local and reversible.

In one of the few studies conducted in children, a 12-week withdrawal of inhaled corticosteroids resulted in a significant increase in bronchial hyperreactivity and a decrease in neutrophil apoptosis but no change in sputum inflammatory markers in the children.[29] An overview of all the studies documenting the effects of inhaled corticosteroids in patients with bronchiectasis is demonstrated in **Table 1**. The studies all had differing end points, and only the positive findings of the individual studies are indicated in the table.

A Cochrane database systemic review of inhaled corticosteroid use for bronchiectasis,[30] undertaken in 2009, identified no pediatric studies and only 6 adult studies. Although some short-term benefits were documented in adults treated with high-dose inhaled corticosteroids, there were no benefits documented when only the placebo-controlled trials were included. The investigators concluded that based on all available studies no recommendations could be made regarding the use of inhaled corticosteroids in children with bronchiectasis because of lack of studies. The investigators indicated that there was insufficient evidence for the routine recommendation of inhaled corticosteroids in adult patients with bronchiectasis in the stable state, although a therapeutic trial may be considered for the control of difficult symptoms in certain subgroups, which needed to be balanced against potential side effects, especially if high doses were used.[30] Furthermore, no recommendations could be made for use of inhaled corticosteroids in adults during an acute exacerbation.[30]

Although the studies of inhaled corticosteroids reviewed earlier were undertaken with the aim of addressing the airway inflammation in patients with bronchiectasis, one research group indicated that a significant proportion of patients with bronchiectasis have adrenal suppression, especially when inhaled corticosteroids are used concomitantly.[31] These investigators indicated that an impaired cortisol response to stimulation was associated with a poor health status. It is also important to remember that the use of inhaled corticosteroids may be associated with other adverse effects, particularly when used in higher doses and for long periods. Although several side effects are mild, others, such as the loss in bone mineral density, especially in postmenopausal women, may be significant. These effects can be lessened by the use of low-dose inhaled corticosteroids, but the studies documenting benefit from corticosteroids in patients with bronchiectasis were those using higher doses of these agents.[10]

Oral Corticosteroids

A Cochrane database systemic review[32] documented no randomized controlled trials of oral corticosteroids in patients with bronchiectasis, either in the stable state or during exacerbations. One case study documented the resolution of severe bronchiectasis in a young infant after prolonged treatment with antibiotics together with a tapering course of oral corticosteroids.[33]

MACROLIDES

In addition to their antibacterial activity, 14- and 15-membered macrolide antibiotics (ie, erythromycin, roxithromycin, clarithromycin, and azithromycin) are known to have considerable antiinflammatory and immunomodulatory activities that may have beneficial effects in several chronic inflammatory airway disorders, including bronchiectasis.[34–39] Although solid evidence to justify this form of therapy in many of these airway disorders is still lacking, beneficial effects of long-term macrolide use has been found in smaller clinical trials of patients with bronchiectasis.[39] Many of these studies show consistent evidence of a decrease in sputum volume, and some studies have documented a decrease in exacerbation frequency.[37,40] Aside from these documented beneficial effects, it is important to recognize that side effects, such as gastrointestinal upset and cardiac arrhythmias (especially prolonged QT interval related), may occur with macrolide use and there remains the risk of development of macrolide resistance among respiratory pathogens, of uncertain clinical significance.[10,39] One particular area of concern regarding resistance is the empiric use of macrolides in patients with bronchiectasis who may be infected with *Mycobacterium avium-intracellulare.* In such cases, the use of macrolides on their own would, in effect, constitute monotherapy and may hasten the development of macrolide resistance in these pathogens. Therefore, in such patients, careful evaluation and investigation for the possible presence of such infections should be undertaken before macrolide initiation. Thus although routine use of long-term macrolide therapy for patients with non-CF bronchiectasis is not currently recommended, there is a case for their use in carefully selected individuals.[34,39,40] For example, one clinician's practice is to try macrolide treatment in selected cases for 3 to 6 months and to discontinue therapy if there is no clear evidence of benefit to the patients in terms of improvement in quality of life or a reduction in the frequency of exacerbations.[18]

Much recent research has investigated the mechanisms underlying the antiinflammatory immunomodulatory activities of macrolide antibiotics, which are quite considerable and encompass effects both in the human host as well as in the microorganisms associated with these conditions. These are described in detail elsewhere.[35,36,38] These effects in the human host include downregulation of cytokine responses, via effects on nuclear transcription factors and other signaling pathways; a reduction in adhesion molecule expression, oxidative stress, and neutrophil function, involving chemotaxis, degranulation, and elastase release; cytoprotection against bioactive phospholipids; and alterations in the production and rheology of airway mucus. In the microorganisms, these may involve modulation of quorum-sensing pathways, with a decrease in bacterial mobility and adherence, virulence factor expression, and biofilm production.[35,36,38]

Erythromycin

Two clinical studies have investigated the potential benefit of erythromycin in patients with bronchiectasis.[41,42] The earlier study was a double-blind, placebo-controlled pilot investigation of 21 patients with bronchiectasis, in which the treatment group (11 cases) received 500 mg of erythromycin twice daily. The investigators documented a significant improvement in FEV_1, FVC, and 24-hour sputum volume after 8 weeks ($P<.05$), with no associated change in sputum pathogens, leukocyte density, or proinflammatory cytokine (IL-1α, IL-8, and tumor necrosis factor α) or LT-B4 levels. The more recent study was an uncontrolled evaluation of the occurrence of exacerbations in 24 subjects with bronchiectasis completing 12 months of therapy with oral erythromycin 250 mg daily. Such treatment was documented to halve both the median (range) number of infective exacerbations ($P<.0001$) as well as the annual days of antibiotic use ($P<.0001$). Additional studies have investigated effects of erythromycin on human neutrophil and elastase function as well as mucous rheology and mucociliary transportability.[43–45]

Roxithromycin

Two older studies were undertaken with roxithromycin: one in children with bronchiectasis showing a decrease in airway hyperresponsiveness (methacholine challenge testing) after 12 weeks of dosing at 4 mg/kg twice daily and the second in patients with chronic lower respiratory tract infections, documenting decreases in the levels of IL-8, neutrophil elastase, and LT-B4 in epithelial lining fluid, also after 3 months.[46,47]

Clarithromycin

One clinical study of clarithromycin (15 mg/kg daily) investigated 34 children with steady state non-CF bronchiectasis, randomized to either the treatment group or placebo, together with supportive therapy, for 3 months.[48] The treatment group showed a significant decrease in IL-8 levels, total cell count, and neutrophil ratios in bronchoalveolar lavage (BAL) fluid and daily sputum production at the end of the study. Also the macrophage count in the BAL fluid of the treatment group increased significantly. There were no significant changes in lung function parameters. Another case study of a patient with chronic obstructive pulmonary disease and bronchiectasis documented an improvement in the clinical condition (no exacerbations, increased quality of life) after introduction of clarithromycin (500 mg twice daily) for a year.[49] Other studies have documented that oral administration of clarithromycin in patients with bronchiectasis results in rapid penetration into respiratory mucus with persistence of drug concentrations that would exceed the minimum inhibitory concentration of many respiratory pathogens[50]; that short-term administration reduces chronic airway hypersecretion, presumably by inhibition of chloride and resultant water secretion across the airway mucosa[51]; and that clarithromycin is effective against biofilm and bacteria associated with biofilm formation.[52]

Azithromycin

Three clinical studies of azithromycin use in patients with bronchiectasis have been undertaken. The first was a study of azithromycin prophylaxis in 39 patients with non-CF bronchiectasis and frequent exacerbations.[53] Dosing used was 500 mg once daily for 6 days, followed by 250 mg once daily for 6 days, and then 250 mg on Monday, Wednesday, and Friday of each week for 4 months. Overall 33 patients completed the course, and, among these, a significant reduction in exacerbations requiring either oral or intravenous antibiotic therapy ($P<.001$); some improvement in lung function in the 25 cases tested before and after treatment, of which only the carbon monoxide transfer factor reached significance ($P = .01$); and a significant decrease in symptoms were documented. Cymbala and colleagues[54] investigated the use of azithromycin (azithromycin, 500 mg, on Monday and Thursday of every week for 6 months) ultimately in 11 patients with non-CF bronchiectasis using a randomized, open label, crossover design. The use of azithromycin was not associated with any change in lung function parameters, but there was a significant reduction in the incidence of exacerbations ($P = .019$). The mean 24-hour sputum volume decreased significantly in the active treatment phase ($P = .005$), which remained decreased in the subsequent control phase ($P = .028$). The most recent study was that of azithromycin, 250 mg thrice weekly, in adult patients with non-CF bronchiectasis, who had had 3 exacerbations requiring rescue antibiotics in the past 6 months.[55] The clinical records of 56 such cases were reviewed retrospectively. The mean length of treatment was 9.1 months. In 29 patients who received 3 or more months of treatment, spirometry showed a significant increase in FEV_1 ($P<.001$). There was also a significant decrease in exacerbations in the patients ($P<.001$), as well as a clinically significant decrease in sputum microbial isolates. Two additional single case studies documented benefit of azithromycin in either idiopathic bronchiectasis or bronchiectasis associated with chronic rejection in a heart-lung transplant recipient.[56,57]

An overview of all the studies documenting the effects of macrolides in patients with bronchiectasis is demonstrated in **Table 2**. The different studies all had differing end points, and only the positive findings of the individual studies are indicated in the table.

OTHER ANTIINFLAMMATORY AGENTS

As indicated earlier, several different cells and mediators play a role in chronic airway inflammation in patients with bronchiectasis, and therefore several additional agents that have, or are perceived to have, a diverse range of antiinflammatory activities have been considered for use in these patients. The overall conclusion is that all the additional antiinflammatory strategies that are currently available lack sufficient evidence to support their use and further controlled trials with carefully chosen end points need to be conducted to determine their potential benefit.[17] In addition, there are several novel antiinflammatory agents that need further evaluation to determine their possible role in the future management of the disease.[11]

LT Receptor Antagonists

A Cochrane Database systemic review[58] concluded that there were no randomized controlled trials with LT receptor antagonists identified, and the investigators concluded that further research was required before the establishment of whether these agents may be of benefit in patients with bronchiectasis.

NSAIDs

The rationale for the use of NSAIDs in patients with bronchiectasis is that elastase, derived from the neutrophils, is significantly involved in the pathogenesis of bronchiectasis, and therefore agents that inhibit neutrophil function and consequently elastase release may be of benefit. Lewellyn-Jones and coworkers[59] investigated the effects of indomethacin on neutrophil function in 9 patients with stable bronchiectasis, and, although the study documented major effects on neutrophil function, there was no adverse change in bacterial colonization of the airway. Other investigators have documented that inhalation of indomethacin was of value in decreasing bronchorrhea in patients with chronic airway disease, including bronchiectasis, probably through an inhibition of prostaglandin-induced airway secretion.[60]

Table 2
Studies documenting the effects of macrolide use in patients with bronchiectasis

References	Macrolide Type (Dose and Duration)	Patient Population (Number Included/Completed or Evaluated)	Type of Study	Significant Positive Findings
Tsang et al,[41] 1999	Erythromycin (500 mg bid × 8 wk)	Adults (21 cases)	Double blind, placebo-controlled, pilot study	FEV_1 ↑, FVC ↑, 24-h sputum ↓
Serisier and Martin,[42] 2011	Erythromycin (250 qd × 12 mo)	Adults, ≥2 infective exacerbations in previous 12 mo (24 cases)	Open label	Number of exacerbations ↓, annual days of antibiotic use ↓
Koh et al,[46] 1997	Roxithromycin (4 mg/kg bid × 12 wk)	Children with airway hyperreactivity (25 cases)	Randomized, double blind, parallel group	Airway hyperresponsiveness ↓
Yalcin et al,[48] 2006	Clarithromycin (15 mg/kg qd × 3 mo)	Children (34 cases)	Randomized controlled	BAL levels of IL-8, total cell count, neutrophil ratios ↓, daily sputum production ↓, BAL macrophage ratio ↑
Davies and Wilson,[53] 2004	Azithromycin (500 mg daily × 6 d, followed by 250 mg daily × 6 d, followed by 250 mg thrice weekly for a total treatment duration of ≥4 mo)	Adults, >4 exacerbations past 12 mo (33 cases)	—	Infective exacerbations requiring antibiotics (oral/intravenous) ↓, carbon monoxide transfer factor ↑, symptoms improved
Cymbala et al,[54] 2005	Azithromycin (500 mg twice weekly × 6 mo)	Adults (11 cases)	Pilot, randomized, open label, crossover	Infective exacerbations ↓, mean 24-h sputum volume ↓
Anwar et al,[55] 2008	Azithromycin (250 mg thrice weekly × 9.1 mo [mean])	Three exacerbations past 6 mo (56 cases)	Retrospective record review	Exacerbations ↓, positive sputum cultures ↓, mean FEV_1 ↑ (in 29 cases completing ≥3 mo)

A Cochrane Database systemic review[61] identified no studies of inhaled NSAIDs in children and only one small study in 25 adults with chronic lung disease (including bronchiectasis and other conditions either linked to the development of bronchiectasis or associated with chronic sputum production). This review reported that the study comparing inhaled indomethacin with placebo documented a significant reduction in sputum production over a 14-day period in the treatment group and a significant improvement in dyspnea. There were no significant differences identified in lung function parameters or in the blood indices indicative of a systemic inflammatory response, and there were also no adverse events noted. The investigators of this review concluded that there was insufficient evidence to support or refute the use of inhaled NSAIDs in the management of bronchiectasis in either adults or children.

A single case study documented decreased sputum production in a 67-year-old woman with bronchiectasis who received indomethacin suppositories and inhaled aspirin for lumbar pain.[62] In addition, a Cochrane Database systemic review[63] investigating the potential role of oral NSAIDs in children and adults with bronchiectasis failed to identify any randomized controlled studies. However, based on some positive data with inhaled NSAIDs, the investigators suggested that a randomized controlled trial of oral agents was needed.

Oral Methylxanthines, Long-Acting β-Agonists, Anticholinergics

No randomized controlled trials of oral methylxanthines were identified by a Cochrane Database systemic review,[64] and the investigators concluded that further research was required to establish any role for these agents in patients with bronchiectasis. Similarly, there have been no randomized controlled trials of either long-term or short-term long-acting β-agonists.[65] However, uncontrolled studies of the long-acting anticholinergic tiotropium in patients with bronchiectasis documented that it reduced daily symptoms and improved quality of life with short-term use.[19] No long-term studies have evaluated the potential role in this agent in reducing exacerbation rates, decreasing lung function decline or improving radiographic changes.[19]

Other

Several novel antiinflammatory agents are in the developmental phase, which tackle inflammation from several different mechanisms, and these may possibly be found to play a role in the future in the management of patients with bronchiectasis.[11]

SUMMARY

Despite an increasing understanding of the role and mechanisms of airway inflammation in patients with bronchiectasis, studies of the potential role of the various antiinflammatory agents, used to break the pathophysiologic cycle of the disease process, have been somewhat disappointing.[2] It remains true that many studies of the different agents include small patient numbers, are uncontrolled or retrospective in design, and/or have other potential methodological flaws.[18]

The major effect of inhaled corticosteroids noted is a decrease in sputum volumes,[10] and, although corticosteroids, both inhaled and oral, have long been used in patients with bronchiectasis, an overall summary of available data suggests that evidence for their benefit appears to be marginal.[18] In contrast, macrolides seem to have benefit, particularly in patients with bronchiectasis and chronic mucous hypersecretion, and their use may be associated with improved lung function and clinical status, associated with a decrease in sputum volume and lung inflammatory marker levels.[10] However, their use is not recommended routinely but rather in carefully selected patients who need to be followed up closely along with therapy for 3 to 6 months, and the macrolides can be withdrawn if no clear-cut evidence of benefit is documented.[18] Although the potential rationale for the use of many of the other antiinflammatory therapies is clear, data are either lacking or inconclusive. Newer antiinflammatory agents in development hold a potential promise for the future.

REFERENCES

1. King P. Pathogenesis of bronchiectasis. Paediatr Respir Rev 2011;12:104–10.
2. Stafler P, Carr SB. Non-cystic fibrosis bronchiectasis: its diagnosis and management. Arch Dis Child Educ Pract Ed 2010;95:73–82.
3. Wilson R. Bronchiectasis. In: Niederman MS, Sarosi GA, editors. Respiratory infections. 2nd edition. Philadelphia: Lippincott Williams & Wilkins; 2001. p. 347–59.
4. Cole PJ. Bronchiectasis. In: Brewis RA, Corrin B, Geddes DM, et al, editors. Respiratory medicine. 2nd edition. London: WB Saunders; 1995. p. 1286–317.
5. Tsang KW, Bilton D. Clinical challenges in managing bronchiectasis. Respirology 2009;14:637–50.
6. Kharitonov SA, Wells AU, O'Connor BJ, et al. Elevated levels of exhaled nitric oxide in bronchiectasis. Am J Respir Crit Care Med 1995;151(6):1889–93.
7. Horvath I, Loukides S, Wodehouse T, et al. Increased levels of exhaled carbon monoxide in

bronchiectasis: a new marker of oxidative stress. Thorax 1998;53(10):867–70.

8. Loukides S, Horvath I, Wodehouse T, et al. Elevated levels of expired breath hydrogen peroxide in bronchiectasis. Am J Respir Crit Care Med 1998;158(3):991–4.

9. Gaga M, Bentley AM, Humbert M, et al. Increases in CD4+ T lymphocytes, macrophages, neutrophils and interleukin 8 positive cells in the airways of patients with bronchiectasis. Thorax 1998;53(8):685–91.

10. King P. Is there a role for inhaled corticosteroids and macrolide therapy in bronchiectasis? Drugs 2007;67(7):965–74.

11. Loebinger MR, Wilson R. Pharmacotherapy for bronchiectasis. Expert Opin Pharmacother 2007;8(18):3183–93.

12. O'Donnell AE. Bronchiectasis. Chest 2008;134:815–23.

13. Prasad M, Tino G. Bronchiectasis, part 2: management. J Respir Dis 2008;29(1):20–5.

14. ten Hacken N, Kerstjens H, Postma D. Bronchiectasis. Clin Evid (Online) 2008;2008:1507.

15. Ilowite J, Spiegler P, Kessler H. Pharmacological treatment options for bronchiectasis. Focus on antimicrobial and anti-inflammatory agents. Drugs 2009;69(4):407–19.

16. Pappalettera M, Aliberti S, Castellotti P, et al. Bronchiectasis: an update. Clin Respir J 2009;3:126–34.

17. Goeminne P, Dupont L. Non-cystic fibrosis bronchiectasis: diagnosis and management in 21st century. Postgrad Med J 2010;86:493–501.

18. Metersky ML. New treatment options for bronchiectasis. Ther Adv Respir Dis 2010;4:93–9.

19. Redding GJ. Update on treatment of childhood bronchiectasis unrelated to cystic-fibrosis. Paediatr Respir Rev 2011;12:119–23.

20. Pressler T. Targeting airway inflammation in cystic fibrosis in children: past, present, and future. Paediatr Drugs 2011;13(3):141–7.

21. Chang AB. Bronchiectasis: so much yet to learn and to do. Paediatr Respir Rev 2011;12:89–90.

22. Pasteur MC, Bilton D, Hill AT; British Thoracic Society Bronchiectasis (non-CF) Guideline Group: a subgroup of the British Thoracic Society Standards of Care Committee. British Thoracic Society Guideline for non-CF bronchiectasis. Thorax 2010;65:i1–58.

23. Subie HA, Fitzgerald DA. Non-cystic fibrosis bronchiectasis. J Paediatr Child Health 2010. DOI:10.1111/j.1440–1754.2010.01871.x.

24. Elborn JS, Johnston B, Allen F, et al. Inhaled steroids in patients with bronchiectasis. Respir Med 1992;86(2):121–4.

25. Tsang KW, Ho PL, Lam WK, et al. Inhaled fluticasone reduces sputum inflammatory indices in severe bronchiectasis. Am J Respir Crit Care Med 1998;158(3):723–7.

26. Tsang KW, Tan KC, Ho PL, et al. Inhaled fluticasone in bronchiectasis: a 12 month study. Thorax 2005;60(3):239–43.

27. Tsang KW, Lam WK, Sun J, et al. Regression of bilateral bronchiectasis with inhaled steroid therapy. Respirology 2002;7(1):77–81.

28. Martinez-Garcia MA, Perpina-Tordera M, Roman-Sanchez P, et al. Inhaled steroids improve quality of life in patients with steady-state bronchiectasis. Respir Med 2006;100:1623–32.

29. Guran T, Ersu R, Karadag B, et al. Withdrawal of inhaled steroids in children with non-cystic fibrosis bronchiectasis. J Clin Pharm Ther 2008;33(6):603–11.

30. Kapur N, Bell S, Kolbe J, et al. Inhaled steroids for bronchiectasis. Cochrane Database Syst Rev 2009;1:CD000996.

31. Holme J, Tomlinson JW, Stockley RA, et al. Adrenal suppression in bronchiectasis and the impact of inhaled corticosteroids. Eur Respir J 2008;32(4):1047–52.

32. Lasserson T, Holt K, Greenstone M. Oral steroids for bronchiectasis (stable and acute exacerbations). Cochrane Database Syst Rev 2001;4:CD002162.

33. Crowley S, Matthews I. Resolution of extensive severe bronchiectasis in an infant. Pediatr Pulmonol 2010;45(7):717–20.

34. Jaffe A, Bush A. Anti-inflammatory effects of macrolides in lung disease. Pediatr Pulmonol 2001;31(6):464–73.

35. Bush A, Rubin BK. Macrolides as biological response modifiers in cystic fibrosis and bronchiectasis. Semin Respir Crit Care Med 2003;24(6):737–48.

36. Giamarellos-Bourboulis EJ. Macrolides beyond the conventional antimicrobials: a class of potent immunomodulators. Int J Antimicrob Agents 2008;31:12–20.

37. Crosbie PA, Woodhead MA. Long-term macrolide therapy in chronic inflammatory airway diseases. Eur Respir J 2009;33:171–81.

38. Friedlander AL, Albert RK. Chronic macrolide therapy in inflammatory airways diseases. Chest 2010;138(5):1202–12.

39. Altenburg J, de Graaff CS, van der Werf TS, et al. Immunomodulatory effects of macrolide antibiotics—part 2: advantages and disadvantages of long-term, low-dose macrolide therapy. Respiration 2011;81(1):75–87.

40. Bochet M, Garin N, Janssens JP, et al. [Is there a role for prophylactic antibiotic treatment with macrolides in bronchiectasis?] Rev Med Suisse 2011;7(280):308, 310–312 [in French].

41. Tsang KW, Ho PI, Chan KN, et al. A pilot study of low-dose erythromycin in bronchiectasis. Eur Respir J 1999;13(9):361–4.

42. Serisier DJ, Martin ML. Long-term, low-dose erythromycin in bronchiectasis subjects with frequent

infective exacerbations. Respir Med 2011;105(6): 946–9.

43. Mikami M. [Clinical and pathophysiological significance of neutrophil elastase in sputum and the effect of erythromycin in chronic respiratory diseases]. Nihon Kyobu Shikkan Gakkai Zasshi 1991; 29(1):72–83 [in Japanese].

44. Shibuya Y, Wills PJ, Cole PJ. The effect of erythromycin on mucociliary transportability and rheology of cystic fibrosis and bronchiectasis sputum. Respiration 2001;68(6):615–9.

45. Gorrini M, Lupi A, Viglio S, et al. Inhibition of human neutrophil elastase by erythromycin and flurythromcyin, two macrolide antibiotics. Am J Respir Cell Mol Biol 2001;25(4):492–9.

46. Koh YY, Lee MH, Sun YH, et al. Effect of roxithromycin on airway responsiveness in children with bronchiectasis: a double-blind, placebo-controlled study. Eur Respir J 1997;10(5):994–9.

47. Nakamura H, Fujishima S, Inoue T, et al. Clinical and immunoregulatory effects of roxithromycin therapy for chronic respiratory tract infection. Eur Respir J 1999;13(6):1371–9.

48. Yalcin E, Kiper N, Ozcelik U, et al. Effects of clarithromycin on inflammatory parameters and clinical conditions in children with bronchiectasis. J Clin Pharm Ther 2006;31:49–55.

49. Vila-Justribo M, Dorca-Sargatal J, Bello-Dronda S. Bronchiectasis and macrolides. Arch Bronconeumol 2006;42(4):205–6.

50. Tsang KW, Roberts P, Read RC, et al. The concentrations of clarithromycin and its 14-hydroxy metabolite in sputum of patients with bronchiectasis following single dose oral administration. J Antimicrob Chemother 1994;33(2):289–97.

51. Tagaya E, Tamaoki J, Kondo M, et al. Effect of a short course of clarithromycin therapy on sputum production in patients with chronic airway hypersecretion. Chest 2002;122(1):213–8.

52. Ohgaki N. Bacterial biofilm in chronic airway infection. Kansenshogaku Zasshi 1994;68(1):138–51.

53. Davies G, Wilson R. Prophylactic antibiotic treatment of bronchiectasis with azithromycin. Thorax 2004;59: 540–1.

54. Cymbala AA, Edmonds LC, Bauer MA, et al. The disease-modifying effects of twice-weekly oral azithromycin in patients with bronchiectasis. Treat Respir Med 2005;4(2):117–22.

55. Anwar GA, Bourke SC, Afolabi G, et al. Effects of long-term low-dose azithromycin in patients with non-CF bronchiectasis. Respir Med 2008;102: 1494–6.

56. Carro LM. [Long-term treatment with azithromycin in a patient with idiopathic bronchiectasis]. Arch Bronconeumol 2005;41(5):1–2 [in Spanish].

57. Verleden GM, Dupont LJ, Vanhaecke J, et al. Effect of azithromycin on bronchiectasis and pulmonary function in a heart-lung transplant patient with severe chronic allograft dysfunction: a case report. J Heart Lung Transplant 2005;24(8):1155–8.

58. Corless JA, Warburton CJ. Leukotriene receptor antagonists for non-cystic fibrosis bronchiectasis. Cochrane Database Syst Rev 2000;4:CD002174.

59. Llewellyn-Jones CG, Johnson MM, Mitchell JL, et al. In vivo study of indomethacin in bronchiectasis: effect on neutrophil function and lung secretion. Eur Respir J 1995;8(9):1479–87.

60. Tamaoki J, Chiyotani A, Kobayashi K, et al. Effect of indomethacin on bronchorrhea in patients with chronic bronchitis, diffuse panbronchiolitis, or bronchiectasis. Am Rev Respir Dis 1992;145(3):548–52.

61. Pizzutto SJ, Upham JW, Yerkovich ST, et al. Inhaled non-steroid anti-inflammatories for children and adults with bronchiectasis. Cochrane Database Syst Rev 2010;4:CD007525.

62. Inoue H, Aizawa H, Koto H, et al. Effect of cyclooxygenase inhibitor on excessive sputum. Fukuoka Igaku Zasshi 1991;82(4):177–80.

63. Kapur N, Chang AB. Oral non steroid anti-inflammatories for children and adults with bronchiectasis. Cochrane Database Syst Rev 2007;4: CD006427.

64. Steele K, Greenstone M, Lasserson JA. Oral methylxanthines for bronchiectasis. Cochrane Database Syst Rev 2001;1:CD002734.

65. Sheikh A, Nolan D, Greenstone M. Long-acting beta-2-agonists for bronchiectasis. Cochrane Database Syst Rev 2001;4:CD002155.

Antimicrobial Therapy for Bronchiectasis

Anne E. O'Donnell, MD

KEYWORDS

- Bronchiectasis • Antibiotics • Maintenance • Antimicrobial therapy

KEY POINTS

- Antibiotics have a role in the management of acute exacerbations of bronchiectasis and as a part of a long-term maintenance strategy.
- Clinical trials are underway to determine the efficacy and safety of various inhaled antibiotics for chronic therapy for bronchiectasis.
- Clinicians need to tailor their therapies to the individual patient based on their best clinical judgment and informed by the data and guidelines that are currently available in the published literature.

INTRODUCTION

Patients with non–cystic fibrosis (non-CF) bronchiectasis are commonly infected with microorganisms that contribute to the chronic cycle of infection and inflammation that may ultimately lead to progressive airway and lung parenchymal dysfunction.[1,2] Nonenteric gram-negative bacteria, Staphylococcus aureus, and nontuberculous mycobacteria (NTM) are common pathogens in bronchiectasis. Fungal organisms may be colonizers or may contribute to progressive disease. Approximately one-third of the patients with adult bronchiectasis are chronically infected with Pseudomonas, and these patients experience a more accelerated decline in lung function and more frequent exacerbations than those infected with other organisms.[3] In contrast, patients with no pathogens isolated from their sputum generally have the mildest disease.[4] Hence, antibiotic therapy is an important component of care for many patients with bronchiectasis. The goals of antibiotic therapy include reduction in frequency and severity of bronchiectasis exacerbations, improved quality of life, and possibly slowing of disease progression. Coupled with other treatment modalities described in this issue of Clinics in Chest Medicine, antibiotics play an important role in the therapeutic regimen of patients with bronchiectasis. However, there are no antibiotics specifically approved by regulatory agencies for treatment of non-CF bronchiectasis. There are only a few randomized clinical trials of antibiotics in bronchiectasis, most of which are not sufficiently powered to inform clinical decision making. Hence, careful clinical judgment coupled with an understanding of the available literature and expert panel guidelines are needed to guide antibiotic prescribing for individual patients with bronchiectasis.

MICROBIOLOGY OF BRONCHIECTASIS

Four studies of patients with adult bronchiectasis (conducted in Australia, the United States, and the United Kingdom) have demonstrated that Haemophilus influenza and Pseudomonas aeruginosa are the 2 most common pathogens cultured from sputum specimens.[4–7] Moraxella catarrhalis is also seen, as well as Streptococcus pneumoniae and S aureus. NTM were cultured from approximately 20% of patients in a cohort from Texas,[5] but these are less common and/or rarely detected in non-US subjects. The rate of fungal colonization versus infection in patients with bronchiectasis is

Division of Pulmonary, Critical Care and Sleep Medicine, Georgetown University Hospital, 4 North Main Hospital, 3800 Reservoir Road NW, Washington, DC 20007, USA
E-mail address: odonnela@georgetown.edu

Clin Chest Med 33 (2012) 381–386
doi:10.1016/j.ccm.2012.03.005
0272-5231/12/$ – see front matter © 2012 Elsevier Inc. All rights reserved.

unknown. **Table 1** summarizes the microbiological profile of patients with bronchiectasis.

Sputum culture results and antibiotic sensitivity data are important in ultimately choosing the appropriate antibiotic treatment in patients with bronchiectasis. One study from Scotland explored the utility of a sputum color chart to assess the reliability and predictive value of sputum characteristics to assess bacterial colonization.[8] The finding of purulent sputum was associated with bacterial colonization, cystic or varicose bronchiectasis, and reduced lung function. However, to completely assess infection status, formal laboratory culture methodology is required. Routine laboratory antibiotic sensitivity testing is also used to assess potential antibiotic therapies, but at least one investigation has suggested that some patients with bronchiectasis have complex populations of bacteria that result in variable antibiotic susceptibility.[9] In addition, the utility of antibiotic susceptibility for antibiotics other than macrolides appears to be unreliable for guiding therapy for patients infected with *Mycobacterium avium* complex organisms.[10]

INDICATIONS FOR ANTIBIOTICS IN BRONCHIECTASIS

It is difficult to decide when to initiate antibiotic therapy for a patient with bronchiectasis. Many patients have daily cough with sputum production, and cultures often show pathogenic organisms even when the patient is clinically well.[11] Antibiotic therapy is generally indicated when the patient has an acute exacerbation of symptoms characterized by an increase in cough, change in quantity or quality of sputum, dyspnea, fever, and malaise.[12] The choice of antibiotic should be guided by sputum microbiology testing. The optimal dosing and duration of therapy are not known and are generally decided based on clinical response.

Historically, some patients with frequent infectious exacerbations have been treated with chronic oral antibiotics, but there is a paucity of data to support that practice. There are a few published series on using long-term inhaled antibiotic therapy to reduce exacerbations in patients chronically colonized with gram-negative bacteria, a practice that is now considered the standard of care in the treatment of CF bronchiectasis. Clinical trials are currently underway to better assess the efficacy of maintenance inhaled antibiotic therapy in non-CF bronchiectasis.[13]

ANTIBIOTICS FOR ACUTE EXACERBATIONS OF BRONCHIECTASIS

Mild to moderate exacerbations of bronchiectasis should be treated with an oral antibiotic targeted at the suspected infecting organism; the optimal duration of therapy is unknown, but most patients should receive the antibiotic for 10 to 21 days.[14] Therapy is aimed at reducing the sputum microbiological load; the patient should show improvement in clinical symptoms at the end of treatment.[11,12] Ideally, a sputum culture should be submitted to the microbiology laboratory before initiation of antibiotic therapy. Empiric therapy can be chosen based on the patient's prior culture history. If there are no prior cultures performed, the likely infecting organism can be suspected on the basis of clinical findings. Patients with milder disease (forced expiratory volume in the first second of expiration >60% predicted) and relatively low volume of daily sputum production (<20 mL/d) can be started on a nonpseudomonal antibiotic; those with more severe disease should be empirically treated with an antipseudomonal agent pending culture results.[11] When the patient presents with a severe infectious exacerbation, identification of the pathogenic organism is particularly important. When the patient has an organism such

Table 1				
Bacteriology of bronchiectasis				
	Study/Year (n)			
Organisms	**Nicotra et al,[5] 1995 (n = 123)**	**Pasteur et al,[6] 2000 (n = 150)**	**King et al,[4] 2007 (n = 89)**	**Li et al,[7] 2005 (n = 136)**
H influenza	30	35	47	39
P aeruginosa	31	31	12	11
M catarrhalis	2	20	8	2
S pneumoniae	11	13	7	22
S aureus	7	14	4	4
No organism	Not specified	23	21	Not specified
Mycobacterium	17	0	2	Not specified

as drug-resistant *P aeruginosa* or methicillin-resistant *S aureus*, intravenous (IV) antibiotic therapy may be required. Depending on the exacerbation severity and local practice, IV antibiotic therapy may require hospital admission. Home administration of IV antibiotics is an option for the patient who has an exacerbation due to one of the earlier-mentioned organisms and who is able to manage the required treatments without ancillary support.

Tsang and colleagues[15] evaluated the efficacy of oral levofloxacin versus IV ceftazidime for 10 days in 35 patients with acute exacerbations of bronchiectasis; both therapies were effective. Darley and colleagues[16] reported microbiological efficacy in 9 patients treated in an open-label trial with 7 to 10 days of IV meropenem. There has been one study that evaluated the role of inhaled antibiotic therapy in addition to oral ciprofloxacin in acute exacerbations of bronchiectasis due to *P aeruginosa*; that trial showed improved microbiological outcomes with combination therapy but no additional clinical benefit.[17]

Patients with acute infectious exacerbations of bronchiectasis likely benefit from other therapies, including airway clearance. They require careful microbiological and clinical monitoring. Improper use of antibiotics for acute exacerbations may have adverse consequences. Macrolide and fluoroquinolone antibiotics may mask coexisting infections with mycobacteria, which can result in delayed treatment or development of resistant organisms.[10,18]

ANTIBIOTICS FOR CHRONIC MAINTENANCE THERAPY IN BRONCHIECTASIS

The utility of chronic maintenance antibiotic therapy in non-CF bronchiectasis is unknown. Patients with frequent exacerbations and debilitating symptoms, especially copious daily sputum production, may be candidates for maintenance antibiotic therapy. The recent British Thoracic Society guidelines recommend consideration of long-term antibiotic therapy for patients with 3 or more exacerbations per year.[12] Chronic antibiotic therapy should be part of a multimodality treatment approach to patients with significant bronchiectasis. Airway clearance, exercise, and other therapies should also be included in the daily treatment regimen.

Rotating or prolonged oral antibiotic strategies have been used in patients with bronchiectasis for many years but with little supporting evidence. A retrospectively reported cohort of 26 patients who were treated with repeated scheduled cycles of oral antibiotics, including quinolone, for 6 to 84 months demonstrated radiographic disease

stability.[19] Ten patients given prolonged oral ciprofloxacin (≥90 days) had decreased exacerbations, but 2 of the patients developed resistant organisms.[20] Hence, standard maintenance oral antibiotics are not currently recommended in non-CF bronchiectasis. However, of note, oral macrolide antibiotics may have a role (see later) when used for their immunomodulatory benefits rather than for their anti-infective properties.

Inhaled antibiotics have a potential role as maintenance therapy for non-CF bronchiectasis. The theoretical advantages include the high concentration of antibiotic delivered into the airway and the reduced systemic absorption and systemic side effects. Several studies have investigated the role of inhaled antibiotics for chronic use in bronchiectasis. Orriols and colleagues[21] reported on 17 patients who were randomized to treatment with inhaled ceftazidime (1000 mg twice per day) and inhaled tobramycin (100 mg twice per day) versus routine care. The treated patients had reduced hospital admissions but no change in oral antibiotic use. Two studies have shown microbiological benefit with the administration of cycled inhaled tobramycin, but these studies were not designed to assess clinical results.[22,23] In the first study, Barker and colleagues[22] randomized 74 subjects to receive tobramycin, 300 mg twice daily, or placebo for 4 weeks; the treated subjects showed a significant decrease in *Pseudomonas* density 2 weeks after completion of the study drug. The second study was an open-label trial of 41 patients who received 3 cycles of inhaled tobramycin administered on a 2 weeks on/2 weeks off schedule. This study also had a positive microbiological end point.[23] Of note, some subjects in both these trials developed adverse respiratory events, including cough and wheeze. A year-long trial of inhaled gentamicin, 80 mg twice daily, versus placebo was recently reported; 65 subjects were enrolled in the study and 57 completed the protocol. Positive clinical end points included decreased exacerbations, increased time to next exacerbation, and improved quality of life, and there were no significant adverse events.[24] A small retrospective report of 17 British patients with non-CF bronchiectasis who received nebulized colomycin was published in 2010; the patients had a mean time on colomycin therapy of 21 months with good results and no toxicity.[25] Steinfort and Steinfort[26] reported similar findings from a US cohort treated with inhaled colisitin. A recent retrospective review of 30 patients who were treated with a combined regimen of systemic antibiotics (IV gentamicin and ceftazidime for 2 weeks or oral ciprofloxacin for 3 months plus nebulized colistin for 3 months) documented a *Pseudomonas* eradication rate after therapy of 80%, although approximately half of the patients were reinfected within a mean of 6 months.[27]

Chronic oral macrolide therapy may have a role in the maintenance regimens of patients with bronchiectasis. Macrolides have antiinflammatory and immunomodulatory properties, and they have been demonstrated to reduce exacerbations in CF bronchiectasis[28] and chronic obstructive pulmonary disease.[29] Small, mostly retrospective clinical trials have also suggested benefit in non-CF bronchiectasis. Fifty-six patients treated with 250 mg of azithromycin 3 times per week for a mean length of 9 months showed decreased exacerbation frequency.[30] A retrospective review of 24 subjects who received daily erythromycin, 250 mg, also showed decreased exacerbations; all subjects completed a minimum of 12 months of therapy.[31] An open-label trial of azithromycin, 500 mg twice weekly, for 6 months also showed clinical benefit.[32] The potential benefits of maintenance macrolide therapy must be weighed against the risks, including the development of resistant organisms (particularly *M avium* complex), or drug-related side effects, including hearing loss.

Chronic antibiotic therapy must also be considered for patients with bronchiectasis infected with NTM. The decision to initiate NTM antibiotic therapy requires careful consideration; not all patients infected with NTM organisms need treatment.[33] Antibiotic therapy is warranted when infection is documented by 2 or more positive sputum cultures or one bronchoalveolar lavage culture and evidence of significant clinical and radiographic findings suggesting active disease.[33] Although some patients with bronchiectasis may be infected with NTM organisms alone, many patients are coinfected with gram-negative or gram-positive organisms. The decision about which organisms to target with antibiotic therapy can be difficult; many expert clinicians suggest treating the gram-negative or gram-positive organisms first with 2 to 3 weeks of antibiotic therapy and assessing clinical response. If the patient has improvement in symptoms and radiographic abnormalities, NTM antibiotics may then be withheld. The patient then needs ongoing close follow-up to assess for recrudescence of the infections. See Chapter XX for further details on evaluating and treating patients with NTM and bronchiectasis.

At present, there are several phase 2 and 3 clinical trials underway to evaluate the role of maintenance antibiotic therapies in non-CF bronchiectasis. Dry powder ciprofloxacin and tobramycin are under study, as well as nebulized liposomal ciprofloxacin, liposomal amikacin, levofloxacin, and aztreonam.[34–39] Fosfomycin/tobramycin inhaled combination therapy is also being evaluated.[40]

There are no approved chronic maintenance antibiotic therapies for bronchiectasis. The clinical trials and expert recommendations discussed earlier suggest that there may be a role for these therapies in a select group of patients with non-CF bronchiectasis. Select patients may benefit from a maintenance inhaled antibiotic regimen (continuous or cyclic) and/or thrice weekly oral macrolide administration. However, given the current lack of data, the practitioner must be cautious and selective about the use of such therapies. If these therapies are prescribed, the patient needs to be instructed in proper administration techniques and in the care and maintenance of their nebulizers and other delivery devices. The time commitment/burden of treatment needs to be assessed with each individual patient. Discussion of potential side effects and the off-label nature of this prescribing is required. Patients should be referred for clinical trials when possible.

SUMMARY

Antibiotics have a role in the management of acute exacerbations of bronchiectasis and may also benefit selected subsets of patients with bronchiectasis as a part of a long-term maintenance strategy. At present, there are no Food and Drug Administration–approved antibiotics for either acute or chronic management of bronchiectasis. Clinical trials are underway to determine the efficacy and safety of various inhaled antibiotics for chronic therapy for bronchiectasis. Until those results are available, clinicians need to tailor their therapies to the individual patient based on their best clinical judgment and informed by the data and guidelines that are currently available in the published literature.

REFERENCES

1. Morrissey BM. Pathogenesis of bronchiectasis. Clin Chest Med 2007;28:289–96.
2. Cole PJ. Inflammation: a two-edged sword: the model of bronchiectasis. Eur J Respir Dis Suppl 1986;147:6–15.
3. Martinez-Garcia MA, Soler-Cataluna JJ, Perpina-Tordera M, et al. Factors associated with lung function decline in adult patients with stable non-cystic fibrosis bronchiectasis. Chest 2007;132:1565–72.
4. King PT, Holdsworth SR, Freezer NJ, et al. Microbiologic follow up study in adult bronchiectasis. Respir Med 2007;101:1633–8.
5. Nicotra MB, Rivera M, Dale AM, et al. Clinical, pathophysiologic, and microbiologic characterization of bronchiectasis in an aging cohort. Chest 1995;108:955–61.

6. Pasteur MC, Helliwell SM, Houghton SJ, et al. An investigation into causative factors in patients with bronchiectasis. Am J Respir Crit Care Med 2000; 162:1277–84.

7. Li AM, Sonnappa S, Lex C, et al. Non-CF bronchiectasis: does knowing the aetiology lead to changes in management? Eur Respir J 2005;26:8–14.

8. Murray MP, Pentland JL, Turnbull K, et al. Sputum colour: a useful clinical tool in non-cystic fibrosis bronchiectasis. Eur Respir J 2009;34:361–4.

9. Gillham MI, Sundaram S, Laughton CR, et al. Variable antibiotic susceptibility in populations of Pseudomonas aeruginosa infecting patients with bronchiectasis. J Antimicrob Chemother 2009;63: 728–32.

10. Griffith DE. Nontuberculous mycobacterial lung disease. Curr Opin Infect Dis 2010;23:185–90.

11. Tsang KW, Bilton D. Clinical challenges in managing bronchiectasis. Respirology 2009;14:637–50.

12. Pasteur MC, Bilton D, Hill AT, et al. British Thoracic Society guideline for non-CF bronchiectasis. Thorax 2010;65:i1–158.

13. Metersky ML. New treatment options for bronchiectasis. Ther Adv Respir Dis 2010;4:93–9.

14. O'Donnell AE. Bronchiectasis. Chest 2008;134:815–23.

15. Tsang KW, Chan WM, Ho PL, et al. A comparative study on the efficacy of levofloxacin and ceftazidime in acute exacerbations of bronchiectasis. Eur Respir J 1999;14:1206–9.

16. Darley ES, Bowker KE, Lovering AM, et al. Use of meropenem 3 g once daily for outpatient treatment of infective exacerbations of bronchiectasis. J Antimicrob Chemother 2000;45:247–50.

17. Bilton D, Henig N, Morrissey B, et al. Addition of inhaled tobramycin to ciprofloxacin for acute exacerbations of Pseudomonas aeruginosa infection in adult bronchiectasis. Chest 2006;130:1503–10.

18. Chang KC, Leung CC, Yew WW, et al. Newer fluoroquinolones for treating respiratory infection: do they mask tuberculosis? Eur Respir J 2010;35:606–13.

19. Biewend ML, Waller EA, Aduen JF, et al. Radiographic evolution and antimicrobial resistance patterns in patients with bronchiectasis treated with cyclic antibiotics [abstract]. Proc Am Thorac Soc 2005;2:A176.

20. Rayner CF, Tillotson G, Cole PJ, et al. Efficacy and safety of long-term ciprofloxacin in the management of severe bronchiectasis. J Antimicrob Chemother 1994;34:149–56.

21. Orriols R, Roig J, Ferrer J, et al. Inhaled antibiotic therapy in non-cystic fibrosis patients with bronchiectasis and chronic bronchial infection by Pseudomonas aeruginosa. Respir Med 1999;93:476–80.

22. Barker AF, Couch L, Fiel SB, et al. Tobramycin solution for inhalation reduces sputum Pseudomonas aeruginosa density in bronchiectasis. Am J Respir Crit Care Med 2000;162:481–5.

23. Scheinberg P, Shore E. A pilot study of the safety and efficacy of tobramycin solution for inhalation in patients with severe bronchiectasis. Chest 2005;127:1420–6.

24. Murray MP, Govan JR, Doherty CF, et al. A randomized controlled trial of nebulized gentamicin in non-cystic fibrosis bronchiectasis. Am J Respir Crit Care Med 2011;183:491–9.

25. Dhar R, Anwar GA, Bourke SC, et al. Efficacy of nebulized colomycin in patients with non-cystic fibrosis bronchiectasis colonized with Pseudomonas aeruginosa. Thorax 2010;65:553.

26. Steinfort DP, Steinfort C. Effect of long-term nebulized colistin on lung function and quality of life in patients with chronic bronchial sepsis. Intern Med J 2007;37:495–8.

27. White L, Mirrani G, Grover M, et al. Outcomes of pseudomonas eradication therapy in patients with non-cystic fibrosis bronchiectasis. Respir Med 2012;106:356–60.

28. Cai Y, Chai D, Wang R, et al. Effectiveness and safety of macrolides in cystic fibrosis patients: a meta-analysis and systematic review. J Antimicrob Chemother 2011;66:968–78.

29. Alberts RK, Connett J, Bailey WC, et al. Azithromycin for prevention of exacerbations of COPD. N Engl J Med 2011;365:689–98.

30. Anwar GA, Bourke SC, Afolabi G, et al. Effects of long-term low dose azithromycin in patients with non-CF bronchiectasis. Respir Med 2008;102: 1494–6.

31. Serisier DJ, Martin ML. Long-term low dose erythromycin in bronchiectasis subjects with frequent infective exacerbations. Respir Med 2011;105:946–9.

32. Cymbala AA, Edmonds LC, Bauer MA, et al. The disease modifying effects of twice-weekly azithromycin in patients with bronchiectasis. Treat Respir Med 2005;4:117–22.

33. Griffith DE, Aksamit T, Brown-Elliott BA, et al. An official ATS/IDSA statement: diagnosis, treatment and prevention of nontuberculous mycobacterial diseases. Am J Respir Crit Care Med 2007;175:367–416.

34. Wilson R, Welte T, Polverino E, et al. Randomized, placebo-controlled, double-blind, multi-center study to evaluate the safety and efficacy of ciprofloxacin dry powder for inhalation (ciprofloxacin DPI) compared with placebo in non-cystic fibrosis bronchiectasis [abstract]. Eur Respir J 2011;38(Suppl 55): 334S.

35. Newhouse MT, Hirst PH, Duddu SP, et al. Inhalation of a dry powder tobramycin PulmoSphere formulation in healthy volunteers. Chest 2003;124:360–6.

36. Bilton D, DeSoyza A, Hayward C, et al. Effect of a 28-day course of two different doses of once a day liposomal ciprofloxacin for inhalation on sputum Pseudomonas aeruginosa density in non-CF bronchiectasis [abstract]. Am J Respir Crit Care Med 2010;181:A3191.

37. O'Donnell AE, Swarnakar R, Yashina L, et al. A placebo-controlled study of liposomal amikacin for inhalation once daily in the treatment of bronchiectasis patients with chronic Pseudomonas aeruginosa lung infection [abstract]. Eur Respir J 2009;34:23S.

38. Geller DE, Flume PA, Staab D, et al. Levofloxacin inhalation solution (MP-376) in patients with cystic fibrosis with Pseudomonas aeruginosa. Am J Respir Crit Care Med 2011;183:1510–6.

39. Barker A, O'Donnell A, Daley C, et al. Microbiological results of a phase 2 open-label study of aztreonam for inhalation in patients with bronchiectasis and gram-negative bacteria in the airways [abstract]. Chest 2010;138:512A.

40. MacLeod DL, Barker LM, Sutherland JL, et al. Antibacterial activities of a fosfomycin/tobramycin combination: a novel inhaled antibiotic for bronchiectasis. J Antimicrob Chemother 2009;64:829–36.

Pulmonary Resection and Lung Transplantation for Bronchiectasis

David C. Mauchley, MD[a], Charles L. Daley, MD[b],
Michael D. Iseman, MD[b], John D. Mitchell, MD[a],*

KEYWORDS

- Bronchiectasis • Lobectomy • Segmentectomy • Pulmonary infections
- Video-assisted thoracic surgery • Lung transplantation

KEY POINTS

- The incidence of non-CF bronchiectasis appears to be rising worldwide.
- Surgical resection of focal areas of parenchymal damage remains an important adjunct in the treatment of non-CF bronchiectasis, breaking the cycle of recurrent pulmonary infections.
- Surgical resection of the most severe areas of lung destruction in diffuse bronchiectasis (debulking) may lead to symptom improvement and slow the progression of the disease process.
- The majority of surgical resections for focal bronchiectasis may be accomplished with minimally invasive (thoracoscopic) techniques, with minimal morbidity and mortality.
- Rarely, diffuse non-CF bronchiectasis may treated with bilateral lung transplantation, with acceptable results.

INTRODUCTION

First described by Laennec in 1819, bronchiectasis continues to be recognized as a cause of considerable respiratory illness. Bronchiectasis is characterized by abnormal dilation of bronchi and is usually the result of recurrent pulmonary infections. Patients suffer from symptoms such as chronic cough, excessive sputum production, and hemoptysis, and may eventually develop a progressive decline in respiratory function. Most patients can be treated medically, but those who fail or become intolerant of medical treatment may be eligible for surgical management.

Initial attempts at surgical resection for bronchiectasis were fraught with complications. Postoperative bronchopleural fistula and empyema occurred in up to 50% of cases,[1,2] and perioperative mortality was as high as 46%.[2] The introduction of effective antibiotics in the 1950s as well as improvements in surgical technique led to a dramatic decline in perioperative morbidity. At present, surgical resection is reserved for patients with focal disease who remain symptomatic despite optimal medical management. Diffuse bronchiectasis is usually treated with bilateral lung transplantation, and is mainly limited to patients with cystic fibrosis (CF). Occasionally selected patients with diffuse

Funding sources: Dr Mauchley: None. Dr Daley: None. Dr Iseman: None. Dr Mitchell: None.
Conflicts of interest: Dr Mauchley: None. Dr Daley: None. Dr Iseman: None. Dr Mitchell: None.
[a] Section of General Thoracic Surgery, Division of Cardiothoracic Surgery, University of Colorado School of Medicine, 12631 East 17th Avenue, C-310 Aurora, CO 80045, USA
[b] Division of Mycobacterial and Respiratory Infections, National Jewish Health, 1400 Jackson Street, Denver, CO 80206, USA
* Corresponding author.
E-mail address: John.Mitchell@ucdenver.edu

Clin Chest Med 33 (2012) 387–396
doi:10.1016/j.ccm.2012.04.001
0272-5231/12/$ – see front matter © 2012 Elsevier Inc. All rights reserved.

bronchiectasis will undergo a debulking procedure to remove the most pathologic focus. Patients who would benefit from such an approach include those with severe medically refractory symptoms or massive hemoptysis.

GENERAL PRINCIPLES

Once thought to be in decline, the incidence of non–CF-related bronchiectasis is now believed to be on the increase in North America and throughout the world.[3] The typical presentation includes recurrent pulmonary infections accompanied by sputum production and occasional bouts of hemoptysis. Traditional medical treatment consists of rotating schedules of targeted antibiotic therapy along with maneuvers to promote secretion clearance. Surgical resection is reserved for patients who demonstrate disease progression despite optimal medical treatment, or become intolerant of medical therapy. Failure of such treatment represents the most common reported indication for surgical resection.[4–8]

The basic concept behind surgical resection for bronchiectasis is to remove permanently damaged areas of lung parenchyma that antibiotics penetrate poorly, and thus serve as a reservoir for microbes leading to recurrent infection. Resection of diseased segments will alter the pattern of repeated bouts of infection, and provide significant relief of cough and sputum production. Operative intervention may also benefit patients with concomitant cavitary lung disease or recurrent bouts of hemoptysis.

The ideal candidate for surgical therapy should have truly localized disease that is amenable to anatomic lung resection (lobectomy, segmentectomy). Nonanatomic (wedge) resections should be avoided, as this approach frequently results in incomplete removal of the affected area. Incomplete resection has overwhelmingly been found to be the greatest predictor of symptomatic failure in these patients.[4,5,7,9,10] The use of anatomic resection techniques infrequently has a significant effect on the patient's overall lung function, as the diseased areas of lung tend to contribute little to gas exchange.

Medical therapy should always be attempted before entertaining the idea of surgery, as the majority of patients will improve. Prospective randomized trials evaluating the additional benefit of surgical resection in the medical treatment of bronchiectasis have not been conducted. Retrospective studies comparing patients with bronchiectasis requiring hospitalization found that those treated surgically were more likely to be symptom-free at long-term follow-up. These patients also had fewer yearly hospital days and had an overall trend toward decreased mortality.[11,12]

PREOPERATIVE ASSESSMENT

The typical clinical presentation of a patient with bronchiectasis is as already described. Although most patients present with a productive cough, the presence of a nonproductive cough does not rule out bronchiectasis, and often indicates upper lobe involvement. Preoperative pulmonary reserve is determined through standard preoperative pulmonary function testing, and occasionally split function perfusion testing when appropriate.

The diagnosis and location of bronchiectasis is made using standard radiographic techniques. Chest radiographs are often abnormal but rarely assist in surgical planning. Common findings include focal areas of consolidation, atelectasis, and occasional evidence of thickened bronchi. High-resolution computed tomography (HRCT) scanning has replaced contrast bronchography as the gold standard for radiologic diagnosis of bronchiectasis. This imaging modality can detect the distribution of bronchiectatic alterations with a 2% false-negative and 1% false-positive rate.[13] Findings on HRCT suggestive of the disease include a lack of bronchial tapering on sequential slices, as well as bronchial dilation such that the internal diameter of the affected bronchus is greater than the accompanying bronchial artery.[3] The extent of disease seen on HRCT has been correlated to quality of life and subsequent functional decline.[14,15] The left lung is more commonly affected than the right, and the dependent lower lobes tend to harbor more disease than the upper lobes. Middle lobe and lingular disease is often associated with nontuberculous mycobacterial disease (**Figs. 1** and **2**). Upper lobe involvement is suggestive of several lung diseases including CF, sarcoidosis, or allergic bronchopulmonary aspergillosis.

Bronchoscopy is performed preoperatively, primarily to identify the involved microbial pathogens through collection of sputum and bronchoalveolar lavage specimens. Culture results should include in vitro susceptibility testing, when appropriate, for the cultured organism to assist in preoperative antimicrobial therapy. Bronchoscopy can also identify concomitant obstructive endobronchial abnormality or an unexpected foreign body, and localize the source of active hemoptysis to the segmental and even subsegmental level.

Many patients who have been suffering with chronic lung infections will have lost weight and can be significantly malnourished at presentation.

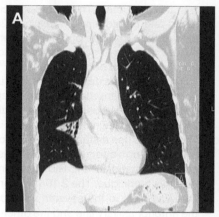
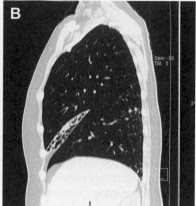

Fig. 1. Coronal (*A*) and sagittal (*B*) computed tomography images of a patient with right middle lobe bronchiectasis. Note the collapse/consolidation of the lobe in the sagittal plane.

If this is the case, an aggressive preoperative regimen of nutritional supplementation is recommended. In the most extreme cases, this may require the placement of a nasojejunal feeding tube or a percutaneous gastrostomy. This approach is typically not necessary for those with limited, focal parenchymal disease. Preoperative evaluation for gastroesophageal reflux disease should be performed in all patients. If it is present and is thought to be contributing to the patient's chronic pulmonary disease, antireflux surgery with or soon after pulmonary resection should be considered.

The authors have used multimodality treatment approach in their practice, where patients appropriate for surgical therapy are discussed at a weekly multidisciplinary conference attended by surgeons, pulmonologists, and infectious disease physicians with specialization in respiratory infectious disease. This approach ensures that the patients receive the appropriate antimicrobial therapy, and assists in optimal timing of surgical intervention. The timing of surgical resection is usually predicated on the duration of the preoperative antimicrobial treatment, allowing enough time to produce a bacterial nadir at the time of surgery. The authors consider that this aspect is crucial in minimizing the risk of complications in the perioperative period.

SURGICAL TECHNIQUE
Anesthesia

A standard anesthetic technique used for thoracic surgical procedures is used. Single-lung ventilation is accomplished with the use of a double-lumen endotracheal tube, or rarely a single-lumen endotracheal tube with the assistance of a bronchial blocker. Early lung isolation may also limit dispersion of purulent secretions to uninvolved areas of the lungs. A thoracic epidural is recommended for postoperative analgesia when a thoracotomy is planned. However, this is usually not necessary in the event of a thoracoscopic approach whereby initial postoperative analgesia is provided by intercostal administration of 0.25% bupivacaine at multiple levels placed at the end of the procedure by the operative team. An arterial line and urinary catheter are placed, and intraoperative fluid administration is limited as with other forms of extensive lung resection. Extubation at the end of the procedure is planned.

Surgical Approach

Bronchoscopy is routinely performed immediately before initiation of the surgical procedure, clearing the airway of secretions to optimize ventilation during the operation. If severe airway inflammation

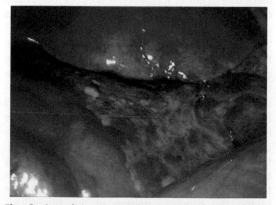

Fig. 2. Actual intraoperative image of the patient shown in **Fig. 1**, with discoloration and collapse of the involved lobe in comparison with the adjacent upper lobe.

is found at the time of bronchoscopy, surgical therapy may be delayed until infection control is optimized. Lastly, there is always the possibility that the patient may have normal variations in bronchial anatomy, knowledge of which would be helpful before attempting anatomic resection.

Historically, surgical resection for bronchiectasis was always approached via lateral thoracotomy, tailored for the targeted segment or lobe. These incisional techniques have largely been replaced by video-assisted thoracoscopic surgery (VATS). The decision to use an open or VATS approach is usually determined preoperatively based on extent of disease on radiologic imaging, particularly with respect to the degree of pleural obliteration. If using an open thoracotomy, mobilization of muscle flaps should be accomplished at the onset of the procedure, for transposition into the hemithorax later after resection is complete. An extrapleural dissection plane, if needed, may be initiated before placement of the rib spreader.

Several important differences exist between anatomic resection for infectious lung disease and resection for malignancy. Pleural adhesions are frequently present, and in some cases can be extensive and vascular in nature. Adhesions are typically more dense around the involved segment(s) of lung, but can be scattered throughout the hemithorax. In upper lobe–predominant disease, the adhesions to the overlying parietal pleura can be significant and quite difficult to lyse. Presence of pleural adhesions can usually be predicted on the preoperative computed tomography scan, but the amount of pleural symphysis may be underestimated. Adhesions are usually divided safely with a thoracoscopic approach, often with improved visibility compared with open thoracotomy. Care must be taken to avoid adjacent vital structures such as the phrenic nerve or great vessels during this part of the dissection.

The bronchial circulation is frequently hypertrophied in cases of long-standing infectious disease, and particular care must be taken to assure hemostasis. Bronchial arteries should be ligated with clips if enlarged. Significant lymphadenopathy is also usually present, and in the setting of chronic granulomatous disease can make dissection at the pulmonary hilum and around vessels hazardous. When dividing pulmonary fissures with stapling devices, the authors advocate a line of division just on the side of the uninvolved lobe, which ensures complete resection and helps prevent staple-line dehiscence.

The pulmonary vessels and bronchus are divided and sealed using standard stapling devices. Once the resection is completed, the diseased segment or lobe should be removed in a bag, unless the incision is generous enough to avoid contamination with the specimen. The intrathoracic space is irrigated and then drained with 1 or 2 28F thoracostomy tubes. Portions of the specimen are sent for culture, and the remainder for pathologic analysis.

Although most published series[4–7,9,10] of surgery for bronchiectasis describe resection using an open (thoracotomy) approach, a VATS approach has been successfully used in some studies and is the preferred approach at the authors' institution.[8,16] The authors use a standard VATS technique using 2 10-mm ports and a 4-cm utility incision centered over the anterior hilum. Rib spreading is avoided with this technique. The 2 10-mm ports are placed first, with one in the seventh intercostal space in the anterior axillary line and the other just posterior to the scapular tip. Once the feasibility and safety of a VATS approach are confirmed, the utility incision is made. A wound protector is placed in the utility incision to avoid contamination and retract the soft tissues of the chest wall. Modifications can be made to this technique to better serve the specifics of the planned resection. Adhesions are well visualized, and are typically easier to divide thoracoscopically, although the presence of dense adhesions or complete pleural symphysis may warrant conversion to thoracotomy. The planned resection is then completed in a manner analogous to an open approach.

Use of Tissue Flaps

Although not performed routinely in resection for bronchiectasis, tissue transposition should be considered when there is increased risk for breakdown of the bronchial stump. Factors that increase this risk include poorly controlled infection before surgery, resection in the setting of significant drug resistance, or the rare case of pneumonectomy for bronchiectasis.[17] The authors favor use of either a latissimus dorsi or intercostal muscle flap for coverage of a bronchial stump, and omentum for use after a right pneumonectomy.[18] Serratus muscle flaps should be avoided, as there tend to be problems with wound healing in these characteristically thin patients related to the winged scapula that results from serratus transposition. Mobilization of the latissimus is performed at the initiation of the procedure, and the muscle is transposed through the second or third intercostal space. When an omental flap is warranted, the omentum is mobilized via a midline laparotomy before thoracotomy and tacked to the undersurface of the right hemidiaphragm for retrieval later during the thoracic portion of the procedure. Significant intrathoracic space issues may result occasionally after resection, and may be at least partially addressed with latissimus transposition.

Postoperative Management

Management of patients after surgery for bronchiectasis is not significantly different from that of any patient who has undergone anatomic lung resection. Emphasis is placed on early mobilization, aggressive pulmonary toilet, chest physiotherapy, and nutritional supplementation. Chest-tube management is routine. Appropriate antimicrobial therapy is maintained in the postoperative period and is often continued for several months, depending on the organism isolated. Bronchoscopy may be necessary to help with mobilization and clearance of secretions, particularly in patients who present with bilateral disease and are consequently left with unilateral disease postoperatively. Those who are treated with a thoracoscopic approach can leave the hospital as early as the second or third postoperative day, whereas those who undergo thoracotomy are often hospitalized for up to a week.

COMPLICATIONS

The complications that accompany lung resection for bronchiectasis mirror those that follow lung resection for other indications, with a few exceptions. Reported morbidity following resection ranges from 9% to 19% depending on the series (**Table 1**). The most common complications after surgery for bronchiectasis include atelectasis requiring therapeutic bronchoscopy, prolonged air leak, space problems, empyema, bronchopleural fistula (BPF), and wound infection.[4–7] Absence of preoperative bronchoscopy, forced expiratory volume in 1 second of less than 60% of the predicted value, and incomplete resection have all been associated with the development of postoperative complications.[19] The complications are similar after resection with a VATS approach (**Table 2**).

Although rare after lobectomy or segmentectomy, the development of a postpneumonectomy BPF is a source of significant morbidity. It occurs more frequently on the right side, after completion pneumonectomy, and in the setting of patients who have persistently positive sputum cultures for organisms such as multidrug-resistant *Mycobacterium tuberculosis*.[18,20] Prevention of BPF formation is of paramount importance when presented with a high-risk patient. Appropriate antimicrobial treatment of adequate duration should be given before surgery, a tension-free technique used to close the bronchus, and muscle or omentum used to buttress the closure. BPF formation after pneumonectomy is suggested by fever, cough productive of serous followed by purulent sputum, contralateral lung infiltrates, and a dropping air-fluid level on chest radiograph. Management begins with prompt drainage of the infected space to prevent further damage to the remaining lung. If diagnosed very early after resection, primary repair of the bronchial stump with rebuttressing may be attempted. In the setting of delayed diagnosis, management usually requires rib resection and creation of an open thoracostomy window (Eloesser flap), followed by surgical closure of the fistula and subsequent closure of the chest with instillation of antibiotic solution (Clagett procedure).

As mentioned, intrathoracic space problems are somewhat more common after surgery for bronchiectasis, mainly because the remaining lung often will not fully expand. This situation leaves residual space that is typically not problematic, but can lead to development of empyema in cases that involve parenchymal injury or significant pleural soilage. Again, prevention is key, and patients with these potential problems should be anticipated. Liberal use of muscle flaps to minimize the space can help prevent complications.

OUTCOMES

Perioperative mortality after resection for bronchiectasis is very low, with contemporary rates ranging from 0% to 1.7% (see **Table 1**). Completion pneumonectomy remains a highly morbid procedure, and leads to much of the mortality related to surgical treatment of this disease.[9,18] Renal failure and advanced age (>70 years) are also associated with postoperative mortality in this group of patients.[20] Mean age at the time of surgery ranges from 24 to 59 years, and women seem to be more frequently affected than men.[4–8,20,21] The most common reported indication for surgical intervention is failure of medical therapy. Left-sided disease predominates, and complete resection of disease is possible 80% to 90% of the time. The most commonly performed procedure is lobectomy, followed by segmentectomy, lobectomy with segmentectomy, and pneumonectomy. Very few patients undergo bilobectomy for bronchiectasis alone, although this is not uncommon in patients infected with nontuberculous mycobacteria. The most common reported reason for incomplete resection is bilateral disease, although most of these patients should be candidates for contralateral resection at a later date. The great majority of patients are either asymptomatic or have symptomatic improvement at follow-up. Lack of symptomatic improvement is most commonly associated with incomplete resection,[4,5,7,9,10,19,20] but has also been associated with saccular bronchiectasis, history of sinusitis, and tuberculous infection.[10,20]

Table 1
Summary of patients' characteristics, hospital stay, and operative mortality after surgical resection for bronchiectasis

Surgical Approach	Reference (Y)	Study Period	No. of Patients	Mean Age, Years (Range)	Hospital Stay, Days (Range)	Complication Rate (% Total Patients)	Operative Mortality (%)
Thoracotomy	Kutlay et al,[4] 2002	1990–2000	166	34.1 (7–70)	NR	11.4	1.7
	Balkanli et al,[5] 2003	1992–2001	238	23.7 (15–48)	9.4 (5–24)	8.8	0
	Gursoy et al,[6] 2010	2002–2007	92	38.7 (10–67)	8.5 (NR)	16.3	1.1
	Bagheri et al,[7] 2010	1985–2008	277	34.7 (8–65)	NR	15.8	0.7
	Zhang et al,[20] 2010	1989–2008	790	41.6 (6–79)	9.8 (6–120)	16.2	1.1
VATS	Weber et al,[21] 2001	1992–1999	64	54.5 (20–81)	8.5 (4–41)	18.7	0
	Zhang et al,[20] 2010	2005–2009	52	41 (NR)	11 (NR)	15.4	0
	Mitchell et al[8]	2004–2010	171	59 (26–82)	3.7 (1–23)	8.9	0

Abbreviations: NR, not reported; VATS, video-assisted thoracoscopic surgery.

Table 2
Summary of morbidity after surgical resection for bronchiectasis

Surgical Approach	Reference (Y)	Prolonged Air Leak/Space Issues	Atelectasis	Empyema/BPF	Wound Infection	Bleeding	Arrhythmia	Overall Morbidity
Thoracotomy	Kutlay et al,[4] 2002	1.7	2.3	1.2	0	1.7	0	11.4
	Balkanli et al,[5] 2003	2.5	2.9	1.7	0	1.7	0	8.8
	Gursoy et al,[6] 2010	9.8	3.2	0	3.3	0	0	16.3
	Bagheri et al,[7] 2010	3.2	3.6	3.2	5.7	0	0	15.8
	Zhang et al,[20] 2010	2.7	2	1	0	1.1	4	16.2
VATS	Weber et al,[21] 2001	9.3	NR	0	0	1.5	3.1	18.7
	Zhang et al,[20] 2011	1.9	3.8	1.9	0	0	3.8	15.4
	Mitchell et al[8]	5.6	0.5	0	0.5	0	1.4	8.9

All values represent percentage of all patients in each reference.
Abbreviations: BPF, bronchopleural fistula; NR, not reported; VATS, video-assisted thoracoscopic surgery.

Three series in the last decade have specifically analyzed the outcomes of patients who undergo a VATS resection for bronchiectasis. Weber and colleagues[21] describe a 5-trocar method of performing thoracoscopic lobectomy in 64 patients with benign lung disease, 49 of whom had bronchiectasis or chronic lung infection alone. A mortality rate of 0%, morbidity rate of 18.7%, and conversion to open procedure in 15.3% were reported. Conversion was mainly due to dense pleural adhesive disease or upper lobe–predominant disease. Compared with a cohort of patients who underwent planned open lobectomy during the same time period, those who underwent a VATS resection suffered fewer postoperative complications, had less blood loss, and had a shorter hospital stay. Zhang and colleagues[22] reported 52 patients who underwent VATS lobectomy using 2 ports and a utility incision. Their results echo those of Weber and colleagues, with no mortality, a morbidity of 15.4%, and a conversion rate of 13.5%. Again, compared with a matched control cohort of patients undergoing open lobectomy from the same time period, the thoracoscopic group had a lower rate of morbidity and shorter hospital stay. Pain was also assessed with an 11-point scale in these patients, and was significantly lower in the thoracoscopic group.

The authors have recently reported the experience in VATS resection for bronchiectasis at their institution.[8] A total of 212 anatomic resections were performed in 171 patients over a 6-year period. The majority of infections were due to nontuberculous mycobacterial species, although 33% had a mixed infection. Mortality was 0%, the complication rate was 9%, and conversion to thoracotomy occurred in 4.7% of cases. The mean hospital stay was 3.7 days. The results of the aforementioned reports in selected patients suggest that pulmonary resection for bronchiectasis can feasibly be performed with a VATS approach, with negligible mortality, similar morbidity, shorter hospital stay, and less pain when compared with open thoracotomy.

LUNG TRANSPLANTATION

Lung transplantation in patients with bronchiectasis is only indicated for those with diffuse disease that is not amenable to segmental surgical resection combined with declining lung function despite maximal medical therapy. The vast majority of transplants for bronchiectasis are performed on patients with CF. Bronchiectasis develops in nearly all cases of CF leading to chronic cough, expectoration of abnormal mucus, progressive airflow obstruction, and persistent respiratory tract infections. Quality of life is poor in those with advanced bronchiectasis, and they are at increased risk of death secondary to declining lung function. Lung transplantation has been shown to both improve quality of life and prolong survival in appropriately selected patients.[23,24]

CF is the third most common indication for lung transplantation overall and is the most common indication for bilateral lung transplant.[25] Bilateral lung transplant is preferred in those with suppurative lung disease secondary to CF, even in those with heterogeneous disease. Single-lung transplantation risks contamination of the new graft by the old lung in the setting of an immunocompromised patient. Some centers will perform a single-lung transplant in conjunction with contralateral pneumonectomy to avoid this risk.

The guidelines for referral of patients with CF and bronchiectasis for transplantation are listed in **Box 1**. Furthermore, patients should be considered for transplantation if there is less than a 50% likelihood of survival over 2 years without transplant, if quality of life will likely be improved with transplant, there are no contraindications to transplant, and if they are committed to proceeding with the evaluation and listing after a concrete understanding of the risks and benefits of the operation. Young female patients with CF are considered for

---

Box 1
Guidelines for lung transplantation in diffuse bronchiectasis (both CF and non-CF)

Guidelines for Referral to a Transplant Center

- FEV_1 below 30% predicted/rapid decline in FEV_1, particularly in young female patients

- Exacerbation of pulmonary disease requiring ICU stay

- Increasing frequency of exacerbations requiring antibiotic therapy

- Refractory and/or recurrent pneumothorax

- Recurrent hemoptysis not controlled by embolization

Guidelines for Transplantation

- Progressive decline in lung function
- Oxygen-dependent respiratory failure
- Hypercapnia
- Pulmonary hypertension

Abbreviations: CF, cystic fibrosis; FEV_1, forced expiratory volume in 1 second; ICU, intensive care unit.
    Data from Loebinger MR, Wells AU, Hansell DM, et al. Mortality in bronchiectasis: a long-term study assessing the factors influencing survival. Eur Respir J 2009;34:843–9.

early referral if they suffer rapid deterioration in pulmonary status, as they have a particularly poor prognosis.[25] Several studies in the 1990s showed that infection with *Burkholderia cepacia* in prospective CF transplant candidates was associated with significant posttransplantation infectious complications and poor outcomes.[26,27] This finding has led to the recommendation that the presence of *B cepacia* infection be a relative contraindication to lung transplantation in the CF population, although some centers continue to offer transplantation therapy in this setting. More recent evidence suggests that some, but not all subspecies within the *B cepacia* complex confer increased perioperative risk.[28] Infection with *Mycobacterium abscessus* before transplantation has been associated with significant morbidity also, and this has made some centers reticent to transplant such patients.[29]

Complications after lung transplantation for CF and bronchiectasis include hemorrhage, pulmonary edema, primary graft dysfunction, anastomotic dehiscence, and various infectious complications. Bacterial infections are common after transplant for bronchiectasis, as numerous pathogens chronically reside in the respiratory tract secretions of these patients. Antibacterial regimens guided by preoperative and perioperative cultures are used postoperatively in addition to the standard prophylactic medications given for viral and fungal pathogens.[30]

Patients with CF and bronchiectasis can expect a dramatic improvement in pulmonary function after lung transplant as well as the ability to perform activities of daily living without limitations. Long-term survival has been demonstrated in a review of 123 patients with CF who underwent either bilateral lung transplantation or bilateral lower lobe transplant from living donors.[31] Survival rates were 81% at 1 year, 59% at 5 years, and 38% at 10 years. A sustained improvement in quality of life after transplantation can be expected for at least 1 to 3 years.[30]

Transplantation for non-CF bronchiectasis is rare, and specific referral guidelines have not been developed. For this reason, the guidelines used for those with CF bronchiectasis are generally used.[25]

REFERENCES

1. Lindskog GE, Hubbell DS. An analysis of 215 cases of bronchiectasis. Surg Gynecol Obstet 1955;100: 643–50.
2. Ochsner A, DeBakey M, DeCamp P. Bronchiectasis; its curative treatment by pulmonary resection; an analysis of 96 cases. Surgery 1949;25:518–32.
3. O'Donnell AE. Bronchiectasis. Chest 2008;134:815–23.
4. Kutlay H, Cangir AK, Enon S, et al. Surgical treatment in bronchiectasis: analysis of 166 patients. Eur J Cardiothorac Surg 2002;21:634–7.
5. Balkanli K, Genc O, Dakak M, et al. Surgical management of bronchiectasis: analysis and short-term results in 238 patients. Eur J Cardiothorac Surg 2003;24:699–702.
6. Gursoy S, Ozturk AA, Ucvet A, et al. Surgical management of bronchiectasis: the indications and outcomes. Surg Today 2010;40:26–30.
7. Bagheri R, Haghi SZ, Fattahi Masoum SH, et al. Surgical management of bronchiectasis: analysis of 277 patients. Thorac Cardiovasc Surg 2010;58: 291–4.
8. Mitchell JD, Yu JA, Bishop A, et al. Thoracoscopic lobectomy and segmentectomy for infectious lung disease. Ann Thorac Surg 2012;93:1033–40.
9. Agasthian T, Deschamps C, Trastek V, et al. Surgical management of bronchiectasis. Ann Thorac Surg 1996;62:976–8 [discussion: 979–80].
10. Fujimoto T, Hillejan L, Stamatis G. Current strategy for surgical management of bronchiectasis. Ann Thorac Surg 2001;72:1711–5.
11. Annest LS, Kratz JM, Crawford FA. Current results of treatment of bronchiectasis. J Thorac Cardiovasc Surg 1982;83:546–50.
12. Sanderson JM, Kennedy MC, Johnson MF, et al. Bronchiectasis: results of surgical and conservative management. A review of 393 cases. Thorax 1974; 29:407–16.
13. Young K, Aspestrand F, Kolbenstvedt A. High resolution CT and bronchography in the assessment of bronchiectasis. Acta Radiol 1991;32:439–41.
14. Eshed I, Minski I, Katz R, et al. Bronchiectasis: correlation of high-resolution CT findings with health-related quality of life. Clin Radiol 2007;62:152–9.
15. Sheehan RE, Wells AU, Copely SJ, et al. A comparison of serial computed tomography and functional change in bronchiectasis. Eur Respir J 2002;20:581–7.
16. Mitchell JD, Bishop A, Cafaro A, et al. Anatomic lung resection for nontuberculous mycobacterial disease. Ann Thorac Surg 2008;85:1887–92 [discussion: 1892–93].
17. Shiraishi Y, Nakajima Y, Katsuragi N, et al. Pneumonectomy for nontuberculous mycobacterial infections. Ann Thorac Surg 2004;78:399–403.
18. Sherwood JT, Mitchell JD, Pomerantz M. Completion pneumonectomy for chronic mycobacterial disease. J Thorac Cardiovasc Surg 2005;129:1258–65.
19. Eren S, Esme H, Avci A. Risk factors affecting outcome and morbidity in the surgical management of bronchiectasis. J Thorac Cardiovasc Surg 2007;134:392–8.
20. Zhang P, Jiang G, Ding J, et al. Surgical treatment of bronchiectasis: a retrospective analysis of 790 patients. Ann Thorac Surg 2010;90:246–50.

21. Weber A, Stammberger U, Inci I, et al. Thoraco-scopic lobectomy for benign disease–a single centre study on 64 cases. Eur J Cardiothorac Surg 2001;20:443–8.

22. Zhang P, Zhang F, Jiang S, et al. Video-assisted thoracic surgery for bronchiectasis. Ann Thorac Surg 2011;91:239–43.

23. Courtney JM, Kelly MG, Watt A, et al. Quality of life and inflammation in exacerbations of bronchiec-tasis. Chron Respir Dis 2008;5:161–8.

24. Loebinger MR, Wells AU, Hansell DM, et al. Mortality in bronchiectasis: a long-term study assessing the factors influencing survival. Eur Respir J 2009;34: 843–9.

25. Orens JB, Estenne M, Arcasoy S, et al. International guidelines for the selection of lung transplant candi-dates: 2006 update–a consensus report from the Pulmonary Scientific Council of the International Society for Heart and Lung Transplantation. J Heart Lung Transplant 2006;25:745–55.

26. Egan JJ, McNeil K, Bookless B, et al. Post-transplan-tation survival of cystic fibrosis patients infected with Pseudomonas cepacia. Lancet 1994;344:552–3.

27. Snell GI, de Hoyos A, Krajden M, et al. Pseudo-monas cepacia in lung transplant recipients with cystic fibrosis. Chest 1993;103:466–71.

28. Murray S, Charbeneau J, Marshall BC, et al. Impact of Burkholderia infection on lung transplantation in cystic fibrosis. Am J Respir Crit Care Med 2008; 178:363–71.

29. Daley CL. Nontuberculous mycobacterial infec-tions in transplant recipients: early diagnosis and treatment. Curr Opin Organ Transplant 2009;14: 625–36.

30. Hayes D, Meyer KC. Lung transplantation for advanced bronchiectasis. Semin Respir Crit Care Med 2010;31:123–38.

31. Egan TM, Detterbeck FC, Mill MR, et al. Long term results of lung transplantation for cystic fibrosis. Eur J Cardiothorac Surg 2002;22:602–9.

Index

Note: Page numbers of article titles are in **boldface** type.

Clin Chest Med 33 (2012) 397–404
doi:10.1016/S0272-5231(12)00050-0
0272-5231/12/$ – see front matter © 2012 Elsevier Inc. All rights reserved.

Moving?

Make sure your subscription moves with you!

To notify us of your new address, find your **Clinics Account Number** (located on your mailing label above your name), and contact customer service at:

Email: journalscustomerservice-usa@elsevier.com

800-654-2452 (subscribers in the U.S. & Canada)
314-447-8871 (subscribers outside of the U.S. & Canada)

Fax number: 314-447-8029

Elsevier Health Sciences Division
Subscription Customer Service
3251 Riverport Lane
Maryland Heights, MO 63043

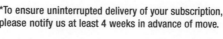
*To ensure uninterrupted delivery of your subscription, please notify us at least 4 weeks in advance of move.

ELSEVIER

Printed and bound by CPI Group (UK) Ltd, Croydon, CR0 4YY
03/10/2024
01040350-0019